P9-CKK-877

Risk-Benefit Analysis

Richard Wilson
Department of Physics
Center for Risk Analysis
Harvard University

and

Edmund A. C. Crouch
Cambridge Environmental Inc.

Published by the Center for Risk Analysis
Harvard University

Second Edition
Distributed by Harvard University Press

Distributed by Harvard University Press
© Copyright 2001 The President and Fellows of Harvard College.
All rights reserved.

ISBN 0-674-00529-5
Library of Congress Control Number: 2001094318
Full Cataloging-in-Publication (CIP) Data available through the Library of
Congress.

Design and production: Digital Design Group, Newton, MA 02460
Cover Carton: © 2001 The New Yorker Collection from cartoonbank.com. All Rights
Reserved.

Printed in Canada

Table of Contents

Preface   xi

1. Introduction: Perspective on Risk   1
  Perception is Crucial   3
  Definition of Risk   8
  Risk Changes as Events Unfold   10
  Measures of Risk   11
  Different Measures Can Lead to Different Decisions   14
  Absolute or Incremental Risk   17
  Defining the System Boundary   18
  Layout of the Book   21

2. Methods of Risk Calculation and Estimation   25
  Evaluation of "Historical" Risks   27
  "New" Risks: (1) Factorization of an Engineering System
    with an Event Tree   38
  "New" Risks: (2) of Epidemiology and Its Ambiguities   46
  Risks of Doses Less than Background: The "Linear Default"   49
  Beneficial Effects and Hormesis   53
  New Risks: (3) The Use of Animal Data to Estimate Risks to Humans   57
  Probability of Causation   64
  Elicitation of Expert Opinion   67
  Exposure and Dose Estimation   68
  The Risk of a System—the Impact Pathway Approach   75
  Risk of the Impossible   77
  Large and Immeasurable Risks   78
  The Chimera of Zero Risk—Predictable but Irrelevant   79

3. Uncertainty and Variability   81
   Risk Implies Uncertainty   81
   Different Types of Uncertainty   83
   As Risk Changes with Time, So Does Uncertainty   85
   Stochastic Uncertainties   85
   Variability vs. Uncertainty   86
   Uncertainty vs. Error   89
   Independence of Uncertainties   90
   Uncertainty in Cancer Risk Assessment   90
   Monte Carlo Models   92
   Model Uncertainty   93
   Uncertainty in Expert Elicitation   95
   Overconfidence in Uncertainty Estimates   96

4. Perception of Risks   99
   Tversky's Analyses   100
   Other Attributes and Dimensions   102
   Managers and Decision Makers Consider Public Perception   107
   Comparing Risks (Risk-Risk Comparisons)   114
   Comparing Risks for the Same Benefit (Cost Effectiveness)   122
   Expression of Risks   124
   Public Misconceptions   125
   Common Public Misconceptions   126
   Recipe for Communication   131

5. Formal Comparison of Risk and Benefit   135
   Distributional Inequity   138
   Deriving Suitable Value Functions   139
   Choice of Discounting Rates   143
   Approximations and Simplified Schemes   145

6. Risk Management: Managing and Reducing Risks   147
   We Calculate Risks in Order to Reduce Them   148
   Schemes for Analyzing Risk Management Options   148
   Criteria for Risk Management   152
   The Ban or Taboo   155
   Best Available Control Technology   157
   Risk-Cost-Benefit Analysis   158
   The Precautionary Principle   159

Regulation on Upper Limit of Risk   159
Risk versus Certainty of Information   161
The "De Minimis" Risk   164
Risk-related Decisions of the U.S. EPA   165
Probability of Causation   167
Management by Avoiding Precursors   172
Asbestos and Dioxin   174
Reducing Risk by Technological Improvement   176
Radiation Protection   178
Economic Incentives   179
The Multiple Uses of a Risk Assessment   180
Use of Comparisons to Guide a Manager   181
Safety Culture and the Importance of Incentives 183
Congress as the Filter for Societal Values   183
The Dual Role of the Courts   184

7. **Lists of Risks**   **191**
Some Examples of Risk Calculations   192
The Risk (of Death) in Living   192
Life Expectancy   194
A Selection of Risks: Historically Calculated   195
Time (or Action) to Reach One in a Million Risk 208
Loss of Life Expectancy (LOLE)   210
A Partial List of Catastrophes   218
Amounts Paid to Avert Deaths   218
Variation and Uncertainties   223
Detailed Discussions of Some Risks   223

8. **Bibliography**   **265**
Books   265
Journals   278
Websites   279
Specific References   283

Appendix 1: Some Famous Quotations   **311**

Appendix 2: Application of EPA's Hazardous Waste Identification Rule   317
   1. Variability   318
   2. Uncertainty   319
   3. Legislative Mandate and its Interpretation   220
   4. Precise Definitions   223

Appendix 3: Procedure Used for Age Adjustment by NCHS   333

Appendix 4: Are Mushrooms Safe to Eat, or Should They Be Considered Toxic Waste?   335
   The Problem   335
   Materials and Methods   335
   Results   336
   Implications   337
   Modifying Comments   339

Appendix 5: Evaluating the Lung-Cancer Risks Due to Smoking, Exposure to Asbestos, and Their Combination   341
   Smoking   342
   Asbestos   350
   Assigning Causation of Lung Cancer to Smoking and Asbestos— the Logic of the Approach   355
   Interaction between Smoking and Cigarettes   358

Epilog   363

Index   365

About the Authors

Richard Wilson is Mallinckrodt Research Professor of Physics at Harvard University. He helped to start the Energy and Environmental Policy Center in 1973 and served as its director from 1975 through 1978. For the last twenty-five years he has been involved with environmental concerns, especially with various environmental risks about which he has written many articles. He was awarded the Forum Award of the American Physical Society in 1990 for communications with the public (on physics and applications, and especially on risk) and the Distinguished Achievement Award of the Society for Risk Analysis in 1993. His website is *phys4.harvard.edu/~wilson*

Edmund A. C. Crouch is a Senior Scientist at Cambridge Environmental, Inc., where he has been for over eleven years since its founding. He became interested in risk assessment after a Ph.D. in theoretical physics from Cambridge University and three years as a Research Assistant at the Cambridge Energy Research Group. He spent eight years in the Department of Physics at Harvard University, working in the Energy and Environmental Policy Center. His main interest is improving the scientific content of risk assessments. His website is: *www.cambridgeenvironmental.com/people/crouch/edmund.htm*

Acknowledgements

Each separately and both of the authors together have been stimulated by friends and colleagues too numerous to mention. We had extremely helpful advice and encouragement, from Dr. Allan Bromley, Dr. John Evans, Dr. Dade Moeller, Dr. Howard Raiffa, William Ruckelshaus Esq. and Dr. Arthur Upton, particularly in the early days of our work on Risk Analysis. In particular we would like to thank the following who have critically reviewed some or all of the manuscript and made useful calculations, comments and suggestions. Dr. T. J. Carrothers, Dr. Sam Napolitano, Mr. Anton Yakovlev, Dr. Ari Rabl, Dr. John Graham (Colorado), Dr. John Graham, (Harvard Center for Risk Analysis), Dr. Laura Green, Martin Kaufman Esq., and Dr. Thomas McKone. Without their help the book would have many more errors than it has.

Preface

Each day citizens, opinion leaders, and policy makers are confronted with information about previously unrecognized threats to health and safety. If families with young children live near electric powerlines, will they suffer an increased risk of childhood leukemia? Does inhaling particles in outdoor air increase the risk of adverse cardiopulmonary events? If pregnant women eat foods with trace amounts of dioxins and PCBs, will their children suffer increased rates of developmental problems? If a community's public water system has elevated concentrations of the chemical chloroform, should that be cause for health concerns? Although media headlines often raise these questions, it is often not apparent what the answers are, what the uncertainties are, and what should be done to address public concerns.

A relatively new field of scholarship called risk analysis has emerged to provide the best possible answers to these kinds of questions. Many lay people associate the term "risk analysis" with a technical assessment of whether a hazard may exist and, if so, how likely or serious it could be. Among professionals, however, the term has a broader meaning that also encompasses analysis of strategies to control risk and to provide information to the lay public about risk.

In this book by Richard Wilson and Edmund Crouch, the reader is provided a clear yet rigorous introduction to the entire field of risk analysis. Students and faculty at the Harvard Center for Risk Analysis are grateful that the materials that Professor Wilson has used in his years of teaching at Harvard will now be available, in book form, to students and professionals throughout the world. Professor Wilson's perspective as a scholar, teacher, consultant and expert witness is nicely complemented by Dr. Crouch's extensive experience as a practicing analyst for clients in business and government.

The book should be understood in the context of a field that is growing in importance throughout the developed and developing world. Although many of the leading scientists in the field are based in the United States, there are also active communities of risk analysts in Europe, Japan, the former Soviet

Union, China and elsewhere in the world. In fact, the Society for Risk Analysis (SRA), an international association of 2,500 scientists and engineers, was established in 1980 (with Dr. Wilson as a charter member) to advance the tools and applications of risk analysis. SRA has sections in North America, Europe and Japan that each hold annual meetings where scientists and students present their work. The first World Congress on Risk Analysis is being organized as this book goes to press.

The scientific literature on risk analysis is exploding. The publication *Risk Analysis: An International Journal*, sponsored by SRA and in the first issue of which Dr. Crouch and Dr. Wilson published a paper, is the best known peer-reviewed journal in the field. Other relevant journals include *Journal of Risk Research; Human and Ecological Risk Assessment; Risk: Health, Safety, and the Environment; Journal of Risk and Uncertainty;* and *Risk and Decision Policy.* Although these journals are all interdisciplinary, there are also many important risk-related articles published in leading disciplinary journals in fields such as engineering, toxicology, economics and psychology.

The role of risk analysis in public policy is much more developed in the United States than it is in many other parts of the world. I can pinpoint several milestones in the progression of America's risk-oriented approach to questions of health, safety, and environmental policy. First, the nuclear energy issue in the 1970s spawned significant scientific interest in the development of the technical tools of risk analysis. What became the U.S. Nuclear Regulatory Administration built risk concepts into standard regulatory procedures for the licensing and operation of nuclear power plants and thus risk assessments are now commonplace at nuclear power plants in the USA and abroad. Second, concerns about the safety of food and color additives caused the US Food and Drug Administration to develop technical procedures for determining what is a "safe" or negligible amount of contaminant in food. These procedures, rooted in a subfield called regulatory toxicology, exerted a powerful influence on the evolution of chemical risk assessment. Third, public concerns about pesticides and hazardous wastes caused the U.S. Environmental Protection Agency to develop guidelines for human health and ecological risk assessments. Finally, concerns about the costs of risk regulation have caused every U.S. President since Richard Nixon to issue an executive order compelling agencies to perform economic evaluations of major rules. these executive orders have increased the role of cost-benefit analysis in us agency decision making. Finally, the U.S. Congress has required various uses of risk analysis in diverse laws governing drinking water, pesticides, and oil pipeline safety.

As important as these developments were, I have always felt that the U.S. Supreme Court decision in the 1980 benzene case (Industrial Union, 1980) was the pivotal stimulus for risk analysis in U.S. policy making. In this case, the U.S. Occupational Safety and Health Administration argued that the permissible exposure limit for benzene in the workplace should be reduced from 10 to 1 parts per million in air, even though OSHA had not performed a quantitative risk assessment. The affected industry challenged this rule. A plurality of the Court, led by Justice John Paul Stevens, ruled that OSHA's position was untenable and that, prior to regulating a risk, an agency must perform a risk assessment, demonstrate that a significant risk may exist, and further demonstrate that the proposed rule would significantly reduce that risk. Although lawyers will say that this ruling applies only to chemicals in the workplace, the logic of the Stevens opinion was so compelling that it has stimulated interest in risk analysis in many other fields. Interestingly, Justice Stevens notes in his opinion that it was preliminary analytic work by Professor Richard Wilson of Harvard that helped persuade the Court that quantitative risk assessment was feasible.

In light of this history of risk analysis, I can think of no more appropriate authority to offer an introduction to the field than Richard Wilson. As Director of the Harvard Center for Risk Analysis, I am honored that the Center has played a modest role in encouraging the completion of this book.

John D. Graham, Ph.D. Director Harvard Center for Risk Analysis
February 7, 2001

1

Introduction: Perspective on Risk

Life is a risky business. We all continuously face risks of some sort or another. Sometimes we face risky monetary decisions; sometimes we face dangers to life and limb. Not only do we face these dangers, we make decisions daily about them and compare, even if only implicitly, the risk to the benefit. Each morning we decide to get up, face the world and the boss and forgo the benefit of a day in bed, but avoid the risk of being fired and the cost of lost salary. We decide when it is safe to cross the road, and when it is wiser to wait; we may choose to ride by auto rather than bicycle or walk; we may use safety glasses while home woodworking, or decide to quit smoking.

In these everyday choices that we make consciously or unconsciously, we assess the risk more or less crudely, assess the benefits of monetary gain, pleasure, or other objectives, and make our own trade off. This rapid risk-cost-benefit analysis is based on a host of factors, such as reasoning, guess-work, and past experience. In many obvious cases, the actual risks are small, and the risk assessment need be done only crudely and perfunctorily to be adequate. Individuals may reach different decisions on the timing for crossing roads since different individuals may not agree on the values they apply to different risks. In the old aphorism: "one man's meat is another man's poison." Moreover, these values may not remain constant over time in even one individual.

In this book we introduce a few of the ideas and difficulties associated with attempts to formally perform risk assessments and make risk benefit comparisons. The risks that we discuss are to health and human welfare. While it is plausible that other species are of interest, usually it is the survival and welfare of the whole population of such species that are of concern, not individuals or specific groups. Risks to such other species may be included in a risk-cost-benefit analysis, but we will assume that such effects are included in the monetary or non-monetary analysis of benefits and costs—while noting that our concern may ultimately in fact be for the indirect effects on humans of the direct effects on other species.

We will endeavor to put the analysis in commonplace terms as much as possible. We maintain that if the risk assessor cannot express the risk simply enough to be understood by others, it is likely that he does not understand the risk himself. We therefore argue that words used in risk assessment should follow common parlance rather than have a specialized meaning. That is not to downplay the role of the expert, however, nor to suggest that technicalities are not appropriate in technical documentation.

The word risk implies uncertainty. We do not discuss situations with outcomes that are definite and certain, although uncertainties can arise in many different ways. The uncertainty about involvement in auto accidents does not arise because we do not know whether cars are involved in accidents, but because we do not know whether our particular car will be involved in an accident. There are other cases where the risks are hypothetical—we do not know whether the event actually occurs—and much of our uncertainty arises from this. Trichloroethylene given repeatedly at high doses causes liver cancer in some strains of mice, but there is no strong direct evidence that it causes cancer in humans at low doses, although it is often considered prudent for regulatory policy to make the hypothetical assumption that it does. Individuals exposed to trichloroethylene are faced with an uncertainty of a different kind from that in the automobile example above. This is discussed in Chapter 3 under "Model Uncertainty." The important distinction between variability and uncertainty is also discussed in Chapter 3.

Events or actions, which may pose a risk to humans are perceived through the filter of our senses. Perceptions are further modified by experience, time of occurrence, culture, religion, and other variables that make each person unique. We cannot, a priori, expect the assignment of the same values to similar risks by different persons. The experience of attempting to cross a street in an unfamiliar city is an example—an inhabitant may clearly recognize a "safe" situation, where the visitor hesitates. The results are differences of opinions, each opinion based on perceptions of risk, but differing from all others with different perceptions. We include a discussion of risk perception in Chapter 4.

Perception is Crucial

The importance of perceptions of risks is illustrated by Table 1-1 (Marsh-McLennan, 1978), which summarizes results of a public opinion survey of twenty years ago. Most people seem to believe that life was becoming more dangerous, even though most objective measures show the contrary to be true. Figure 1-1 (from the Vital Statistics of the U.S.) shows how in almost every age group the risk of dying has steadily fallen in the last 100 years. This figure shows the dramatic bump in 1919 due to the worldwide influenza epidemic which killed more people than the First World War. The increases in death rate among the 15–35 year olds in 1965 to 1975 are attributable to car accidents, and from 1975 to 1990 to AIDS.

One standard inverse measure of the probability of dying is the expectation of life, or life expectancy. This has been steadily increasing in the U.S. since about 1900. This is shown in U.S. statistics in Figure 1-2. There is a difference (fortunately decreasing) in life expectancy between black and white Americans. Life expectancy has changed slowly throughout the millennia. Half the skeletons in the Beijing caves, 7,000 years ago, were young, suggesting a life expectancy of 13 years. Roman writers talked about 23 years. Life expectancy slowly rose and reached 35 years in Sweden in 1750, from which time more accurate records were kept. Figure 1-3 shows the rapid rise in life expectancy for Sweden since about 1850 reaching 80 years recently. Figure 1-3 shows that life expectancy in Japan and France has almost caught up, as it has in the United States. Until 1980, life expectancy in the USSR was about 1 year less than in the United States, France, Japan and Sweden, but fell to

---

TABLE 1-1

Public Opinion Survey from Marsh-McLennan Companies

Thinking about the *actual amount of risk* facing our society, would you say that people are subject to more risk today than they were twenty years ago, less risk today, or about the same amount of risk as twenty years ago?

	Top Corporate Executives ($N = 401$)	Investors, Lenders ($N = 104$)	Congress ($N = 47$)	Federal Regulators ($N = 47$)	Public ($N = 1,488$)
More risk	38	60	55	43	78
Less risk	36	13	26	13	6
Same amount	24	26	19	40	14
Not sure	1	1	0	4	2

FIGURE 1-1

Death Rates from 1900 to 1998 for Various Age Groups: United States

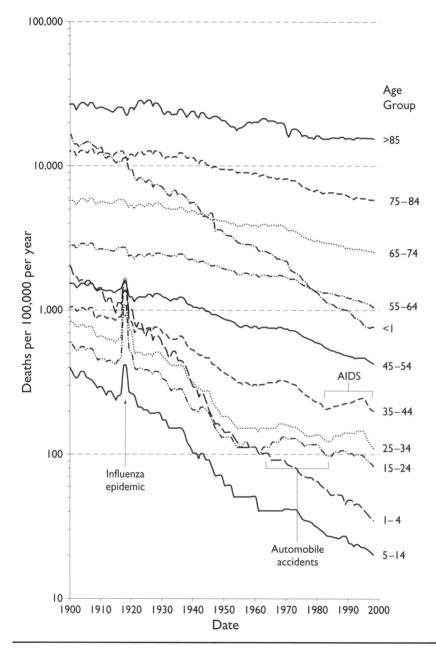

FIGURE 1-2

Expectation of Life at Birth in the United States
(1900–1928, Death Registration States Only)

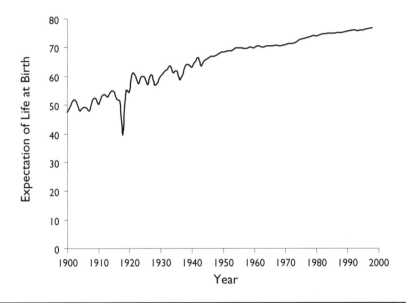

---

about 67 for Russian males in the mid 1990s, rose again in 1997, and is slowly decreasing again. As also shown in Figure 1-3, life expectancy in some developing countries is still substantially shorter than for the other countries shown in Figures 1-2 and 1-3.

This increase in life expectancy in developed countries has been brought about by the elimination of many large risks to life, such as many infectious and contagious diseases, poor working conditions, and inadequate nutrition[1] (Doll, 1979). Improved medical technology is now making small improvements, at high cost. This, in itself, leads to problems. The issues that these concepts address are illustrated both by a cartoon and by a quotation from H. Daly in 1982:

"As far as we know, God is not impatient for our lives to be lived soon"

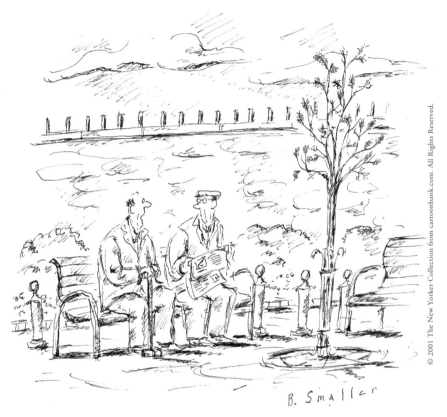

© 2001 The New Yorker Collection from cartoonbank.com. All Rights Reserved.

"My goal is to die before there's a technology breakthrough that forces me to live to a hundred and thirty."

Western societies now concentrate on the many smaller risks, many of which are poorly understood, in order to further reduce total risks. Perhaps the fact that many more risks, even though smaller, are now being discussed, has caused the apparent alarm of those whose opinions are summarized in Table 1.1. The problem may also be a question of a different understanding of the word risk. We have, for example, not found anyone who thinks that life expectancy in the U.S. is going down or is about to go down, in spite of the fact that many people believe that life is riskier! This different understanding of the word "risk" is one of the issues in perception of risks discussed in Chapter 4. The problem is very deep seated. Mankind is used to dealing with decisions in a binary manner: "yes, it is safe" or "no, it is dangerous." Yet

FIGURE 1-3

Expectation of Life from 1700–2000 in Sweden/France/Japan

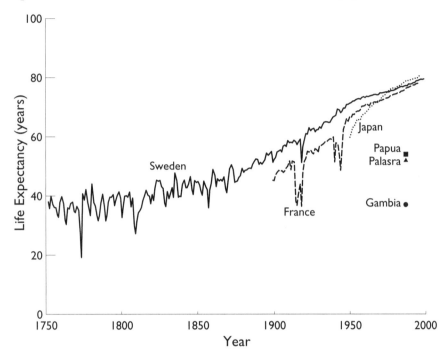

the world rarely works that way, and chance events are inherent. We therefore suggest that it is a role of a specialist to interpret for the general public and guide them as to which risks are acceptable and which are not.

But even if a risk is *acceptable* (worthy of acceptance) it may not be *accepted.* Decisions are clearly never based on actual risks but (at best) on the decision maker's perception of them. In this book we make an assumption, most of the time, that an expert's calculation of the magnitude of a risk is likely to be more accurate than a lay person's perception, and that societal decisions are more likely to lead to a general good if the expert's calculation is used in an analysis than if a lay person's perception is used. But a failure of a decision maker to recognize the perception of a lay person can lead to a public revolt—and a negation of the decision. The effectiveness and correctness of any decision is usually judged by lay persons. This point is discussed further in Chapter 7.

It is the differing perceptions, opinions, and sometimes political agendas, of individuals and groups that control their differing actions. When an individual action has a small possible consequence—ranging from no harm to a maximum of one death at a time—and the action is repeated by large numbers of individuals, typically these differences lead to a spectrum of results, good, bad and indifferent, but typically, no single action is likely to have a catastrophic effect.[2] Individuals can see not only the results of their own actions, but also the results of the ill-conceived actions of others. They can then adjust their future behavior to reduce the harmful effects. Recently we have built large technological systems, so that a single decision can now result in large harmful effects—several thousands of deaths. In such circumstances, there is much less opportunity for this feedback to limit harmful effects, since the first wrong action could be disastrous, when compared with historical precedents. We therefore often want to find out how risky an action is before anyone has performed it, and so we attempt to introduce some objectivity into the analysis of risk, instead of relying on imperfect and uninformed direct perception. We introduce objectivity in an attempt to modify a priori perceptions by the use of objective evidence. Furthermore, it is necessary always to bear in mind that any such attempt at analysis of risks only attacks one aspect of any problem—the risks of any event or action have always to be weighed against costs and benefits.

Definition of Risk

Risk is a word used in many different ways by different disciplines. Indeed, so varied is its use that some authors have avoided the word entirely. Accordingly we consider it necessary to define precisely what we mean by a risk and by its numerical measurement. There are three meanings of the noun in the Oxford English Dictionary: (1) "hazard, endanger, exposure to mischance or peril" and (2) "the chance of hazard or commercial loss," (3) "as in Risk-Money, an allowance paid to a cashier to cover accidental deficits." The quantitative meaning we use in this book is close to (2).

Although there are uses of the word risk that are more inclusive, in this book we associate risks with events or actions. It is an often overlooked fact that inaction, whether it is conscious or unconscious, can also be risky and is susceptible to analysis. For example, society has so far decided to take no action to prevent a meteor or comet from striking the earth, and society is so far taking few actions to reduce the CO_2 buildup in the atmosphere. The events and actions may be small or large, from digging one shovel of dirt to creating new seas, from creating a one-way street to decisions on whole highway construction programs. For each event or action we associate some units of risk, leading to a risk per street crossing for example, or a risk per ton of copper ore mined. Thus in some way we have a visualization:

$$\text{Total risk} = \begin{pmatrix} \text{How much} \\ \text{or how often} \end{pmatrix} \otimes \begin{pmatrix} \text{Some risk per} \\ \text{unit of action,} \\ \text{or per event} \end{pmatrix} \qquad (1\text{-}1)$$

In more useful form we can write:

$$\text{Risk} = \text{Probability} \otimes \text{Severity} \qquad (1\text{-}2)$$

In a decision-making context we are concerned with a perception of a risk. This is an approximation of the risk itself so that we initially interpret the terms in this equation as being perceptions (either of the decision maker or of his expert consultant or his employer), so that the equation thus reads:

Our perception of the magnitude of risk from some event depends on some form of product of how often we think the event will occur and how serious we consider each occurrence to be in its effects.

To illustrate, consider the following cases:

(a) The risk of a broken leg is greater for an inexperienced skier than for an experienced skier.

(b) The risk of death or injury in auto accidents is greater for those not wearing restraint harnesses (seat belts) than for those who are.

In (a), the severity of injury (broken leg) is the same, but we expect the probability, per day of skiing, to be higher for the inexperienced skier. In (b), we expect the probability of accidents is approximately the same, but the severity to be markedly higher for the unrestrained auto occupants.

Notice that we have refrained from putting an ordinary multiplication sign ($\times$) in the above equation, since in some practical cases risk perceptions may not be truly multiplicative (Tversky et al., 1990). Nevertheless, it appears that most risks do have some multiplicative features, and we shall use this below in our first attempt to introduce objectivity. Others have defined risk less objectively (Fischoff, 1984).

Thus far, the discussion has been concerned mainly with single events or actions. Of course, the definition was left open, so that such "single" events/ actions could cover most cases, but in essence they consist of the most elementary actions we are to analyze with respect to their risk content. To associate a risk with more complex events or actions, it is necessary to break down the actions into individual smaller actions. Then we usually assume that summation is possible and write:

$$\text{Risk} = S \{\text{probability} \otimes \text{severity} \otimes \text{weight}\} \qquad (1\text{-}3)$$

where the S stands for whatever form of addition (unknown) is actually used by individuals. The weight factor is included separately here—it could perhaps be included in the "severity" term if the equation relates perceptions, but it is convenient for later discussion to isolate it. It is included to account for the possibility that in evaluating a problem consisting of many different parts, risks of apparently similar magnitude may be accorded very different weights in consideration of the totality. Any inappropriate assignment of weight, or erroneous perception of the risk of any section of a problem, may lead to inappropriate ("incorrect") actions or decisions. That is, such actions or decisions would result in end results different from those planned, and thus not optimal from some point of view. One attempt at reducing such non-optimal results is the objective analysis of risk, which we pursue throughout this book. A technical reader will recognize that we are describing a Bayesian approach to a discussion of probability: that is, a perceived probability is a prior probability modified by subsequent data.

Risk Changes as Events Unfold

It is important to realize that the concept of risk is not static in time. As events develop, the risk changes. When I start to cross a road there is a risk that I will be killed by an oncoming car. If I reach the other side the risk will have dropped to zero. If I fail to reach the other side and the car does me in, the risk reaches 100% and is no longer called a risk. This point also holds for the assessment of risks of exposure to radiation or to a chemical. Whereas there is a risk that anyone will develop cancer as a result of exposure to radiation that is not a sensible concept for a person who already has that cancer. Instead we can ask "what is the probability that his cancer was caused by radiation." This is often called "The Probability of Causation" (POC) (Mettler and Upton, 1975; NIH, 1985) and can be related quantitatively to the risk by the equation derivable from Bayes' theorem:

$$\text{POC} = \frac{(\text{Risk from Radiation})}{(\text{Risk due to all causes})} \qquad (1\text{-}4)$$

It is important to distinguish clearly the two concepts of Risk and Probability of Causation. For example, although the risk of developing angiosarcoma from vinyl chloride exposure is small, the incidence of angiosarcoma is itself small, so that the fraction of angiosarcomas caused by agents other than vinyl chloride can also be small, so that the Probability of Causation is high when someone even with a small exposure to vinyl chloride develops an angiosarcoma.

Measures of Risk

To make any start on objective assessments it is necessary to realize what is being measured. Death is one clear, objective, measure.[3] The total annual risk of death at any age is the probability of dying within one year. In the absence of any extra causes, population averages for this measure are obtained from national mortality tables (see Chapter 7). But in risk assessments we are interested in additional risks of death (or components of the total risk of death) due to some specific actions that we undertake—either of our own volition or involuntarily. More often, we are interested in how much of an action to undertake, so that we wish to evaluate measures such as "extra probability of death per unit of action"—for example, extra probability of death per cigarette smoked, or deaths per ton of coal mined.

Death is not the only measure of risk which may be of interest, for although it is probably the most objective one, and for this reason is often used, it may not capture large components of what are perceived as "risks." For balanced decisions involving risks, a consideration of other measures of risk may be vital. A matrix of a few possible measures, which may be evaluated, is:

Deaths	by age (e.g., deaths of children, of working men, of senior citizens)
	by cause
Injuries	by cause
	by type (e.g., acute, physical, loss of limb, reduction in IQ)
	by some sort of severity index
Per	year
	lifetime
	unit operation
	event
	ton
	unit output

Other measurement units have been proposed or evaluated in some circumstances and may be useful in some decisions, some of the common ones being:

Loss of life expectancy (LOLE) [sometimes listed as years
    of life lost (YOLL or YLL)]
Man days lost (MDL)
Working days lost (WDL)
Public days (days for individual enjoyment) lost (PDL)
Quality adjusted life years (QALY)
Disability adjusted life years (DALY)

Death is one measure commonly used in current risk assessment, although rarely properly discussed. We all die eventually: indeed the largest single cause of death is birth! What is meant here is "premature death," and it is usually very important to distinguish between deaths at different ages. Since Life Expectancy is one of the few statistical concepts understood by nonspecialists, Loss of Life Expectancy (LOLE) can be an important measure to explain the risk to the public. But in general the appropriate measures of risk to use in any given risk assessment will depend on the specific details of the question the risk assessment is designed to illuminate—presumably they will be those corresponding as nearly as possible to the way in which the risks are perceived.

Morbidity has only recently been discussed systematically. In a monumental work, Murray and Lopez (1996) discuss how to calculate Quality of Life Years or Disability Adjusted Life Years for diseases and injuries. Disability Adjusted Life Years (DALY) is the Years of Life Lost (YOLL) plus Years Lived with Disability (YLD) adjusted for severity of the disability. For an individual whether there is death or whether there is merely a disability is very important. In calculating a risk, however, many early (1975–1995) risk assessors took account of the fact that pollutants cause morbidity as well as mortality either by arbitrarily increasing the risk estimate, or by insisting on a smaller value of the acceptable risk. Early analysts of black lung disease among coal miners belittled it by calling it a mere disability. But a victim of black lung disease can die of it, after a delay but still prematurely, just as surely as cancer can kill after a long latent period. It has therefore been a common practice, which will be adopted in much of this book, to include such disabling diseases among mortality. Recent comprehensive risk studies (European Com-

FIGURE 1-4

Three Different Metrics of Occupational Risk in Coal Mining, U.S.

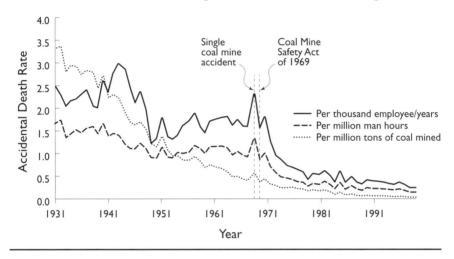

mission, 1999) have begun to use the more advanced concepts of Murray and Lopez and their followers.

Currently, the commonest types of risk assessment are probably those produced by or for the U.S. EPA or similar state agencies, in connection with Superfund sites (or similar chemically contaminated sites addressed by state statutes). Such risk assessments generally are supposed to evaluate estimates of two measures of risk, a lifetime probability of cancer and a "hazard index." The former is an estimate of the increment in the probability for an individual of any type of cancer arising at any time in their lifetime. The usual estimates evaluated are upper bounds on this probability, obtained by extrapolation from experiments on laboratory animals at high dose rates or from epidemiological studies of exposed human populations. The "hazard index" is less well-defined. It is made up of a sum over chemicals of "hazard quotients," each being the ratio of potential dose rate for a particular chemical (usually deliberately evaluated at the upper end of what might be possible on a particular site) to a "reference dose" for that chemical. The "reference dose" for a chemical (defined by U.S. EPA) is a dose rate for that chemical estimated to be unlikely to cause any harm to any member of the population.

Accidental Death Rates by Type of Coal Mine, U.S.

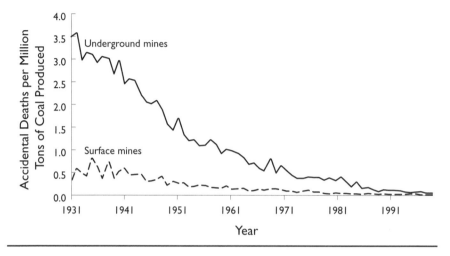

Different Measures Can Lead to Different Decisions

In this book we will usually be limiting ourselves to risks of death—probabilities of dying or expected excess numbers of deaths—due to various actions, although other risks will be occasionally mentioned. Although we shall not concern ourselves much with it, the distinction introduced above between risks and measures of risk is not totally academic. We illustrate it with a simple example given by risk of working in the U.S. coal industry, taken as a whole, between 1950 and 1970. Figure 1-4 displays three measures of risk in this industry vs. calendar year. The first, the number of accidental deaths per ton of coal mined declined throughout this period (and indeed for over a century). By this measure the industry appears to be getting safer. But the number of accidental deaths per person employed increased slightly over the period 1950–1970. From this perspective one might assert that the industry was getting more dangerous, not safer. However, after 1970 both measures improved considerably.

Neither measure taken alone is "right" or "wrong," nor are they even contradictory. The first might be the view of a coal industry executive, or even the President of the United States responsible for the overall well being of the country. The second might be the perspective of a trade union leader interested in the welfare of his members. Any risk assessment that attempted to be complete would have to draw attention to both aspects of the risk of coal mining expressed by the different measures used above, and attempt to take both into account, depending on the purpose of that risk assessment. In addition, it is likely that other factors, such as the distinction shown in Figure 1-5 between underground mines and surface mines, would have to be explicitly considered.

The best steps to take to reduce the risk might also depend on which of the two measures we use. If we doubled the number of miners, each working on alternate days, the risk per miner might decrease by a factor of about 2, but the risk per ton of coal mined (Figure 1-4) would stay roughly constant. In a decision process both measures and both points of view will usually have to be considered. Although a politician is primarily interested in the total societal impact (risk per ton mined), it is not consistent with a just society to have one group with a much larger total risk than another group. In comparing risk and benefits we naturally consider both groups; those engaged in particularly hazardous occupations get (or should get) hazard pay to compensate for the increased risk by an increased benefit.

In the above paragraph we have completely ignored many issues that may be important in particular assessments and decisions. These include:

- risk to the public (as distinct from risk to the workers) from dust and water emissions, from subsidence and from coal transport, for example.

- variations between groups within the industry. Coal face (underground) workers and surface workers endure different hazards in the "underground" part of the industry, and similarly the hazards to those in strip mining (surface) operations differ.

- other risks of death from, e.g., pneumoconiosis (black lung disease), and other components of risk ranging from the risks of traveling to work, through injuries and illnesses.

We also ignored still other measures of risk. Death is only a partial measure of risk and for the best understanding of risk as many such partial measures as possible should be evaluated. While it is possible to (arithmetically) aggregate all such measures in some way, they would have to be added together with some weighting factors relating different measures (as in the formulae quoted earlier, except using arithmetic summation and multiplication). This is done in the evaluation of QALYs and DALYs mentioned briefly above. However, any such weighting of different measures is necessarily somewhat arbitrary and furthermore may obscure or usurp clear perceptual differences. The arbitrariness is easy to illustrate by attempting to find a weighting factor to relate deaths, Man Days Lost (MDL) and Working Days Lost (WDL).

Accidents occur at all ages, but the average age of persons dying of accidents is 42 years compared with an average age of death of 79 years for American nonsmokers as a whole. The loss of life expectancy is thus 37 years and the loss of working life expectancy is about 25 years (taking account of retirement at age 67), leading to $37 \times 365.25 = 13,514$ Man Days Lost (MDL) or $25 \times 300 = 7,500$ Working Days Lost (WDL) per death. But the average age for cancer deaths is about 54, so the loss of life expectancy is about 25 years and of working life expectancy about 13 years which leads to or 9,131 MDL per death and 3,900 WDL per death. Any weighting factor would thus strictly have to depend on the cause of death—although an average of 6,000 WDL per death is often used—and whether such an average is adequate will depend on the particular case. However, these estimates do not usually assist in a practical risk-benefit calculation, since we do not necessarily perceive death as being simply equivalent to a loss of a certain number of working days. Many people take more account of non-working (or "public") days.

With these caveats on measures of risk in mind we return to our "objective" risk assessment. Having chosen measures, they must be evaluated for the action or event under study. The straightforward way of doing this is to break down each action or event into component parts until each component may be taken as a whole, to evaluate the risk measure for each such component and then to sum to obtain the resultant measure of risk for the original action or event. The depth of analysis can obviously vary, depending on the problem and on the analyst, but the first essential for any analysis is identification of component parts, which may be individually treated. Our previous example of coal mining accidents has been treated as such a component and averaged over all employees, although of course it would be possible to "take it apart" further and separately analyze risks to coal face workers, surface workers, office workers, etc., and include other risks. It would appear obvious that, having broken the action or event into components, analyzed each component and summed up again, the measure of risk for the complete action or event has been obtained. This is, however, not quite true, or rather, this is an incomplete statement. Consider a single action, with the possibility of either carrying it out or not. In the first case, the procedure above will evaluate some measure(s) of risk for performing the action. However, even if the action is not carried out, it is likely that there will be still some risks to the persons who would otherwise be affected by the action. There is thus an arbitrary choice in a risk assessment—should such a "background" level of risk be subtracted from each evaluated measure to account for the risks which would be present even in the absence of the action or event which is being assessed? There is an even greater difficulty in decomposing a risk into its parts and adding all of the parts. As discussed further in Chapter 4, Tversky and colleagues have shown that when a risk is so decomposed into its parts, the magnitude of the perceived risk increases, although the true risk, what-ever it is, must remain the same.

Absolute or Incremental Risk

The problem we have posed refers to the case of a simple decision: do or refrain. If the decision is among two or more alternatives, a similar problem arises as soon as any attempt is made to make any comparison—should the comparison be based on absolute or incremental measures of risk? This question becomes acute when one realizes that comparisons based on the first may give different results from those based on the second. An example shows this.

Consider two alternative actions, A and B, either of which involves chang-ing the status of some of the N people in the population. Prior to any action the populace is subject to some background risk with a measure X per person. If action A involves increasing the risk for N/2 people to 1.1 X, whereas action B increases the risk for N/3 people to 1.2 X we have a case in which results differ depending on whether absolute risk or incremental risk is ana-lyzed.

$$\text{For A the absolute risk is} \quad N/2 \times 1.1\, X = 0.55\, NX. \quad (1\text{-}5)$$

$$\text{For B it is} \quad N/3 \times 1.2\, X = 0.4\, NX. \quad (1\text{-}6)$$

Thus, the risk of A is greater than the risk of B. But now look at incremental risks:

$$\text{for A} \quad N/2 \times (1.1\, X - X) = 0.05\, NX, \quad (1\text{-}7)$$
$$\text{for B} \quad N/3 \times (1.2\, X - X) = 0.066\, NX. \quad (1\text{-}8)$$

Thus, with this measure, the risk of B is greater than the risk of A, a result apparently at variance with the one from absolute risk. This example was constructed, of course, to be clear cut and obvious. In practice, one would not treat the whole population as homogeneous and facing similar risks, and similarly, the work forces on the projects would not be homogeneous.

Defining the System Boundary

The problem we have just considered is just one (albeit an important one) of those that arise from lack of definition of system boundaries. In evaluating a measure of risk for any action or event/project, i.e. for any system, the value we obtain will depend on the boundaries we set to that system—which parts will be included and which excluded. In evaluating total risks in the problem above, we were effectively trying to draw a boundary around some set of actions and/or events and/or geographical regions and evaluate the measures of risk of interest within that boundary. In evaluating a differential risk, in the ideal case we draw a boundary around all actions/events, etc., and evaluate the relevant measure(s) of risk for everything in two cases, the first with the project, the second without, and then subtract to obtain a differential measure.

Let us look a little more closely at an example we used before—the coal industry. We showed before graphs of two measures of risk for the coal industry—accidental deaths per ton mined and accidental deaths per person employed—over a twenty-year period. Although we did not explicitly state this, we assumed a certain system boundary in presenting those risk measures. In this case, the system boundary enclosed the U.S. coal industry (defined by a Standard Industrial Classification number), including office workers and coal face workers together, including surface (open pit) and underground mines together, and including bituminous coal and anthracite together, but was limited to deaths among those working in this industry only. To be more complete, it would be necessary to include also accidental deaths in other industries due to the requirements of the coal industry (even if we still limit ourselves to the single measure of accidental deaths). Thus the coal industry uses machinery, which in turn uses iron and steel; and accidental deaths occur in the machinery production industry, in the iron and steel industry, in iron ore mining and in transport between all of these. Some of these accidental deaths may thus be ascribed to coal production. Similarly the coal industry uses some electricity bought from the electrical utility industry, in which there occur accidental deaths also—some of which may thus be ascribed to the coal industry. In some public discussions of the risk from nuclear power, opponents have emphasized that the risk of air pollution (while small) is not (as nuclear proponents, have often claimed) zero, because energy and electricity have been used both in construction and uranium enrichment—and a part of that electricity is generated by burning coal.

There is a complicating factor in this—both the iron and steel industry and the electricity industry use coal, so it would appear that carrying the argument an extra step leads to circularity. But the argument is not circular, since not all the coal is used in iron and steel and electricity production. One way of describing the situation is to say that the series we obtain is convergent. This problem is met also in the discipline of net energy analysis and is similarly solved (mathematically) by solving coupled sets of equations. The result is a change in the evaluated magnitude of our measure of risk—but this is to be expected, since the system we are now analyzing (defined by the system boundaries) has been enlarged to include those portions of the electricity supply industry, and the iron and steel industry, required to keep the coal industry in operation. As in net energy analysis, there may be some ambiguity in performing risk analyses on systems such as that described in the last paragraph. It is usual to assume that all parts of the system are linear (i.e. an increase of output of any industry of x% requires increases of all its inputs by x%) unless better models are available. If some operation has multiple outputs, it is difficult or impossible to unambiguously assign risks to each output. But with suitable choice of system boundary, such ambiguities can perhaps be minimized in their impact on the total measures of risks being sought.

Some apparent ambiguities may be resolved by more precise articulation of the problem actually under study. Consider the problem of evaluating some measure of total societal impact from the production of iron in the U.S., and note that perhaps one-third of the iron ore used is actually imported. Evidently some of the risk in producing iron ore comes from the risk of mining, milling and transporting iron ore, but what risk measure should be assigned to imported iron ore to account for these risks in its production? There are at least three possibilities:

(1) *Assign zero risk.*

This might be appropriate if the measure of risk required is to the total risk to the U.S. population of iron production. Since import of iron ore causes no production-related risk to anyone in the U.S., we can ignore any actual risks incurred in its production. (Note that we will not get a zero risk attribution to imports on a differential risk basis, since paying for the imports would require some actions, which would not be risk free).

(2) *Assign a risk measure equal to that incurred in production of ore in the U.S.*

This is the simplest procedure to follow, and leads to indifference (from the total risk point of view) between imports and U.S. production. This assignation is equivalent to assuming that all variations in production occur in U.S. sources.

(3) *Assign a risk measure equal to that actually incurred in overseas production.*

This is the most difficult option here considered, since it requires much more analysis. It might be appropriate if the total risk to the global population of iron production were required. Such an analysis would be needed were we interested in CO_2 emissions and climate change, for example.

The analysis and the response to the analysis will be different depending upon the persons making the decision. Leaders of a country may wish to take the widest possible boundaries. Even so, the option for iron ore production risk assessment may well be (2), since the measure is available (it has to be computed in analysis of U.S. production anyway), requires no decisions to be made on the domestic/import split (as would be required for (1)) and is an approximation to (3) (if it may be assumed that risks are not too disparate between countries). An individual local utility operator deciding which type of power station to use would not *directly* consider CO_2 emissions from coal mines or accidents in transport. If society wishes these factors to be taken account in local decisions, the costs must be *internalized* by taxation or charges as discussed further in Chapter 5.

It is important to recognize this fact that different decision makers will usually use different boundaries. The position of system boundaries is of crucial concern when attempting to make risk comparisons between different systems (or projects, events, actions). For any use to be made of such comparisons, the systems under consideration should presumably be designed to perform similarly or produce the same or similar results. A particular example is that of relative risks of energy (especially electricity) generating (or converting) systems—especially the comparisons between the "conventional" systems (using coal, oil, gas, hydropower or nuclear energy) and "unconventional" systems (various solar technologies, wind, biomass, etc.) (Crouch and Wilson, 1980, European Commission, 1999). While most of these technologies may be used for generating electricity, comparison of the different systems utilized from a risk point of view may be easily and grossly affected by alteration of system boundaries. The choice of system boundaries should, of course, be predicated explicitly on the exact question required of interest in any such comparison.

We have attempted to define the meaning of risk by discussing risk analysis. Readers will have noticed our firmly held opinion that risk analysis, and more generally, risk-cost-benefit analysis, cannot properly be performed without close attention to the decision at issue. What question are we asking? The risk analysis may be considered as a branch of decision analysis. A classic reference is Raiffa (1968), and there are many other good references available. But there are crucial distinctions in practice. The usual domain of decision analysis, in business, involves choice between options that differ only slightly—consequences may vary by perhaps 5%, but this may be the difference between bankruptcy and a comfortable profit margin.[4] Catastrophes need not be considered explicitly in any business decision, because society takes care (at least to some extent) of the consequences of catastrophe by its bankruptcy laws. Decisions are usually required on short term problems. Risk-benefit analysis, on the other hand, is called upon to deal with decisions involving much greater uncertainty, where catastrophes have to be considered explicitly and may contribute substantially to both uncertainty and expected values. Further, the problems may be very long-term. In cases of large uncertainties, one use of risk analysis may be to set bounds on the possible consequences of decisions—and these bounds may then be used in the risk-cost-benefit analysis as some form of "worst expected case."

Layout of the Book

We regard the introduction of objectivity as essential for a sound decision. Unless a person has calculated a risk, with its uncertainty, outlined his procedure, and highlighted the omissions, we cannot be sure he has made a reasoned, rational decision. This statement has an important consequence. Risk assessment should not be an arcane discipline, carried out by narrowly focused experts in a back room. The assessment should be understood, and preferably carried out, by people responsible for the risky technology. The manager of an oil refinery should understand the details of the risks that the refinery poses. Only then will he know what are the central factors in his technology on which to concentrate. This is particularly important when risk assessment is being used to discover ways of reducing risks. Often (all too often) a risk assessment seems to be merely presented to the public to justify a decision already made. Then the risk analyst appears to be merely an advocate; a sophisticated "hired gun," using more or less arbitrary results to support a pre-ordained policy preference. It need not be thus. Chapter 2 discusses objective, thorough, methods of estimating risks.

The objectivity of analysis inevitably involves an understanding of uncertainty. Physical scientists are used to discussing error in physical measurements, and books have been written on "The Theory of Error." The same mathematical tools are available to discuss uncertainty in the results of a risk assessment. However, words must be carefully chosen. While "error" is often an appropriate word, when a train engineer has run his train off the end of the platform by not stopping in time, it is not usually used in risk contexts because of its pejorative connotations. We have heard it said that when a physician hears the word "error" he calls his lawyer at once! The role of uncertainty is so important in risk analysis that we have devoted a whole chapter to it (Chapter 3).

Having objectively evaluated risks of events or actions, with their uncertainties, what do we do with the results? A lot depends upon how the risks are perceived—a subject we discuss in Chapter 4. The crucial assumption is made that the perception of the expert is closer to the "real" risk than the perception of lay people. This may not always be true. The expert may develop a narrow focus because of this attention to detail whereas a lay person may "get the whole picture" more readily. In order to help bring the perception close to reality it is usually desirable to compare such risks with those of different events or actions designed to achieve the same or similar ends.

In Chapter 5 we describe a straightforward risk-risk comparison, but usually the risks are only one measure of effectiveness, so that the harder job of trying to compare risks with costs and benefits must be essayed. In this chapter we outline some methods of comparing risks with benefits. Firstly, we discuss how much an individual, or society, has paid, is paying or might pay in the future to reduce a risk. In this it is important to phrase the societal problem so that it can be answered and not get stymied by the imponderable "value of a life." Then we proceed to a formal layout, which is more general than that used by many government agencies for discussion of risks. We then show how the approaches of various agencies can approximate, in their context, our more extensive perspective.

Chapter 6 is a brief introduction to managing or mitigating risks. Our perspective is that most risks must be managed because they cannot be entirely eliminated. The most important risk manager is the individual in his or her thousands of everyday decisions. Therefore, the closer the management procedures lie the ordinary personal risk management procedures the more likely they are to be understood and accepted.

Approaches to controlling risky actions range from a complete ban (corresponding to the taboo of ancient societies), through adoption of the best available controls (e.g., the Best Available Control Technology defined by the U.S. EPA), to the use of formal risk-benefit analyses to determine appropriate levels of control (including no control). Decisions are made in spite of uncertainties, which are often large. Carefully chosen *incentives* can reduce the effort of devising and implementing regulatory procedures, and are for that reason a preferred strategy. This chapter also lists some statutory requirements with our comments on their approach to risk management strategy.

Chapter 7 assembles a list of risk estimates that we and others have calculated. The list provides useful comparisons and contrasts, and illustrates the dissimilarities between risks with similar magnitude. Also listed are various expenditures made with the intent of saving lives, and the results of such efforts. You may be disappointed by the omission of your favorite (or most unpleasant) risk. We encourage you to add to this table any risks with which you are familiar. Perform a risk assessment and send us the details, to allow us all to learn by comparison, and allow us to extend the lists.

The last section of the book, Chapter 8, is a bibliography of books and articles on risk and benefit. Some of these are the articles explicitly referenced in the text, and others are articles that the authors consider especially helpful, some of which may be of interest for further reading.

Notes

1 This elimination was largely due to measures of public health, rather than medical practice.

2 The adjective "possible" in this sentence must be construed with imagination. When a Serbian nationalist shot an Austrian Archduke in Sarajevo in July 1914, his small action led to the first world war. War is clearly a "possible" result of any political assassination.

3 Clear and objective with the possible exception of the following actual courtroom exchange between a medical examiner and a cross-examining attorney.

   Q. (From the cross-examining attorney): "Doctor, before you performed the autopsy, did you check for a pulse?"

   A. "No."

Q. "Did you check for blood pressure?"

A. "No."

Q. "Did you check for breathing?"

A. "No."

Q. So then it is possible that the patient was alive when you began the autopsy?"

A. "No."

Q. "How can you be so sure, Doctor?"

A. "Because his brain was sitting on my desk in a jar."

Q. "But could the patient have still been alive nevertheless?"

A. "It is possible that he could have been alive and practicing law somewhere."

4 As Mr. Micawber said to David Copperfield, "Annual income twenty pounds, expenditure nineteen and six—happiness. Annual income twenty pounds—expenditure twenty pounds ought and six, result misery."

2

Methods of Risk Calculation
and Estimation

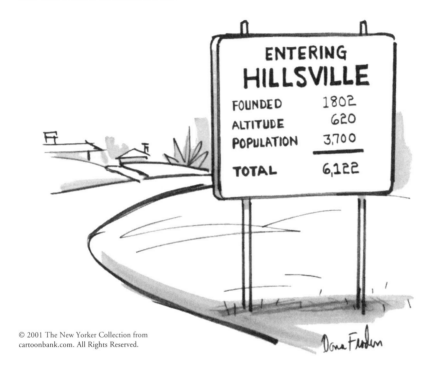

ENTERING
HILLSVILLE
FOUNDED	1802
ALTITUDE	620
POPULATION	3,700
TOTAL	6,122

© 2001 The New Yorker Collection from
cartoonbank.com. All Rights Reserved.

Once the risk measures to use have been decided, as discussed in Chapter 1, and the system boundaries within which they will be used have been mapped, there comes the task of estimating the magnitude of the chosen measures. In practice the analyst must bear this task in mind when evaluating the measures and boundaries, since the methods and data that are available will affect what is possible. The object is to obtain a numerical estimate for both the size of the risk measure and its uncertainty, or equivalent information. As the cartoon illustrates, great care must be taken to discuss the risks in measures that are consistent. The methods adopted will depend to a large extent on the nature of the risk, and of the adverse consequences of the events constituting the risk. Different methods may be appropriate depending on the past occurrences of the risky events (or similar ones), their frequency of occurrence (either expected or observed), their size and severity, and on predictions or expectations for those, which have not previously occurred (or not been observed). The way in which risks are perceived is highly correlated with the way in which they are calculated, and we therefore pay considerable attention to the methods in this chapter.

For ease of classification and discussion, we will distinguish between two classes of risks, which may be called "historical" and "new" respectively. By historical risks, we mean those in which the adverse events associated with them have occurred (and may continue to occur) sufficiently often for a reasonable data set to have been accumulated. In many cases, such risks have aroused sufficient interest that someone has performed analyses already, perhaps leading to a theory or model which is sufficiently detailed to allow useful conclusions about the magnitude of the risk. Examples of "historical" risks include the risks of or from: infectious diseases, motor vehicles, industrial accidents, and effects of weather, such as hurricanes, tornadoes, or lightning strikes.

There are some risks that are historical in the sense that some event has happened in the past which could happen again, and might produce serious adverse consequences if it did, but the frequency of occurrence has been too low to accumulate sufficient data to allow use of the methods commonly used on more frequent historical risks. An example might be the risk of death from a U.S. nuclear plant accident. One may be able to extract a useful "upper limit" to the numerical value risk from historical data but it is often better to proceed as for "new" risks.

"New" risks consist of those risks arising from events, which have not been observed, although they may have happened without our observing them. In many cases some sort of risk may be expected by analogy with historic experience (e.g., exposure to various organic chemicals may be expected to pose some risk), or it may be possible to predict theoretically the possibility of an adverse event (e.g., ignition of the cloud of methane gas released following a collision involving a liquefied natural gas tanker), even though the event has never occurred. New risks may include the whole range from catastrophic but improbable events (e.g., large meteor impacts, dam breaks, reactor meltdowns) to highly probable, low consequence events (e.g., risks arising from exposure to new chemicals). The methods of evaluation may appear to differ for such disparate classes of risk, but the difference is largely in the different emphasis placed on the different parts of the analysis. The basic idea is to break down any new risk into a sequence of events, each of which may be analyzed separately by theory, by analogy with historic risks or from actual occurrence, and then to reconstruct the whole from these parts.

Evaluation of "Historical" Risks

The methods are simple, direct, and obvious, but we go into some detail because the terminology and procedure that has become accepted over the years will be used later when we discuss the "new" risks. All estimates of risk involve some theory or model of how the risk is incurred. The historical data merely tell us what the risk was *last* year, and the model might be that next year will be like last year. A more sophisticated model can take account of the trend of the historical data. In this application, we make no distinction between a model and a theory—each being a description (often in mathematical terms) of how something (e.g., magnitude of risk measure) will change when some "external" variables (e.g., date, quantity of material, number of man hours, size of plant) change.

Historical risks usually arise from events of comparatively high probability, so that an appreciable number of events occur annually in the population at risk, but each event has a comparatively low consequence (less than about 10 deaths per event). We do not discuss high probability, high consequence events, since society has developed in such a way as to eliminate them and ensure that no such events exist. In some cases the consequences of high probability events have been reduced, and in others the occurrence rate of high consequence events has been reduced. The meaning of "comparatively high probability" will vary with the context. For example, an event occurring to an individual with average probability of 10^{-5} per year (1 in 100,000 per year), which would be considered a rare event individually (less than 1 in 1,000 people would experience it in their lifetime), corresponds to a high probability event in the context of the whole U.S. population of more than 281 million people (since it would occur annually about $10^{-5} \times 2.81 \times 10^8 =$ 2,810 times per year). Thus we can have a risk which an individual perceives to be small and will take no action to avoid; but society as a whole might perceive it to be big and spend considerable resources on reducing it.

When a large number of events occurs, one can accumulate a good data base for testing and fitting models, and it is usually sufficient to use the simplest model that fits the data and is physically reasonable for the extrapolations envisaged. It is unnecessary to have a detailed theory on why the event occurs, unless one is interested in estimating the changes in the risk following various specific actions. Examples where this method may be applied are accidents—in traffic, mountain climbing, drowning—and many natural hazards—rain, flood, snow, hail, lightning, and the incidence of some diseases. For these cases we might then assume that the future probability of an event is equal to the past probability, and the consequences of any event similar in the future to those in the past. Alternatively, any time trends observed may be incorporated as approximations to the complicated set of changes in conditions that actually may occur.

A simple case of such a trend might be steady or otherwise predictable, change in the number of potential accident initiators (e.g. autos) or a steady change in conditions affecting the risk (e.g. a steady improvement in the safety of autos). Despite the possibility of such changes in the future, the uncertainty of our risk estimates is comparatively small, because the mechanisms causing risks are many, or are unalterable (either in practice or in theory), even though the mechanisms may be unknown. Figure 2-1 shows

FIGURE   2 - 1

Death Rates for Motor Vehicle Accidents in the United States

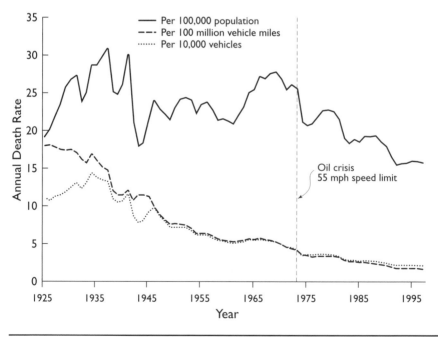

that despite the year-to-year variation, the risk of death in an auto accident has steadily declined over 25 years from 28 to 16 per 100,000 persons per year, with a fluctuation about this steady decline. We can be fairly confident that the rate will, *ceteris paribus*, be 1.6×10^{-4} ±10% for several (perhaps 5) years ahead. Figure 2-1 also shows that, in this case, the death rate per vehicle or per passenger mile shows a smoother trend, so that a model which assumes the number of traffic fatalities proportional to passenger miles traveled or number of cars may give a more accurate estimate of the risk expressed as the death rate per passenger mile or per car—although of course if we were interested in the death rate per 10^4 population, we would require also estimates of the number of passenger miles traveled or the number of cars.

In applications, it is usually necessary to make some sort of extrapolation in order to obtain risk measures relevant to the problem at hand. That is, given a model, which describes how the risk depends on various variables, it is usually necessary to estimate the risk for values of variables that are not included in the data used to set up the model. Perhaps the most common example of such a variable is time. We may have many data on past events to estimate some risk in the past, but to make predictions about the future we have to change the variable <time> in our model. (Naturally, if the risks do not vary with time in our model, changing this variable will not alter the risk estimate.) While auto accident death rates are generally decreasing with time, the fluctuations in these death rates may be due to various causes. For example, a more subtle study shows a sudden drop in auto accidents in calendar year 1974. This drop is relatively greater in deaths per person than in deaths per mile suggesting an effect of the 55 mph speed limit imposed late in 1973. But at least half of this dip is probably due to the reduction in miles per driver—due perhaps to the oil crisis of late 1973. Other common examples include the variables of size, dose, or concentration. Thus we might obtain data on the risk of death or injury in a U.S. industry as a function of the size of the establishment and conceive of a model with size of establishment as a variable. The model would then be "fitted to the data" (i.e. we would choose the model so that it reproduces the data as closely as possible), and might then be used to estimate risks in an establishment size not included in the initial data by changing the variable in the model.

An extension of the procedure outlined above can be used to give us, in many cases, an estimate for the risk of some consequence among some subsection of the population, e.g. the risk of death from pneumoconiosis (black lung disease) amongst miners, in the sense that the subsection of the population involved is described by different values of the variables included in the model(s). We can do this because the subsection differs from the total population. One is then led to ask why this difference occurs, and to inquire what may be done to reduce the higher risk. Further study indicates that the risk of pneumoconiosis depends in some way on the amount of dust inhaled, so that we can, by further investigation, get a relationship between the increase in risk and the amount of dust inhaled (amongst other factors). A risk can then be assigned to a particular cause (inhalation of dust) rather than to the more general and less useful heading of "coal mining."

In other cases we may have many historical data on consequences (e.g. mortality and morbidity) and we may suspect that some action is causing at least some of those consequences, but we have no clear subgroups among the population that differ only in their exposure to the action. A good example is atmospheric air pollution. At very high exposures (doses) in air pollution "incidents," the death rate and morbidity increases dramatically. Figure 2-2 shows the death rates and air pollution in London in December 1952. It is generally accepted that the air pollution at the end of the first week caused the increase in deaths during the first and second weeks of the month. But the effect of exposures ten times smaller is far less certain. Many studies have shown correlations between some measures of air pollution at these lower levels, and mortality (and morbidity), but a correlation is insufficient to prove causality, since there are many other variables (often called confounding variables—income level, smoking habits, occupation, geographical location, psychological stress, etc.) that are or may be correlated with both. The most complete analyses of mortality, attempting to account for as many such other variables as possible, still show some effect from air pollution, so that we can ascribe a yearly risk to this of 2.5×10^{-4} averaged over the U.S. The uncertainty in this estimate is large (±50% at least) Indeed, without evidence of direct cause and effect, the effects we suspect are caused by air pollution may in fact be caused by some other variable which we have missed in the analysis. Other lines of evidence need to be introduced—for example, laboratory evidence shows *acute* morbidity effects for air pollution, but only at levels substantially higher that observed in U.S. cities, although of course this does not preclude a *chronic* effect on mortality. A current hypothesis (Wilson and Spengler 1976) is that morbidity effects are caused in large part by fine particulate air pollution, but this hypothesis has not as yet been adequately tested against alternatives.

FIGURE 2-2

Daily Mean Pollution Concentrations and Daily Number of Deaths During the London Fog Episode of 1952

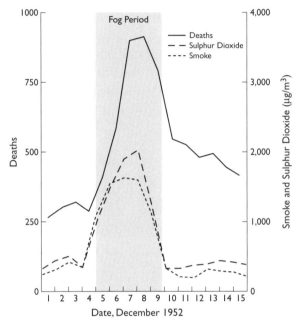

Source: Beaver 1953

The preceding examples illustrate the general rule that, even if there is copious historical data, no risk estimate may be extrapolated into the future without assuming some sort of theoretical model. The air pollution example indicates that even past risks may be uncertain if we lack a sure theoretical framework. Unless there is good reason from any alternative, Occam's razor indicates that the simplest theory that well explains the data should be used, so that in cases where the cause-effect relationship is not well understood the best predictor of future risk is that specific risk which appears to have the smoothest trend in the past. Thus in the auto example, the number of vehicles or the number of passenger miles traveled appear to be more closely related to the death rate than does the total number of people, so that the number of deaths per auto or the number of deaths per passenger mile give less uncertainty in the risk estimates than does the number of deaths per capita. A similar situation obtains in the coal mining industry (Figure 1-4), where it appears that the death rate per ton of coal mined has a smoother time trend than either the death rate per man hour or per person employed, suggesting that the amount of coal mined is a better predictor of the total number killed than are man hours worked or persons employed.

A good analyst will also use any auxiliary information he has to adjust the model and reduce the uncertainty of prediction. In Figure 1-4 we showed the risks due to coal mining. A peak may be noticed in 1968. This was due to a single large accident. This large accident led immediately to new federal laws on mine safety, and incidentally on black lung disease. It is tempting, and may even be correct, to ascribe the continuing subsequent reduction in risk to the implementation of the laws, or to the mind set that the presence of the laws has inculcated.

Using the method above consists basically of adjusting some model to fit past data, and then using the model (which should be physically reasonable) to extrapolate to new situations. Associated with each risk estimate made using this technique will be an uncertainty, which must be evaluated in order to know the confidence, which may be placed in the estimate of risk. This uncertainty arises from two basic sources. The most difficult to deal with is that due to error in the choice of model (choosing a model or theory which is not in accord with physical reality, and thus may give incorrect predictions) while the other, that due to statistical variations, is relatively much simpler.

The model or theory used may actually correspond to "the way things really are"—i.e. it may correspond to the real physical world in some sense. Hopefully the best verified theories do correspond to the physical world, at least over a restricted range of values of the variables. Such theories would include the so-called "laws of physics," many of which, in the form known to and used by non-specialists, are applicable only in restricted ranges of variables (they are usually approximations to more general "laws" valid over a much wider range of variables). Thus, the usual notion of addition of velocities only applies for velocities small compared with that of light; Newton's law of gravity applies only if the gravitational fields are not too large; and classical mechanics is an excellent approximation only for objects that are not too small. We use physical laws as our examples since these have usually been the best verified, but it is necessary to point out that all such laws are simply a codification of observations about the physical world. They may be used for prediction within the range of variables for which they are good approximations, but for extrapolation outside such ranges they may give incorrect results and require modification. (In the cases mentioned above, the ranges of variables for which they are good approximations include almost all the cases likely to be met in everyday situations.)

It has been said that "all models are wrong; some models are useful." The best (most useful) models and theories tend to be those in which causal connections have been established between different events—cause and effect (by "best theories" and "established" we mean those which give consistently accurate predictions and are thus widely accepted as valid). The physical laws mentioned above fall into this category.

One good example of risk assessment with modeling based largely on physical laws is the evaluation of the risk from the impact of a large meteorite or comet on the earth. Small meteorites strike the earth frequently (Solomon et al., 1977; Chapman and Morrison, 1994; Gehrels et al., 1994), and large ones occasionally. The probability of impact by larger meteorites and comets is much smaller than for small meteorites because of the reduced number of such objects, and the variation of this probability with meteorite size can be evaluated from historical observational data of various types. The effect of a meteorite impact depends on its velocity, size, angle of impact, composition, and on where it falls. The smallest meteorites vaporize in the atmosphere, and most of intermediate sizes making it to the surface fall comparatively harmlessly into the ocean or open country. But there is also a small probability of hitting a city (proportional to the relative surface areas of urban versus nonurban areas). The *consequences* of an impact will vary smoothly with the size of the meteorite, at least until the size of the impact becomes large enough to have global effects. Up until that size the impact will be local or regional although may be very serious. Above that size the impact is expected to have catastrophic secondary consequences, including immediate widespread fire due to re-entry of high velocity material "splashed" out of the atmosphere by the initial impact, long-term darkness (months to years) due to loading of the atmosphere with particles, and concomitant effects (crop failure, famine, disease).

On the other hand there are many cases in which no direct or causal connections are apparent, but there are indications that one may exist. There is usually observed, for example, a statistical relation between the size of establishments (in a given industry) and the injury and accident rate for employees working in the establishments. The correlation between establishment size and injury rate is unlikely to be directly causal, although it is easy to speculate about the exact relation between establishment size and the direct causes. Using the correlation as a predictive tool may be an acceptable theory for estimating injury rates, e.g., for a given industry, if a stable relationship between establishment size and injury rate has been observed in the past, it may be acceptable to estimate future injury rates as a function of establishment size on the basis of this relationship.

In the example above, one can postulate an indirect linking between the variable of the theory (size of establishment) and effect (injury rate), e.g. larger establishments may be required to employ safety officers, the actions of whom may reduce injury rates; or contrariwise, larger establishments may be necessary to take on more dangerous jobs. It is possible, however, to use a "theory" in which it is known that no causal connection exists, but merely a correlation. In the analysis of the effects of air pollution on human health, it is not known which, if any, component(s) of the pollution actually cause health effects at the low doses typically encountered, so one cannot be certain that the "effects" are actually caused by that component of pollution which is measured (typical measures may be levels of sulphur oxides, nitrogen oxides, hydrocarbons, ozone, fine particles (PM10 or PM2.5), total suspended particulates, etc.). However, since the different components tend to be generated together, it is reasonable to assume (and for those components so far measured the assumption turns out to be reasonably valid) that all the components vary together—their levels are highly correlated—so that measurement of one (or several) gives an indirect measure of all the others. The theory so constructed, in which health effects are related to the levels of measured pollutants, may then give valid predictions provided the proxy variable used (level of pollutant actually measured) maintains the same relationship (correlation) to the actual harmful pollution constituent. It should be noticed that the previous example (size of establishment versus injury rates) may also be an example of this last type.

Caution is in order. Mortality might also be confounded by another effect not causally related to the air pollution but related to another common variable such as temperature or atmospheric stability. This might, for example, be a disease vector.

This use of proxy variables in theories or models is common in risk assessment, where the variables controlling the magnitude of risks are often not known, or not quantifiable (because, for example, there are many human factors), or so complex as to defy useful analysis. In such cases it is usual to use plausible proxy variables in a theory constructed to fit whatever data are available. Generally the simplest model which fits the data and which permits sensible extrapolation of the required amount will be the most useful and believable—Occam's razor being a useful guide. But the use of proxy variables can also be extremely dangerous, and spurious results can be obtained if an important confounding variable is omitted. The death rate in the U.S. is correlated with air pollution variables, but whether this is a causal correlation or not is a matter still in dispute. The true causal connection may be with some combination of factors quite unrelated to these pollutants, for example, cigarette smoking, occupation and income level. More generally, one must be careful to avoid obviously implausible models. There is a well-known correlation between the declining birth rate and the declining incidence of storks in Germany. Yet few would accept this as evidence that storks bring babies, however charming the notion. This is probably an example of a situation where the correction between two variables exists because each is correlated with a third; an increasing population with its increased pressure on other species, and increasing social pressure for small families.

While the use of proxy variables may enable us to predict risks inaccurately, we caution that these proxy variables may be entirely inappropriate for control of such risks. Attempting to reduce risks by modifying a proxy variable may simply confirm that the variable is a proxy, and have no effect on the risk! For example, while various measures of air pollution may be correlated with mortality, and might be suitable for estimating the effect of pollution, it does not necessarily follow that controls on particular types of pollution will have any effect on mortality unless there is a causal effect of that type of pollution on mortality, or unless the controls introduced simultaneously affect something that is causally connected with mortality. As discussed below, overall reduction of fossil fuel burning is more likely to be effective than merely a control of the fine particles produced by such burning.

The use of a parametric model, as described above, allows a numerical estimation of the magnitude of a measure of risk, and, as explained below, also an estimation of the uncertainty in that numerical value. When comparing such numerical values (examples are given in Chapter 7) it is necessary to give some thought to their interpretation, for the interpretation may vary, depending on the context. In most cases, any such figures will be averages over geographical regions, over populations, over time, and over other variables used in or omitted from the models. Suppose, for example, we have estimates of the magnitudes of the annual probability of death from various events for the whole U.S. population. While these estimates give an accurate picture of total annual deaths in the U.S., they may be wildly inaccurate if applied to any particular subgroup of the U.S. population or to any particular individual. This is easy to see if we consider just the risk of dying (from any cause). An average over the whole U.S. population may be obtained from the average death rate which is about 9×10^{-3} per year (i.e. about 2.5 million people die per year out of a population of about 281 million), but for the subgroup consisting of males over the age of 85 the risk of dying was about 0.17 per year in 1998, substantially higher. Evidently, for any such subgroup we can obtain an estimate of the risk by averaging over just that subgroup, but again this figure cannot be accurately applied to any specific member of the subgroup. If all we know about that specific person is that he is a member of the subgroup this may be the best estimate we can offer.

Another sort of averaging, over long time spans, should be borne in mind when considering certain other risks. There is a class of events which could have annual average risks just as large as the everyday causes of death, but which do not result in deaths being seen every year. These are events which are very unusual (average number less than 1 per year), but which may have very large consequences when they do occur. (If they are both unusual and have small consequences, we are not so interested in them.) Examples of such infrequent and (possibly) large consequence events are earthquakes, dam bursts and meteor strikes. The varied amount and varied type of averaging creates problems in attempting to compare risks, since even when put on an apparently equivalent scale (e.g. annual average), equal risks on that scale may be very different. An extreme example of this problem is to compare the case of auto accidents (probability of death 1.6×10^{-4} per year, resulting in about 44,000 deaths per year in the U.S.) with an (hypothetical) event occurring with probability 1.6×10^{-4} per year (once every 6,000 years on average) but which kills almost everybody in the U.S. The average annual risk is the same, but it seems unlikely that these two risks would, or should, be considered equivalent.

We can perhaps clarify some of the ideas above with a specific example, the risk of death (in the U.S.) from extreme weather conditions (e.g. tornadoes, flooding, hurricanes, lightning). We have reasonably reliable data on these for some time in the past, as shown in Figure 2-3, which is drawn from the original data, both the annual numbers of tornadoes and the annual numbers of deaths. In this figure, we note that the number of deaths by tornadoes has fallen over the years, although the number of reported tornadoes has increased markedly. Many persons looking at such a graph would infer that the reporting of tornadoes without casualties has improved. Over long periods (tens to hundreds of years) we expect the weather to be reasonably constant,

FIGURE 2-3
U.S. Tornadoes by Month

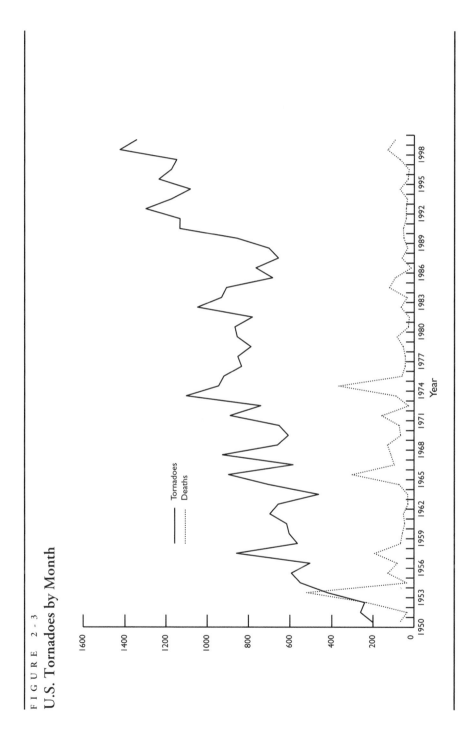

but year-to-year variations in extreme weather conditions will be large. Thus we expect that we can give a value for the expected risk of death, but any model we use must include large year-to-year variability. The simplest model to adopt appears to be that some measure of the mean value of the risk is constant, or perhaps changing slowly with time. By adopting this model, we do not explicitly include causal effects, but hope that the risks are so many and/or unalterable (in the short term) that the model is effectively causal without knowing the causal chains in detail. We use the randomness in this case to advantage to estimate mean values which are reasonably constant or slowly varying, despite the great variations within each possible causal chain (e.g. for the particular sub-set of people being killed by blown projectiles, the probability of a death will involve a complicated product of the number of available projectiles, the population density, the probability of people not taking shelter, etc.). There are very large numbers of people and events, and a small probability of any particular event causing harm to any particular person, and we take an average over these many possibilities, not all of which are likely to be simultaneously affected by changes. If there are cases in which changes may affect all cases, the changes may be taken into account. A good example is injuries from tornadoes. Improved warnings of tornadoes and better advice on what to do have been issued in the past and may be expected to continue—the reduction in the injuries caused by tornadoes has been ascribed to these warnings and advice.

We previously mentioned the U.S. history of auto accident deaths, adopting a model in which we simply assumed constant or decreasing annual risk of death per person or per passenger mile. Sufficient data are available in this case to introduce more complex models. It would be possible to take into account different risks for highway versus urban driving or driving on freeways versus city streets, and include factors such as alcohol consumption. Whether such details would be of use for predictions would depend on the availability and reliability of estimates of the future behavior of such variables.

"New" Risks:

As modern technology was developing two centuries ago, the standard engineering approach was to try it out, and if there were problems, to fix them. New technologies such as railroad travel were risky; indeed there was a fatal accident at the opening of the first passenger railroad—between Liverpool and Manchester (U.K.). But as society learned about the reasons that acci-

FIGURE 2-4
Schematic of Nuclear Power Plant with Emergency Core Cooling System (ECCS)

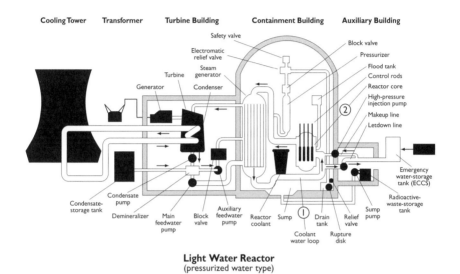

Light Water Reactor
(pressurized water type)

If there is a beak in the coolant water loop ① and a sudden loss of water from the reactor vessel, the core ② could overheat and melt. The ECCS is designed to prevent this catastrophe.

dents occur, hardware and procedures were changed to reduce the accident rate. The number of accidents per passenger mile in railroad travel has dropped by a factor of nearly 100 since 1830. In any technology that developed in this way we can, by using some limited experience, derive *bounds* on the probability of future accidents. Consider the case of the safety of a nuclear reactor where the techniques for dissecting these risks have been most developed. Before discussing this we show in Figure 2-4 a schematic of a reactor with its critical components. The first step is to design the reactor such that it is inherently stable in operation. This was achieved in the light water cooled reactors shown in Figure 2-4. As the reactor gets hotter, the reactivity of the reactor goes down. But the water in the reactor has to be raised to a high temperature (and therefore pressure) to make the efficient energy conversion to electricity. This leads to a possibility, small but finite, that the water will catastrophically leak away. Therefore the second step is to ensure that if the reactor coolant (water) leaks out, then the nuclear reaction shuts off. This occurs in a Light Water Reactor (LWR) by design, because the water is also essential (as a *moderator*) to slow the neutrons down so that the reaction may proceed. These two steps, basic to the design, are the "first line of defense."

In a nuclear reactor heat from radioactive decay of fission products remains for a long time after the nuclear chain reaction has ceased and this heat must be removed or the fuel will overheat, perhaps to melt and release the radioactive fission products. A special cooling system is installed to prevent such overheating. This is a second "line of defense." If the fuel melts, and melts through the steel reactor vessel, the radioactive material may still be held safely inside a reinforced concrete containment vessel. This is a third "line of defense." If the containment vessel fails, and the reactor has been properly sited in a relatively low population area, with an exclusion zone around it, consequences would be limited. Although not often so described, this is effectively a fourth "line of defense." This policy of "defense in depth" has been the policy in the U.S. and most of the developed world from the inception of nuclear power. Imagine the "maximum credible accident" (or set of maximum credible accidents). Then devise a system to prevent the accident from happening. Also, devise a system to cope with the consequences if the accident does happen. In the former Soviet Union, the policy was not so well implemented. The reactors used at Chornobyl, of the "RBMK" type, were *not* inherently stable. Moreover, there was no containment vessel. The basic design was therefore less safe than desirable and possible.

How well does the defense in depth work? As an example, consider the loss of coolant accident (LOCA) in a light water nuclear reactor (LWR). We can first estimate this solely from the considerable experience (8,000 reactor-years world wide) in running such nuclear reactors, in which time one important LOCA (at Three Mile Island [TMI]) has occurred. If we assume that a LOCA is equally likely to occur in any such LWR at any time, we can use this experience to obtain bounds on the probability per unit time (P) of such an accident occurring. With this assumption (which constitutes a model of such events) our best estimate of P is $1/8,000 = 1.25 \times 10^{-4}$ per reactor year, and we say that $p < 6 \times 10^{-4}$ per year with 95% confidence. The rigorous meaning of such a statement is as follows. If the true probability (P) is greater than 6×10^{-4}, there is less than 1 chance in 20 (5%) that we could have had 8,000 reactor years with as few as one LOCA. Similarly we can get a lower bound: 6.5×10^{-5} per year $< P$ with 95% confidence, i.e. if P is less than 6.5×10^{-5} per year, there is less than 1 chance in 20 (5%) that we could have had 8,000 reactor years with as many as one LOCA. We must stress that these numerical values are only correct if the assumptions (model) are correct. In particular it assumes that P does not change with time, whereas it is almost certain that we have learned enough from the Three Mile Island accident to reduce P considerably. Moreover, P is *not* the probability per unit time of adverse health consequences, because a LOCA does not necessarily (and did not at TMI) lead to health hazards. It is only the probability of core damage. At TMI the core damage did not lead to hazardous release of radioactivity off-site. The probability of release given core damage is therefore not unity, although it is probably not zero. It is likely to be about 5% leading to an overall probability (best estimate) of hazardous release of 6×10^{-6} per year if this model is correct.

This limited analysis is inadequate for modern public policy decisions. In modern society we are not content with the "try it and fix it" approach. Individual units in a technology have grown bigger, and the consequences of an individual accident have likewise increased. Society legitimately demands that accidents with large consequences be ruled out, or demonstrated to have a very low probability *before* the technology is allowed to proceed. The upper bound to the risk may well be too high to be acceptable and the simple analysis above gives no clue as to how to reduce any risk that exists. The limitation can be overcome if it is possible to break each event leading to risks into a sequence of well-understood events. This procedure is particularly well suited to discussing nuclear reactor safety with its defense in depth philosophy. The sequences of events form scenarios, which can be discussed in what is called an "event tree" (Rasmussen, 1975). Normally the "tree" is drawn after it has fallen down with the trunk on the left and branches on the right, with time going left to right.

The crucial logical step is identification of all initiating events and all possible sequences of events (event trees) that may lead to serious consequences to public health and safety, and the separation of these sequences into segments that are approximately independent of each other. By analyzing each event in each sequence separately, using theory or past experience or both, the overall probability of occurrence of the whole sequence may be evaluated. It might seem that even a few event trees would end up with a large number of branches to be evaluated. But the process is simplified when it is realized that the hazard of concern is radiation from released radioactivity. Radioactivity will be contained in the fuel elements unless the fuel melts or is otherwise damaged. Therefore, any sequence of events that does not lead to core damage will not be hazardous, and the degree of hazard will be given by

FIGURE 2-5

Simplified Event Trees for a Large LOCA

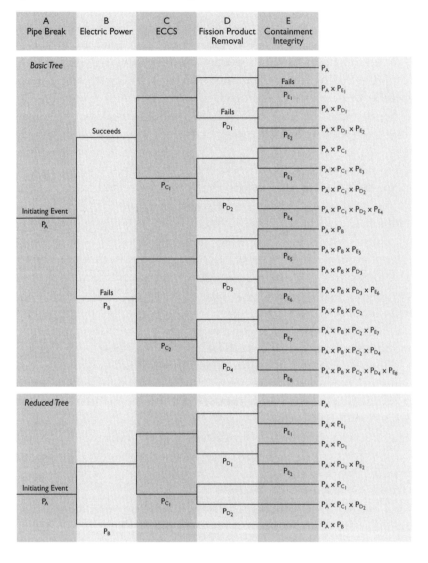

Note: Since the probability of failure, P, is generally less than 0.1, the probability of success (1 – P) is always close to 1. Thus, the probability associated with the upper (success) branches in the tree is assumed to be 1.

the degree of damage (the plant state). Furthermore, all event trees can be terminated at the plant state. Then there will be no release unless the containment fails. The quantity of radionuclides released off-site ("off-site release") will depend on the plant state and characteristics of the containment. A new set of event trees can be constructed leading to the off-site release category. Finally, the radionuclide concentration, the radiation dose there from, and the probability of a fatal cancer can be calculated from the dose in the same way as discussed later in this chapter. This, then leads to a schematic event diagram shown in Figure 2-5. In this diagram time flows from left to right as events unfold.

The crucial step in the logic and the one, which leads to a moderately low figure for the calculated accident probability, is that the steps above are approximately independent of each other. Then the overall accident probability (P) (with the assumptions mentioned below) is equal to:

$$P = P_A \times P_B \times P_{C2} \times P_{D3} \times P_{E8} \qquad (2\text{-}1)$$

FIGURE 2-6
Illustration of Fault Tree Development

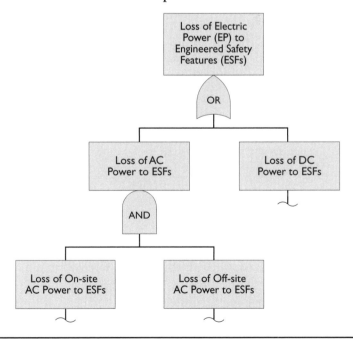

where $P_1 =$ the probability of a pipe break, which may be estimated from historical experience with pipes firstly in other industries, secondly in the limited experience of the nuclear industry and finally with the theory of metal failure

$P_2 =$ is the probability of failure of electric off-site power

$P_{C2} =$ probability of failure of the emergency core cooling system (ECCS)

$P_{D4} =$ is the probability of failure of fission product removal (by containment sprays for example)

$P_{E8} =$ is the probability of containment violation

Even then, the consequences depend upon the population distribution and the weather. A further probability calculation may be performed for major adverse consequences due to unfavorable weather (determined from past data on wind patterns, rainfall etc.).

Failure of the emergency core coolant system (system fault) can occur in a number of ways. Figure 2-6 illustrates part of a "fault tree" that collects all such ways together so that the overall probability of failure (P_2) can be calculated. The figure illustrates two alternative ways of failure, loss of AC power and loss of DC power. Since failure of either will cause failure of the ECCS, they are connected in the diagram by a logical "or" gate. There will only be loss of AC electric power to the engineered safety systems if both on-site and off-site AC power fails. These are therefore connected in a logical "and" gate. Similar elaborations are used for each branch in the tree, until the individual faults can themselves be assigned probabilities from previous experience. The event tree tracks forward — what happens if some initiating event occurs (the example given is the LOCA event). The fault tree tracks backward — what possible ways are there for a particular event to occur.

The basic assumptions of the event tree analysis technique can now be made clear.

1. We assume that the analysis is complete, in the sense that the event trees calculated include, in fact, all those event sequences which exist (or at least all those with a major contribution of risk) and lead to the final outcomes of concern. Also that those event trees analyzed include all, or the major portion, of all possible adverse consequences (outcomes). It is never possible to be absolutely sure about this, but as time passes and no critic has

come up with a forgotten tree, and we do not see any sequences of events actually happen that are not included in the analysis, completeness is more probable.

2. Those probabilities that are assumed to be independent of one another (P_A, P_B, P_{C2}, P_{D4}, P_{E8} in the above example) are in fact independent. If we know of correlations, these can be added as a separate tree. For example, one obvious correlation is by deliberate sabotage of all systems simultaneously.

The validity of these assumptions cannot be proved, and our confidence in their validity for any particular study can only be based on the competence and thoroughness of the analysts, the robustness of the results under criticisms from others and the experience of seeing real event sequences as they happen. The overall probability. P can be small even though the individual probabilities are large enough to be learned from experience (P_A and P_{D4}), or from tests (P_{C2}).

One object of the analysis is to find those areas contributing most to the risk and alters them so as to lower the risk to the point where there would be little likelihood of the overall event sequence occurring during the life of the system. This is best achieved when the analysis is performed by someone who is well acquainted with the plant and its operation.

Event tree calculations have also been performed for the liquefied natural gas (LNG) industry (Keeney, Kulkani and Naii, 1978). In particular, the risk evaluated was a spill from a LNG ship a in a populated estuary, such as the river Thames in the UK, or the Mystic River in Boston, followed by fire or explosion. The principal event tree for large effects is:

a. ship collision;

b. break of tank;

c. wind toward population center;

d. no ignition sources between the spill site and the population center (so that the LNG is not ignited before it reaches major population centers).

In the chemical industry, event trees are used in analyses of plant safety aimed at reducing hazards; they have been used in the estimation of risks from a particular industrial area containing oil refineries, liquefied petroleum gas (LPG) storage, liquid ammonia storage, and ammonium nitrate storage in Canvey Island (Health and Safety Executive, 1978); and they are widely used in reliability analyses of many complex systems (Kletz, 1977). They are also beginning to be used in general procedures by NASA for all their operations (Stamatelatos, 2001), and by the U.S. Army for discussion of the risks of destruction of chemical weapons (Boyd, 2001). However in none of these is the analysis as straightforward as in nuclear reactor safety for which a *defense in depth* policy was built into the design. The principal successes of this technique have been in the nuclear industry. Not in making the technology acceptable to the public, but in helping nuclear power plant operators to prioritize (italics) their possible actions, and thereby to enable the plants to operate more efficiently, and thereby make them both more economic and safer.

"New" Risks: (2) of Epidemiology and Its Ambiguities

The risks calculated by historical methods above have the feature that the effect immediately follows the cause. When an accident leads to immediate death, or even one within a few hours, attribution of death to the postulated cause is usually obvious. But even for automobile accidents there is a small ambiguity. One percent of automobile deaths occur a year after the accident and are still attributable and attributed. But there is a large class of risks in which death follows the postulated cause by a "latent period" of 20 years or more. In these cases, attribution of effect to a particular postulated cause is far more difficult. Typically a group of people "exposed" to a substance under study are compared with another group of "unexposed" people who have similar health prognoses in all other respects. For example, Doll and Peto (1976, 1978) compared the smoking habits and lung cancer rates of an otherwise well defined and fairly homogeneous group—British physicians. Similarly, the health records of atomic bomb survivors in and near Hiroshima and Nagasaki have been compared with the radiation they received (Pierce et al., 1996). More generally, several hundred epidemiological studies have been made of people exposed to chemical agents (e.g. benzene, vinyl chloride, dioxin and asbestos in their work place).

Ideally such studies include (i) information on the nature of the work place exposure; (ii) information on factors outside the workplace (alcohol drinking, diet, cigarette smoking or exposure to other carcinogens) that might affect the medical outcome and "confound" the results and (iii) simultaneous study, in equal or greater depth of a control group matched to have similar non-occupational influences as in (ii). However, the ideal is rarely

FIGURE   2-7
Alternative Dose-Response Models That Fit the Data

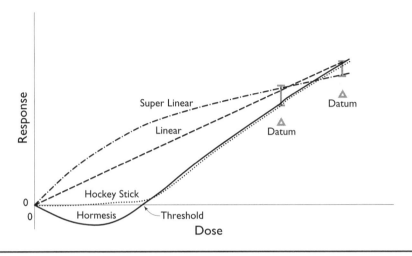

realized as well as it is for cigarette smoking or radiation. The epidemiological studies then provide a statistical "association" between a medical outcome (end point) and the exposure (or surrogate for exposure), rather than a clear-cut causal link. An excellent brief review was given by Cairns (1975).

In a famous presidential address to the Royal Society of Medical Statistics, Sir Austen Bradford Hill (1965) listed a number of attributes of an "association" that enables a scientist to attribute "causality." If causality can be reliably attributed then the risk to a worker can be calculated from this statistical association. The calculated risk for anyone exposed to the same extent is then assumed to be the same as for the exposed worker. But there are a number of complicating factors and as a simple rule of thumb causality would not usually be inferred unless the postulated cause multiplies the probability of the effect by at least a factor of 2 (Taubes, 1995). Technically this is described by saying that the Risk Ratio (or RR) > 2. Nonetheless, epidemiology remains the most important procedure fore assessing health risks (Samet, 1998).

The next issue is what to do with the epidemiological data when it available. The doubling of cancer rates implied by a risk ratio of 2 is unacceptable, in the absence of a clear benefit as might occur in medical treatment for another disease, and steps are taken to avoid the exposure or at least to reduce it. But how much need the exposure be reduced? To address this question it is necessary to understand how risks at lower doses are inferred from those at higher doses using an assumed "dose response" relationship. In most cases, the actual dose response relationship at lower doses (than those examined in the epidemiological study) is not known, and the assumed shape of this relationship is based on theoretical ideas. For cancer in particular, Figure 2-7 illustrates various dose response relationships that have been proposed as potentially applicable in particular cases at low doses. In this figure we draw 4 possible lines connecting data at high doses to the origin—no effect at no dose. The top line is called a supra (or super) linear curve; then the linear dose response; then a dose response with a threshold, or hockey-stick function; and finally a curve showing a beneficial effect at low doses (hormesis). The slope (mathematically, the gradient) of the dose response relationship is variously called the "potency" (here called b), "potency slope," "cancer slope factor," or "unit risk," depending on the units it is expressed in and the person or agency citing it. If the response is assumed to be linear with dose the risk (R) is then related to the dose (d) by:

$$R = \beta \times d \qquad\qquad (2\text{-}2)$$

If the exposure (often an occupational exposure in the "bad old days") is reduced by a factor of a thousand (as is often possible) then according to this equation the risk is reduced by a factor of 1,000. More generally we can consider a third "extrapolation" factor $E(d)$ such that $R = \beta \times d \times E$. If, as some people believe (for at least some cancers and some causal agents), there is a threshold dose, d_t, below which there is zero response, then $E(d < d_t) = 0$ and $R(d < d_t) = 0$. It is important to realize that the assumption that the cancer incidence is proportional to dose has not been proved or denied by direct experiment. It is a conservative assumption in the sense that few people seriously propose anything more pessimistic (i.e., it is difficult to produce plausible theories which produce more pessimistic effects like the supra-linear curve of Figure 2-7).

We must also remember that the parameter of importance in causing cancer (or other health outcome) is not the exposure *per se* but the dose of the substance to the person—and even the dose to a particular organ of interest. The dose is itself derived from exposure and exposure is in turn derived from (and may be multiplicatively related to) the concentration of the chemical and the duration of time the person is exposed.

Risks of Doses Less than Background: The "Linear Default"

"Few issues in health policy are more contentious than the choice of the appropriate dose-incidence model for use in estimating the risks of cancer associated with a carcinogen. The notion that there may be no threshold… seems to contradict everyday experience" (Upton, 1988, 1989). So begins Dr. Arthur Upton, a distinguished physician and former head of the National Cancer Institute, in a review of the subject. But interpretation of everyday experience depends very much on one's training—and for a physicist a linear dose response is a reasonable expectation as will be explained below, although for a biologist or toxicologist a threshold is more usually expected based on observations of other toxic effects. However, in a review paper, Zeise et al. (1987) take several situations where scientists have claimed that the data suggest a threshold or non-linearity, and show that a linear no-threshold theory fits the data equally well.

It is not possible to determine the behavior of cancer rates at low doses of putative carcinogens by historical, epidemiological data. By "low doses" we mean doses small enough that they would increase the rate of a particular cancer by 10% or less — for a common cancer like lung cancer, this would correspond to an increase in overall cancer rate of 1% or less. Although for a very large study (some millions of participants) the statistical accuracy might be sufficient to establish a risk at a level of 10% of the background rate, uncertainties in data that are more than the statistical sampling fluctuations would dominate. By the same token, when an effect is not directly measurable it cannot also be catastrophic with a large risk. However, the public, and the regulatory authorities that follow the directions of the legislators elected by the public, often want to regulate risks 10,000 times smaller than 1%. In place of direct observation, the behavior of cancer rates at such low levels must be determined by some sort of model. Crowther (1924) suggested a simple single stage model for radiation-induced carcinogenesis whereby radiation-induced ionization causes damage in a cell that subsequently replicates, fixing the damage in the genetic material, and leading to cancer. In its simplest form the theory leads to a linear dose response relationship. But his theory was known to be obviously incomplete early on. Cosmic rays ionize tens of millions of atoms in the body each second, and other background radiation contributes even more. While most of these events do not affect cellular genetic material, nevertheless such genetic damage occurs throughout the body thousands of times per second. There must exist some mechanism, repair or excretion, that prevents all but one in a hundred thousand

FIGURE   2-8

Diagram Illustrating the Expected Increment in Disease Resulting from a Low Dose of a Substance

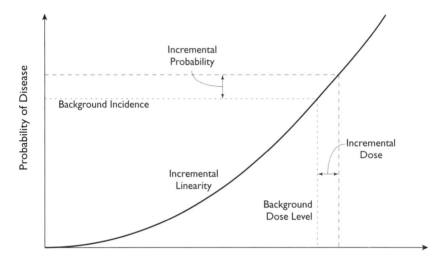

Because cellular effects similar to those produced by the substance may be produced in its absence by "background" mechanisms, the effects resulting from low doses may be additive with those resulting from other "background" risk factors, thus causing an increase in the risk that is proportional to the dose.

billion such cellular damage events from proceeding to form a tumor. Nonetheless it is widely, but erroneously, believed that only genotoxic compounds (that are mutagenic in a laboratory assay) can lead to a linear dose relationship. The initial step of modifying a cell to start a tumor is probably only one step in cancer formation and any step can be modified. Indeed the idea of the 1970s that genotoxic materials are especially carcinogenic and only genotoxic materials can give a low dose linearity runs into many troubles and cannot be sustained as a general principle. It is likely that the major action of even genotoxins in the environment is to promote a cancer already initiated by natural processes.

The multistage models of carcinogenesis, although originating in the 1930s, were developed by Armitage and Doll (1954, 1957) to describe the distribution of cancer as a function of age. These authors assumed that cancers develop in four or five stages and that each stage may be influenced by a different biological mechanism. In applying the model to cancers caused by anthropogenic activity Armitage and Doll suggested that one (or at most two) stages can be influenced by pollutants. Inherent in this description was the assumption that the applied carcinogenic agent and natural processes act similarly at one stage in the carcinogenic process.

As a consequence of this assumption, low doses of pollutants would be expected to increase cancer incidence in direct linear proportion to dose, and effects of different pollutants would add. According to these ideas, therefore, nongenotoxic substances are as likely to lead to a linear dose response as genotoxic substances.

Crump et al. (1976) and Guess et al. (1977) pointed out that the argument for low dose linearity is far more general than the Armitage-Doll theory and depends solely on the fact that cancers caused by the pollutant and natural (background) processes are indistinguishable. They noted that "If carcinogenesis by an external agent acts additively with any already ongoing process then under almost any model the response will be linear at low doses." Crawford and Wilson (1996) showed that the argument is even more general and applies to a wide variety of non-cancer outcomes, including the effects of air pollution in the example earlier. These analyses were used by U.S. EPA 25 years ago as a justification for assuming low dose linearity as a general default for cancer risk assessment. The way in which a non-linear biological dose response can become a linear one in the presence of background is illustrated in Figure 2-8. The arguments of Crump et al. and of Guess et al. were used by the U.S. EPA in the mid 1970s as a justification for assuming low-dose linearity as a general default for cancer risk assessment.

As an example, these general ideas can be used to suggest a linear dose response relationship for the internal cancers produced by arsenic. If this model for induction of cancers by arsenic is correct, then a typical risk-management goal of regulating any (lifetime) risk larger than one in a million runs into difficulties. For example, the concentration of arsenic in water that produces a one-in-a-million risk is between 1 and 5 parts per *trillion* when lung, kidney and bladder cancers are all included. Background levels of arsenic in natural waters (even ignoring dietary sources of arsenic) often exceed this concentration by a factor of 1,000! This then is the core of the problem regulators have faced for the last 14 years in considering the standard for arsenic in drinking water. Either the risk-management goal of one-in-a-million lifetime risk is unattainable, or the model is incorrect, or we should spend enormous sums cleaning up arsenic, by far the majority of which is naturally occurring, in the environment (Wilson, 2000). In January 2001 the EPA promulgated a new standard for arsenic in water of 10 ppb where the risk calculated on a linear basis is 0.1%, but on a more optimistic basis is 1/10,000. But in March 2001, with a new U.S. administration, the U.S. EPA is asking for yet another review of this science and cost calculations that underlie the standard.

The study of toxicological mechanisms has advanced considerably, even since the earliest formulations of the linear-no-threshold theories and the introduction of the general arguments about linearity just discussed. While the general arguments for low dose linearity are rigorous, it may be demonstrated that they do not apply to particular mechanisms of action that can give rise to tumors if those mechanisms do not normally operate to produce "naturally occurring" tumors. The problem that then arises in any particular case is demonstrating to a reasonable degree of certainty (a) that such mechanisms are the only ones acting, and (b) that indeed those mechanisms do not usually operate, and so do not contribute to the naturally occurring background rate of tumors. These questions are usually framed in a policy framework in which simple (yes/no) answers are required; and any risk assessments are then predicated on the correctness of the answers. A more general risk assessment framework will take account of the uncertainties in the answers; but such an approach almost always turns out (at least in 2000) to give results that are dominated by the possibility of linearity at low doses.

FIGURE   2-9

Annual Death Rate vs. Daily Alcohol Consumption

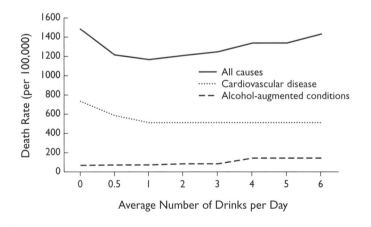

The questions just posed are not new. They were asked by John C. Bridge, Senior Medical Inspector of Factories in the UK, but are often attributed to E. R. A. Merewether, his junior and his successor, "Does silica or asbestos or the fibrosis of the lung they produce tend to inhibit cancer of the lung or to produce it? If the latter, do either of these substances act as specific carcinogenic agents like tar, or is it the disease they produce only prepares the soil for the occurrence of cancer?" (Wilson, 1938). If the former, it is likely that from the argument of Crump et al. that there is a linear dose response. If it only "prepares the soil" then a threshold equal to the observed threshold for the fibrosis (asbestosis) is likely. It is also similar to the question asked about benzene: "are the leukemias caused by benzene always preceded by bone marrow toxicity or not?" For if the former, a threshold for the leukemic action of benzene is probable. Wilson (2000, 2001b) has suggested that the same line or reasoning should be applied to lung cancers from ingestion of arsenic in drinking water. Neither in the asbestos case (Hughes and Weill 1991) nor in the benzene case, (Lamm et al., 1989), has a definitive answer yet been forthcoming. The U.S.EPA usually assumes the linear default.

Beneficial Effects and Hormesis

There is a large literature that suggests that low doses of radiation, and low doses of some toxic substances, may produce beneficial effects. It may be argued, based on experimental observations and some theoretical ideas, that this is a general phenomenon, and the idea has been given the name hormesis. A useful summary of the data supporting the idea of hormesis is given in Calabrese (1999).

Hormesis need not be in conflict with the arguments of Doll, Crump and Crawford discussed in the previous paragraph. These authors argue that there is linearity at low doses but nothing in the argument specifies the sign of the linear slope or how low the dose has to be. The dose response curve might be more complex than usually considered.

We distinguish here two possible types of hormesis. In the first the probability of a specific medical outcome increases (rises), and then decreases (falls), in response to dose. In the second, the probability of one medical outcome increases with increasing dose, possibly in a non-linear fashion, whereas the probability of another medical decreases. The sum of the two probabilities, which we call the total risk of any (perhaps lethal) adverse outcome decreases (falls) and then increases (rises). Since these dose response relationships are derived for a population, and not for an individual the interpretation on a mechanistic level is still unclear.

Damage rates are likely to be identical in all individuals, because of the nature of the damage event. While repair of different types of damage is known to vary between individuals and population groups, and probably depends on other external things such as nutritional status. This implies some differences in the damaging effect of a given dose. The beneficial effect may be due to stimulation of defenses. And it is uncertain how that varies.

A claimed example of the first type of hormesis is the effect of radon gas on the incidence of lung cancer. High concentrations of radon in uranium mines are associated with definite increases in lung cancer rates—and this increase is usually considered to be causal. But at low, the doses found in residential settings, Cohen claims in a controversial "ecological" study that the lung cancer incidence is reduced by the radon exposure (Cohen, 1995, 1997).

An example of the second type of hormesis is the effect of alcohol. For millennia alcohol was considered essential to good health and, indeed, this was well documented by Pearl (1926). Adverse effects of high doses, both on

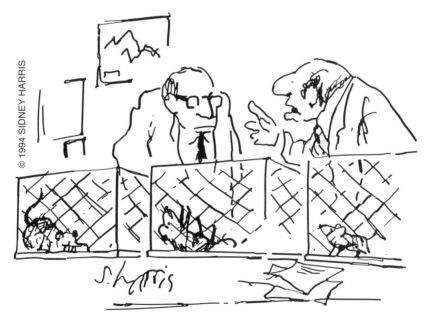

"He is angry that he is not allowed to eat the chemical. He is a control rat."

the individual and on society, were emphasized by the Islamic religion, and by modern society of the last 100 years (leading, for example, to prohibition in the U.S.). Recent research has brought the beneficial qualities back into focus (Moore and Pearson, 1986; Marmot and Brunner, 1991; Poikolanen, 1995; Doll et al., 1994; Thun et al., 1997c). Alcohol in small quantities reduces the incidence of coronary heart disease, and of myocardial infarction. However, at high doses (especially in conjunction with tobacco smoking) it leads to cancer, cirrhosis of the liver and intoxication with all its adverse consequences both to the individual and to society. Data on death rates are reviewed by Doll (1998), from whom we plot Figure 2-9 showing how death from cardiovascular disease diminishes with increasing alcohol consumption even as a death from other causes increases, leading to a hormetic shape to the alcohol consumption versus overall death-rate curve. Since the end-point

FIGURE   2 - 1 0

Scatterplot of Each Agent's LD$_{50}$ Value in Rats and in Mice (4,706 agents plotted)

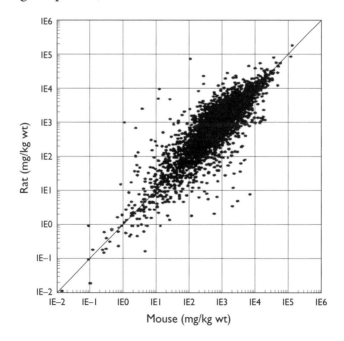

Inscribed line describes the prediction of mg/kg scaling.

considered, death, may be due to many distinct diseases or conditions, and other factors such as lifestyle may affect the outcomes synergistically in different ways it is quite likely that different populations will show different overall dose response curves. Nonetheless, English et al. (1995) summarized 16 studies and found a result for males similar to that found by Doll, but for females the beneficial effect is less evident.

In the text on page 217 and page 232, in Tables 7-2a and 7-3, and in Figure 7-6, we will discuss further the contribution of alcohol to the adverse effects of cirrhosis of the liver, and to automobile and boating accidents.

Doll concludes: "These (conclusions) still need to be refined in detail, but in broad outline they are quite clear—that is, that in middle and old age some small amounts of alcohol (ethanol) within the range of one to four drinks each day reduces (sic) the risk of premature death, irrespective of the medium in which it is taken."

Alcohol therefore provides an interesting example of competing risks from the same substance. We discuss two further possible examples. There is also some evidence, primarily in animals but also in people, that radiation at low doses increases longevity for reasons that are unclear — but maybe due to prevention of infectious disease. If added to the (small) risk of cancer at low doses this, if true, could lead to a U shaped hormesis curve similar to that for alcohol. This possibility has not yet been taken into account by regulatory bodies or scientific committees advising them.

Aspirin seems to work by encouraging the flow of blood. There may well be a linear relationship between blood flow and dose, but it clearly has a "hormetic" dose response curve for much of the population. Low doses, one "baby" aspirin a day, are recommended prospectively for elderly men to reduce the probability of heart attacks. Aspirin clearly reduces headaches and other pain. But sufficiently high doses can cause excessive bleeding and even death as blood vessels burst. For someone who has bleeding problems, such as a peptic ulcer, even a small amount of additional bleeding might make the difference between life and death.

As the example of alcohol shows, society in the last century has vacillated about the best strategy for minimizing risks. Much more difficult are the decisions where one replaces one substance (very risky) by another (slightly risky) or unknown. It is for these that the full analytical treatment and social understanding associated with a complete risk-benefit analysis are needed.

FIGURE 2-11

Comparison of Carcinogenic Potency in Rats and Mice (Crouch 1996)

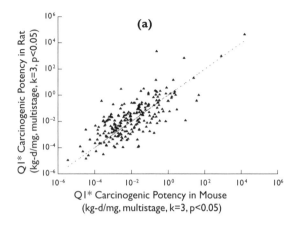

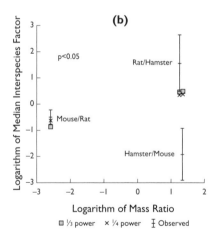

New Risks: (3) The Use of Animal Data to Estimate Risks to Humans

The direct historical method of estimating carcinogenic risks from chemicals and other substances, using the results of epidemiological studies, has only been possible for a handful of substances (about 30). Yet there are thousands of chemicals in nature and in commerce, and exposure of some people to many of these chemicals can be high. For estimating the risks of such expo-

FIGURE 2-12

Human β vs. Animal β Estimates

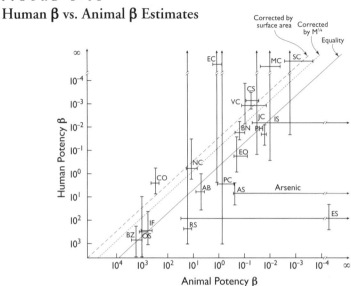

Source: Modified from Allen 1998.

sures, "new" risks in our nomenclature, there is little or no direct historic record.

New risks include those of low probability but large consequence, together with unprecedented ones of both high and low probability and consequence, usually due to the changing nature of society and its actions. Sometimes there may be evidence available on similar risks, or there may be data on investigations that found no evidence of risk. In such cases we can estimate an *upper limit* of risk, but *cannot* show a lower limit of risk or show that the risk is zero. Lack of evidence is not, of course, evidence of lack. Prior investigations may have been insensitive and thus unable to distinguish between zero and a small positive effect. Cairns (1999) expressed this same thought slightly differently by saying that absence of certainty is not absence of risk.

As an example in the estimation of carcinogenic risks from chemicals, the fact that epidemiological studies of humans did not find evidence (by themselves) of a carcinogenic effect from dioxin exposure until recently did not prove a lack of any such risk. It did show that if there is such an effect, it was less than the smallest effect that could have been detected by those epidemiological studies. The small (60%) increase that has recently been seen is still consistent with the earlier studies, which detected no increase.

In order to make estimates of the magnitude of the risk posed by a new chemical or a chemical for which there has, fortunately, been too low an exposure to allow unambiguous epidemiological results, it is necessary to use a model or theory. It would, of course, be desirable to have a complete theory of carcinogenesis, so that we could calculate the risk of a chemical from first principles. Scientists are optimistic that this will eventually be possible, but we cannot wait for its development before making decisions about the use of chemicals. We therefore depend on a battery of short term, *in vitro* tests and tests on animals (usually laboratory animals such as rodents) to guide us. The procedure used for much of the last century to estimate acute toxicity in humans is fairly satisfactory. Acute toxicity is any adverse effect occurring immediately or a short time after a chemical is ingested or inhaled in one single dose or otherwise in a short period of time. Although there are a few ambiguities, it is generally accepted that acute toxicity follows a threshold type dose response. The acute toxic level (often expressed as the dose that is lethal to 50 percent of the test animals, or LD_{50}) will vary somewhat from person to person, and even from time to time, but generally (there are exceptions) a dose 10 times the acute toxic level will kill almost everyone and those exposed to 10 of this the level will usually survive. For most of the 20th century we have used the knowledge from past experience with other chemicals in man and animals, to provide useful estimates of the acute toxicity in people from a measurement of its value in animals. The general procedure for animal to man extrapolation has been described in Calabrese (1983). A recent study (Rhomberg and Wolff, 1998) (Figure 2-10) shows an excellent correlation of acute toxicity between rats and mice which is an approximate equality if the dose of the chemical is measured as a fraction of the animal's body weight. The prediction for people has more uncertainty because rats and mice more similar to each other than to people. But we are all mammals and have many similar tissues. With somewhat greater uncertainty, this correlation can be used to predict acute toxicity for people when direct data on people, or primates, are not available.

The estimate of cancer potency is more complex. Since cancer is a chronic effect usually appearing late in life, animals must be dosed at sub acute levels for a long period, typically 2 years, to develop cancer. The logic of the procedure has recently been summarized by Goodman and Wilson (1991). One of us (Crouch 1996), following earlier work of Crouch and Wilson

(1979), has compared the *carcinogenic* potency of chemicals tested in rats and mice from the data base developed by Gold and Zeiger (1997) (alternatively Gold et al. 1984, 1999). The animals were administered various doses (up to the maximum the animals can tolerate) of the chemical being tested, and watched for their whole lifetime. Figure 2-11a, from Crouch, demonstrates a high correlation of carcinogenic potency between the rat and mouse species used, over a range of 10^{10} in potency—i.e., a chemical, which is a potent carcinogen in one species, is also potent in the other. This correlation is closely coupled to the correlation between acute toxicities above, and the relationship can best be illustrated by a Monte Carlo simulation study (Shlyakhter, Goodman and Wilson 1992). The unit of carcinogenic potency used is the inverse of the units for dose. The dose is expressed as the lifetime average daily dose administered as a fraction of the body weight of the animal. The parameter Q_1^* used is similar to the potency β given in Equation 2-2. The ratio of the potency in the first species (a) to that in the second (b) is defined as an "interspecies potency factor" K_{12}.

$$K_{12} = Q_1^*/Q_2^* \approx \beta_1/\beta_2. \qquad (2\text{-}3)$$

The variation of the interspecies potency factor is shown in Figure 2-11b and the estimate of the mean interspecies factor and its standard error in Figure 2-11c. Given the potency in one species we can estimate it to within a factor of about 10 in the other, although the mean factor between rats and mice, K_{rm}, is also consistent with either unity or a ratio between rats and mice equal to the ¼ power of the ratio of their body masses (M_r and M_m), that is $(M_r/M_m)^{¼}$, a factor presently preferred by EPA.

To derive the potency for people, it is usual to make the assumption that the factor K varies with mass the same way that it does for rats and mice. But since rats and mice live for only two to three years and people live for eighty years, it is necessary to make an assumption about time dependence also. It is usual to assume that if people are given the same dose daily as a rat or mouse (adjusted for body weight) then in a lifetime they will be equally liable to develop cancer. Then using also a factor E(d) to allow for dose response relationships other than linear, the risk in humans R_h becomes:

$$R_h = K_{ah} \times \beta_a \times d \times E(d) \qquad (2\text{-}4)$$

K is assumed to be close to unity *if* the daily dose (given for a lifetime) is measured as a fraction of body weight. This formula with the first three factors was explicitly espoused by Crouch and Wilson (1981).

The attempts to make a similar comparison of potencies between animals and man (Crouch and Wilson, 1979; Allen et al., 1988) are limited by the paucity of data (see Figure 2-12). Chemicals tend to be tested for immediate potential regulation or defense against potential regulation. Human carcinogens will be regulated regardless of the animal data so that there is inadequate incentive to perform modern, standardized experiments with animals! The poor quality of the data leads to a much larger variability for any measurement of K, but nevertheless one can see that the potency in man, and hence the factor K, is predicted within a factor of 10 by the largest measured potency among the animals with one notable exception—arsenic.

Two major cancer bioassays were undertaken in the UK and the United States in an effort to determine once and for all the shape of a dose response relationship. Is it linear or is there a threshold? Some results from the "megamouse" study involving 20,000 BALB/c mice exposed to the chemical 2-acetylaminofluorene (2-AAF) at various doses are shown in Figure 2-13 taken from Littlefield et al. (1979). As any cynic could have predicted the results are equivocal. For bladder cancer (which has a low natural incidence) there is, at low doses of 2-AAF, a very low tumor rate, which can be consid-

---

FIGURE 2-13

Cumulative Incidence of Tumors in Mice vs. Concentration

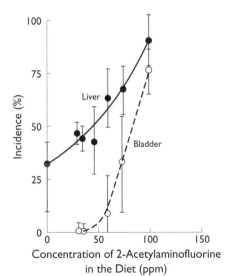

Source: Littlefield et al. 1979.

ered to demonstrate a threshold at 35 ppm. For liver cancer, which has a high natural incidence, the fit to the data of a linear term plus a quadratic term suggests linearity at low doses. More confusing still is that the rate of some other lethal cancers, such as reticular cell sarcoma, which may or may not be relevant for people, is reduced with increasing dose (Pompei, 2001) the risk from all cancers combined will always be dominated by the increase in tumors at that site that displays linearity.

Originally, once a carcinogen was found, often as the incidental result of a rodent bioassay, it was banned, whatever the risk, using legal procedures such as the Delaney clause in the Food and Drug acts (see Chapter 6). This was satisfactory when only a small number of chemicals were known to be carcinogenic. Use of more sensitive animal strains and use of whole life assays have improved the sensitivity so that now about half of both natural and man-made chemicals are found to be carcinogenic in one species and 30% or more in two species in the extensive testing of chemicals by the U.S. National Toxicology Program. Consistent bans are not practical, and risk assessments are therefore necessary. But many of these newly-tested chemicals are found to be carcinogenic only just above the limit of sensitivity set by acute or chronic toxic effects, and there is dispute about the meaning of rodent bioassays carried out at doses that produce overt toxic effects. Ames and collaborators (Ames et al., 1987, 1990, 1995) and later in Table 7-5, list chemicals using a HERP (Human Exposure/Rodent Potency) index. Although many "risky" carcinogens are high on this list, they decline to call their quantity HERP a "risk." While there is a substantial difference in the philosophy, it is nevertheless true that there are approximate numerical relationships between the HERP index and the risk estimates obtained if one assumes low-dose linearity. These are given by: HERP = R (100/ln2) = β d (100/ln2) = (d/VSD)/(10,000/ln2).[1]

Attempts have repeatedly been made to use in vitro short term tests such as an evaluation of mutagenicity in bacteria as an indicator of carcinogenicity (Ames, 1975; Ashby and Tennant, 1991), but all such attempts have substantial problems In the most systematic that were, Ashby and Tennant (1991) pointed out that of 301 chemicals that were tested in the National Toxicology program and satisfied certain reliability criteria, those that are mutagenic have other features that indicate carcinogenicity. The mutagenic chemicals tend to produce cancers in both species (rats and mice) and in multiple organs, and to produce rare tumors. These are attributes that the FDA has long used as indicators of "true" carcinogenicity. Gray et al. (1995) point out that for chemicals in the NTP bioassays the predicitivity of (or ability to predict the) carcinogenicity (carcinogenic potency) in rats from carcinogenicity in mice is also enhanced for the chemicals with these attributes. But Goodman and Wilson (1992) failed to find a correlation between mutagenicity and carcinogenic potency, contrary to an earlier suggestion by Russell and Meselson (1977) based on a limited number of chemicals. Moreover, several established human carcinogens (asbestos, benzene and dioxin) are not mutagens and are regulated by EPA assuming a linear dose response relationship.

Zeise, Crouch and Wilson (1984, 1986) noting the correlation between carcinogenic potency in animals (where measurable) and acute toxicity first noted by Parodi et al. (1982), have suggested that acute toxicity be used as a surrogate for carcinogenicity. This would, in its simplest form, involve assuming that all chemicals are carcinogenic, although many would have low potency, and therefore low risk at typical human exposures. This approach is opposite to the thinking that led to the Delaney clause discussed in Chapter 6. Under it, all chemicals would be regulated according to their assumed potency. Gold et al. (1995) have recently revisited this suggestion. Peto (1985) felt that no procedure for risk analysis is satisfactory, and that all that one can do is make a several lists of chemicals, each ranked according to their "nastiness" by some measure of "nastiness" (toxicity, animal carcinogenicity,

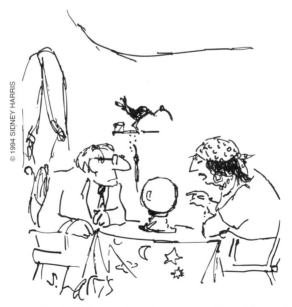

© 1994 SIDNEY HARRIS

"Don't add potassium nitrate to <u>anything</u> this year."

mutagenicity, etc.) and carefully regulate those at the top of each list. However, the standard procedure for cancer risk assessment and management in the U.S. currently remains that based on low-dose-linear extrapolation of risks from high-dose rodent bioassays, or, where available, from human epidemiological studies.

Probability of Causation

Come let us cast lots to find out for whose cause this evil is upon us—Jonah 1:7

The risk that a pedestrian is killed while crossing the road can become unity if and when he or she actually dies. It makes no sense to ask what his risk is. However, when a harmful event has occurred, one can ask: what is the probability that the event, disease or death, was due to a particular action or pollutant? The quantity is often called the Probability of Causation or POC. If a person is lying dead in a road, and traces of his or her clothing are on the bumper of a car that has just stopped, attribution of the death to the cause— automobile accident—is comparatively simple (although investigators must be aware that the collision may not be the "root cause," because for example, an accident might be fabricated to cover up a murder). But when a disease such as cancer follows the postulated cause by many years attribution is harder. This brings to the fore a very important societal issue. How does society assign blame for, or give compensation to, someone who has a disease, which has a number of possible causes? The assignment of causation can then only be expressed on a probabilistic basis. Hopefully it can be achieved in a less random manner than was the selection of Jonah.

For example, it is not now possible, and may be ultimately proven impossible, merely by looking at a cancer to tell whether radiation was the cause or whether other processes, including natural processes, were the cause. It is necessary to understand whether or not there was an exposure large enough to cause the cancer — mere diagnosis of the disease cannot be used to assign a cause. The cause can only be estimated in a probabilistic manner taking account of the exposure and natural incidence of the cancer in question (Bond, 1981; Mettler and Upton, 1995; Rothman, 1987, pp 38–39).

The Probability of Causation (POC) that an outcome O, occurring at a time t, is caused by exposure E_s to a specified substance, s, can be expressed in an equation:

FIGURE   2 - 1 4

Exposure Pathways for a Power Plant or Incenerator

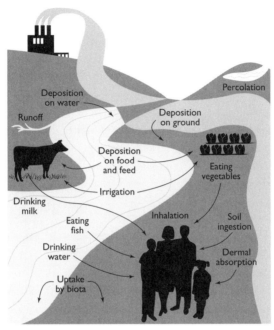

Source: Paustenbach 2000.

$$POC = \frac{(\text{Risk calculated from the estimated exposure to the pollutant})}{(\text{Risk from all causes})} \qquad (2\text{-}5)$$

All causes include both the natural incidence and the incidence calculated from exposure to the pollutant. If the incidence from all causes can be expressed a sum of incidences from k substances i, the calculation follows at once from the theorem, attributed to the Reverend Thomas Bayes in the 18th century, that describes how to change a probability when new information is available. Inserting the exposure variable E_s and the outcome O instead of the variables used in the textbooks:

$$P(E_s|O) = P(E_s)P(O|E_s)/[\sum_{i=1}^{k} P(E_i)P(O|E_i)] \qquad (2\text{-}6)$$

It must be recognized that both the numerator and the denominator vary with a number of characteristics of the person: is he a smoker? Male or female? What is his diet? Is he genetically sensitive? young or old? Although we ask for the POC for an individual, in most cases we can only obtain values of the quantities averaged over a population. This inevitably leads to approximations. The National Cancer Institute has prepared, and is updating, a set of epidemiological tables for such situations (NIH, 1985, 2001). They define excess relative risk [ERR(O|E_i)] as the increase in probability of the outcome due to the dose of the substance s divided by the incidence averaged over the U.S.A. They obtained this incidence from the SEER data. The numerator is derived from models depending mostly tumor rates in Japan. Then they express POC in terms of the "Excess Relative Risk" (ERR) defined by the formula:

$$POC = P(E_i|O)$$
$$= ERR\,(O|E_i)/[(1+ERR(O|E_i)] \qquad (2\text{–}7)$$

Given that a person has received a radiation dose D at age t and developed a cancer at age T, the tables tell us the probability that the cancer was caused by the radiation exposure. To be precise, the excess risk should be derived from a population with the same characteristics as the person under study. But data inevitably are averages, and in this case the numerator and denominator come from countries with different racial characteristics. But there is a much more important assumption in the preparation of these tables. At low doses of radiation these tables assume the Linear-No-Threshold dose response discussed earlier. Just as the risk of the adverse response is uncertain when the dose is small, so is the Probability of Causation. This raises the new issue of what to do when the POC is so uncertain. This makes it essential for scientists and technologists to understand what society is deciding and to use their especial expertise to influence the procedure. For possible exposure to other substances the calculation of POC is less simple and the result is less accurate.

Various authors have discussed the details in discussing these concepts and deriving the relevant values of prevalence and other parameters from epidemiological data. (Lagakos and Mosteller, 1986; Cox, 1987; Greenland and Robins, 1988; Robins and Greenland, 1989). There may be problems with the whole concept. For example, how does one handle a beneficial effect, where the incidence is decreased? It is possible to define a negative "incidence" and negative "risk" in some sense, but a negative POC makes no sense. In these circumstances, POC may be set to zero, but then the usefulness of the concept is debatable. Such details complicate the picture and several authors have suggested that the words "Assigned Share" be used instead of "Probability of Causation." However, even this runs into difficulties when synergistic effects of two substances, such as asbestos and smoking are considered (Chase et al., 1985; Enterline, 1982). Each POC calculated from Equation (2-7) is still below unity, as required for a probability, but the sum of the two POC can exceed unity, because the two are not independent. However, the sum of two "assigned shares" cannot exceed unity, so that the replacement of POC by "assigned share" makes no sense in this case either.

Elicitation of Expert Opinion

Often there exists no satisfactory procedure for calculating a risk or a part of the risk. In such cases, sometimes risk assessors elicit experts and derive some sort of average from their opinions. Such a procedure is often called a "Delphi" study because of the historical procedure for Greek rulers to consult the oracle at Delphi. Unless such an elicitation is performed *very* carefully it will be no more accurate and reliable than the recorded utterances of the oracle. The seminal discussion of the procedure is by Tversky and Kahneman (1975) and is discussed also in Turoff (1970). Cooke describes a number of successes and failures and Kaplan (1992) describes the limitations of the procedure. A group of experts is chosen with a wide range of experience; the data relevant to the problem are collected and the assembled experts are asked to state which of these data they would use to discuss the problem, and what logical procedure the particular expert would use. These data and procedures are then shared among all experts. Not until then are the individual experts asked to provide their assessments that are then compared. Such expert elicitations have been used in reactor safety for such esoteric questions as the probability of an energetic explosion when molten uranium falls upon water (NRC, 1990), for a discussion on the animal to man comparisons and other toxicological issues of chemical carcinogenesis (Evans et al., 1994a, 1994b; Walker et al., 2001a, 2001b), and an abbreviated form, with all information shared but without a face to face meeting, of a discussion of the low dose response to asbestos exposure (D'Agostino and Wilson, 1988). Although not described as Delphi studies, opinions of a expert committees set up the U.S. National

Research Council (National Academy of Sciences) often fall into this category, but are rarely performed as carefully as Kaplan would suggest. We believe there is a great advantage in being very explicit about the procedure used.

Exposure and Dose Estimation

General

In the discussion of cancer risks above, we assumed that the dose of the substance is specified to the risk assessor. But that is rarely the case. In the discussion of reactor accidents we stopped at the quantity of radionuclides released off-site. However, most decision makers want to know the dose to an individual (for personal decisions), to a group, or to the nation as a whole. Much of the early literature on estimation of individual doses was about techniques for evaluating the emission and dispersion of radionuclides from nuclear facilities. Estimating dispersion of chemicals from other power plants, factories, incinerators or waste disposal sites the poses similar problems, and the techniques have developed more generally. The U.S. EPA, state agencies, and others, have made various attempts over the years to construct models that can adequately represent the transport of chemicals through the environment. Most are mathematical representations of simplified versions of the physical processes that occur, generally designed in such a fashion as to overestimate exposures to individuals. Examples range from relatively simple approaches using spreadsheets implementating the EPA's methodology for assessing emissions from combustors (EPA, 1998c), to the complex modeling system of the Hazardous Waste Identification Rule (EPA, 1999). These models generally obtain estimates of concentrations of chemicals in various environmental compartments, for example indoor and outdoor air, water bodies, soil, and foodstuffs. Obtaining human dose estimates requires knowledge of the interaction of people with such environmental compartments — information obtained from observations and surveys of people. A summary of some such information is available in the EPA's "Exposure Factors Handbook" (EPA, 1997).

There are many pathways by which a substance can travel from a source (here assumed to be a chimney stack) to people. Figure 2-14, from an excellent review by Paustenbach (2000), illustrates this. The consuming of contaminated water has been an obvious pathway for centuries, but until recently it was considered a local phenomenon (and probably was). Public health authorities recommended an obvious precaution (still not always taken):

put the sewage and factory effluent outlet downstream from a city and take the drinking water from upstream. (Hopefully the river would clean itself before reaching the next city, but if not it was someone else's problem!) Air pollution from individual coal fires and small factories was also local; and until the last 50 years the dispersion of the pollution by tall chimney stacks was considered adequate. But the old cry "the solution to pollution is dilution" is now considered inadequate. There is a desire to protect against the possibility even of small effects that could only show up in a large population of people. In radiation protection a "collective dose" is defined as the summed product of the radiation dose and the number of people who receive that dose. If there were a threshold below which no harm could be done, then

---

FIGURE 2-15

One Pathway in the Impact Pathway Analysis

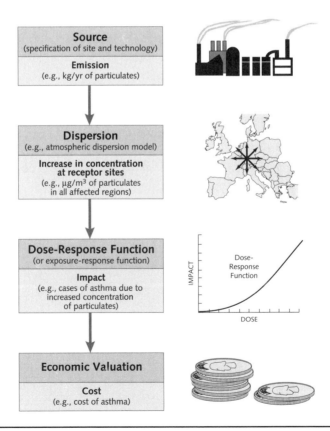

---

dilution to below that level would obviously suffice. But if the linear-no-threshold dose response is correct for radiation, then the collective dose to the whole population is sufficient to define the total effect in that population, provided only that all doses are within the linear part of the dose response curve. In particular, if the probability of cancer is proportional to dose, then the collective dose defines the expected number of cancers. If the effect falls below the linear dose response curve at any dose, the calculation is still useful, because it is an upper-limit to the possible effect. A similar concept applies for other substances, including chemical carcinogens and even the effects of air pollution (Wilson and Spengler, 1996); but while the "collective dose" is a generally accepted concept for evaluation of radiation effects, it is curious that similar definitions of population dose are rarely used in these other cases.

Water

In 1980 the estimation of risks from pollutants in water seemed very simple. Since such pollutants are ingested with the water, all that seemed to be required was to measure the concentration of the substance in the water and estimate the amount of water consumed daily. For setting standards for drinking water, the U.S. EPA deliberately overestimated the amount people drink as two liters per day, based on the quantity of water needed in sunny desert conditions. For accurate risk assessments, and even for some conservative ones, this is an oversimplification for two opposing reasons. Firstly, people vary in their consumption and the mean is smaller than 2 liters a day (Ershow and Cantor, 1989). A substantial fraction of many people's intake of water may come from bottled liquids; and volatile pollutants may easily be driven from tap water when it is heated for use in hot drinks or cooking. On the other hand, dermal contact with water may allow dermal absorption of the pollutants within it; and volatile pollutants in drinking water evaporate into the air, causing additional exposure through inhalation of the vapors (and some dermal absorption of the vapors as well). Although these can occur all over a house, the primary exposure is usually during showering or bathing. Thus, direct ingestion is not the only route of exposure to water-borne pollutants.

There have been many measurements of the concentrations of organic chemicals that were evaporated from the water in experimental showers and showers in residences (Andelman, 1985; Andelman et al., 1992; Giardino and Andelman, 1996) that show that inhalation in a shower can be a major route of entry of water-borne pollutants. McKone (1987) provides a simple model to evaluate inhalation exposures to volatile pollutants in drinking water. The model treats the air in a residence as being in three well-mixed compartments (shower, bathroom, and the rest of the house), with continuous air exchange between these compartments. McKone (1987) originally attempted to estimate the emission of volatile organic pollutants by extrapolation from radon, but that approach can at best be considered heuristic (Little, 1992). Other models have also appeared (Wilkes et al., 1996; Maslia et al., 1996) However, some of the air-exchange rates (e.g. the shower to bathroom air exchange) and other input data to the model (length of time in shower) are likely to be very variable. The model must be "validated" against data. In most cases the input used by McKone (1987) as a default results in a considerable overestimate of the concentrations.

Skin

Before 1970, and for some years thereafter, dermal absorption was studied primarily for short-term occupational exposures by placing some of the pollutant on the skin, and observing how much penetrated within 24 hours. Our understanding of the way in which substances penetrate the skin begins with seminal papers by Scheuplein and Blank (1971), further reviewed by Scheuplein and Bronaugh (1983). They discussed the physical chemistry of skin layers and they showed a marked difference between organic pollutants that are mostly lipid soluble and those materials, which are not. Lipid soluble materials penetrate the skin more rapidly than previously thought and change the structure of the skin as they penetrate. The rapid penetration by organic materials was noticed experimentally by Dutkiewiicz and Tyras (1967, 1968). Indeed for some gases such as benzene, it is likely that dermal absorption is equal to inhalation as a source of human exposure. But dermal absorption has only been systematically included in environmental risk assessments in the last 10 years. But the way in which volatile organic materials penetrate the skin is still not adequately known. The approach of Scheuplein and Blank for estimating penetration rates was to assume a steady state flux across the skin. However, actual conditions of exposure tend to be transient, with the hydration condition of the skin changing (e.g. in showers). Transient absorption is predicted, using theoretical ideas on diffusion, to be considerably higher than would be expected from the steady state (Cleek and Bunge, 1993, Bunge et al., 1995a, 1995b). However, skin is not necessarily a passive diffusive barrier, and recent experiments (Kalia et al. 1996, Pirot et al., 1997 and Bogen et al., 1998) indicate that the simple diffusion model is inadequate.

Air

Air pollution modeling has followed two major approaches. The first and most widely used formulation of atmospheric dispersion , and the basis of most regulatory models, the "Gaussian plume" model, in which the turbulence of the wind spreads pollution from a point source into a plume that has a Gaussian or normal distribution of concentrations about the wind direction. That is, the eddies or turbulence in the air (Taylor, 1922) spread the emitted pollution in such a way that the concentrations will be distributed normally around a peak center-line concentration, with the center-line coinciding with the wind direction. The basic formula for the spread of pollution from a stationary source with a chimney stack of height *h* was developed by Sutton (1932). It relates the concentration C of an emitted substance (a gas, vapor, or particulates) at a point (x,y,z), where the x direction is the direction of the wind, and the z direction is vertical, with the rate of emission (Q) of that substance at the point of origin. C is described by the product of two empirical Gaussian distributions, one for vertical spread and one for horizontal spread perpendicular to the prevailing wind direction, each varying with distance along the plume, x. The plume width parameters (σ_y and σ_z), which are input into the model, are based on empirical correlations and take into account relevant meteorological conditions. These models are adequate for distances up to 10 km.

$$C=\left[\frac{Q}{2\pi u_x}\right]\exp\left[\frac{-y^2}{2\sigma_y^2}\right]\left\{\exp\left[\frac{-(z-h)^2}{2\sigma_z^2}\right]+\exp\left[\frac{-(z+h)^2}{2\sigma_z^2}\right]\right\} \qquad (2\text{-}8)$$

In this formula, u_x is the wind speed in the x direction, and the two exponential z terms account for the reflection of the plume at the ground surface. Slightly more complex forms of this are used in practice, taking account of reflections at inversion layers in the atmosphere, extra mixing that occurs in the wake of buildings, the plume rise that occurs from hot gases exiting stacks, and so forth.

The Gaussian plume model approach is simple to apply, and reasonably accurate in simple situations — in ideal circumstances, it may give concentration estimates accurate within a factor of two or so, particularly for long-term averages. It is extensively used for regulatory purposes, where the increments in concentrations of various relatively non-reactive emitted pollutants is required. At the opposite end of scale are the numerical simulation models derived from the Navier-Stokes equation for fluid flow. Such models requires specification of boundary as well as initial conditions across the spatial array of interest. Wind fields and concentrations are estimated by numerical solutions of the Navier-Stokes differential equations, usually by solving an approximating set of difference equations on a grid. This type of model has been extensively used in photochemical modeling, where the concentrations of a number of reactive pollutants are needed.

While the simple Gaussian plume models are adequate for some regulatory purposes, more complex models may be required. For example, chemical transformations occur to emitted pollutants, and those transformations can be critically important. Examples include the transformation of sulfur oxides (gases and vapors) to sulfates (particles), and the various chemical reactions occurring between nitrogen oxide emissions and vapor and particle phase organic matter to produce smog. Observations demonstrate that these processes occur. For example, McMurry et al. (1981) (Figure 4.6 of Wilson and Spengler, 1996) measured how the particle size distribution changes at a distance from a coal-fired power plant. The coarse fraction of PM_{10} (particles greater than 2.5 million)decreases with distance. The relative amount of the fine particles (around 0.3 m) increases, largely by conversion of SO_2 to sulfates and NO_x to nitrates.

For distances greater than 10 km or a few tens of km, the simple Gaussian plume models become inadequate, and complex numerical codes can be impractical. To fill the gap, long-range transport models have been developed that attempt to track air masses. The first extensive tests of long-range transport was performed for the Office of European Cooperation and Development (OECD, 1977). They carried out two sets of tests. In one set, individual pollutant masses were followed. One air mass, for example, was seen to pick up pollution from sources in the Ukraine, travel over Europe to Spain, move out over the Bay of Biscay, and turn eastwards again over northern Scotland to Scandinavia. Another test confirmed that the OECD model, an early Lagrangian formulation, could predict *average* particulate concentrations over many diverse monitoring stations.

Prediction of air pollution dispersion in extreme accidents is very important because in these situations any threshold for health effects can be exceeded and strong measures such as evacuation may be needed. However, even the best models now available cannot predict the detailed behavior of individual air masses. The U.S. Atmospheric Release Advisory Capability (ARAC) model (Sullivan, et al., 1993) was the best available at the time, did not describe a major feature of the radioactivity deposition after the Chernobyl accident: the deposition 80 miles NE of the plant near Gomel (Belarus) and Briansk (Russia). It was mostly in this region that children ingested or inhaled radioactive iodine and developed thyroid cancers. The deposition occurred during a rainfall, 36 hours after the accident. The model did not include rainfall (many models include both wet and dry deposition, but an adequate treatment of wet deposition usually requires more data than are available) and rainfall was not added in "by hand." It is not certain that U.S. scientists and authorities were aware of the model deficiency and of its' importance. The U.S. ARAC model was very successful in showing that most of the initial plume went eastwards, but some, at a higher altitude, went eastwards toward Japan and Asia (Lange et al., 1988; Gudiksen et al., 1989).

The Kuwait oil fires (February 1991 to October 1991) offered a magnificent opportunity to test long range dispersion models. The main feature of the weather pattern in that period was the prevailing wind from NW to SE, which, most of the time, blew the smoke away from the city of Kuwait and down the Arabian (or Persian) Gulf where it was obvious to the naked eye 300 km away in Bahrain and Dharhan. The heat from the fires caused the smoke to rise and collect an atmospheric temperature inversion layer at about 1,000 m. to 4,000 m Airplanes flew into the plume and recorded concentrations of pollutants. These measurements agreed well with calculations (Sullivan et al., 1994), but the all-important concentration of pollutants on the ground depended upon the more subtle diffusion of pollutants downwards from the inversion layer. The *average* behavior of the plume was reasonably well described. However, some individual deviations, in which for example air masses turned westward over Riyadh in Saudi Arabia, were not well described even after the event (WMO, 1992). These failures of the predictions of the models are not usually considered to be failures of the models themselves, but an indication that the information that is input to the models, wind directions, rainfall etc., is often, inadequate.

Evaluation of the acute impacts of air pollution requires estimating concentrations averaged over short times, and has to take account of the short-term fluctuations in such short-term averages due to variations in wind speed and direction. The complete air dispersion models summarized above are needed for such calculations. In contrast, if all that is required is an estimate of long-term average concentration, then major simplifications are possible. Such long-term average concentrations are relevant, for example, for the discussion of cancer risks, which depend on exposures accumulated over time, and for which short-term fluctuations are generally unimportant. Rather than estimate the speed of the wind that disperses the substance at every place and time, all that is required is a long-term average wind speed (actually the average of the reciprocal of the speed). In most places the wind blows from a variety of directions over a year so that an average over directions is often adequate (and it is fairly simple to improve on this approximation using a long-term average wind-rose; or better, to combine the averaging over wind directions and speeds). Then one can integrate Sutton's equation over y, and for distances where σ_z is greater than the stack height and the plume has reached the ground we find a very simple formula: for long-term average ground-level concentration $C = Q /[(2\pi)^{1.5} \times (u_x \sigma_z)]$. An average of this expression over typical weather conditions (σ_z is different for different weather conditions) will then usually give an estimate of average concentration equal to that from more complex calculations within a factor of four, which is often still more precise than the other factors in the risk calculations. One advantage of this procedure is that it is possible to describe it to lay people.

The Risk of a System—the Impact Pathway Approach

In the above sections of this chapter we have mentioned some procedures for calculation of risks from a specific action or pollutant rather than for a system as a whole. The separate steps must still be combined together. Theogical procedure is illustrated for emissions from a power plant in Figure 2-15. Various authors have emphasized the importance of emissions at every step of the diagram. Pickford (1975) produced materials flow diagrams for various types of power plants, from which impacts may be derived. Kates et al. (1984) emphasized the importance of a diagram not merely to illustrate and understand the process but to understand where intervention may best reduce or avoid emissions. to this logical procedure in the European analysis of impacts of electricity generation, ExternE. The name "Impact Pathway Approach" is attached (European Commission, 1999; IAEA, 1996, 1999; Rabl and Spadaro, 2000). The ExternE program drew such impact pathway diagrams for every type of power plant under discussion. They emphasize the importance of NOT imposing an arbitrary boundary when comparing such cycles.

Although the logic and systematic approach are widely adaptable, the numerical value of the risk at one location cannot easily be transferred to another location. Rabl and Spadaro (2000) argue that the transferability problem arises at two distinct levels:

■ Data, which originate from sources other than those directly related to the application being investigated must be used with caution.

■ Even if the basic data is applicable, the higher level (calculated) results from other studies may be inapplicable.

The following examples considered in the recent ExternE study for the European Commission (1999) illustrate some of the transferability issues:

■ Health and environmental damages are highly location-specific. This means that they depend on country-specific (e.g. overall environmental quality level), site-specific (e.g. baseline level of pollution), and individual (age, sex). How are health and environmental effects going to depend on household size? It is plausible that they might depend on factors like individual susceptibility that might be correlated with household size. A possible entry might be: genetic makeup) characteristics. The degree to which the findings can be credibly transferred to another location, even within a country, depends on the nature of the medical or environmental endpoint.

■ In the evaluations of both the probability of, and consequences of, a severe nuclear accidents, in some earlier studies of external costs, the Chornobyl accident was used as the reference for calculations concerning nuclear plants operating in the Western world. Such an approach is associated with a number of fundamental problems. Firstly, the future probability (per reactor operating year) of an accident in any nuclear power plant was estimated by taking the single Chernobyl accident in the numerator, and the total number of reactor operating years, world-wide, in the denominator. This accident occurred at a reactor (RBMK) with a specific (flawed) design, operating in a specific environment with a low safety culture, and located at a specific site. This clearly overstates the accident probability for a modern plant with safer design and safer operation although it obviously *understates* the risk for the RBMK reactors *before* the post-Chernobyl improvements. Second, with this approach, the estimation of the consequences conditional on a specific type of accident is purely deterministic and equal to the consequences of the one specific major accident, while different weather conditions, accident management strategies, sheltering conditions and the effects of evacuation practices are not considered.

■ In the case of potential effects of hydropower, there is great site-specific and regional variation, with many dams of many different types (e.g., 125 large and many more small dams in Switzerland alone), some over 150 years old and some new, many accidents, no Probabilistic Risk Analyses (PRA), or Probabilistic Safety Assessments (PSAs), and no international standardization of licensing requirements. Consequently, although one may be able to make statements about the general safety of the dams in a specific region, one can not make statements regarding the risk that each dam poses individually without analyzing each one separately[2].

- Should the "value of life" used in the studies carried out by highly developed countries also be used in the studies carried out by developing countries? On economic arguments the answer is probably no, since the "value of a life" can be related to local economic indicators. On ethical arguments there is disagreement. Some people will argue that all persons are equally valuable, but if the "value of life" is replaced by "how much is society prepared to pay to save lives" (discussed further in Chapter 5), there is clearly a large variation. Consequently, any resolution of the problem will depend on the specific objectives of the comparative study.

Risk of the Impossible

In the continual search for substances that have escaped the "net" and may cause a small addition to cancer rate, we must pay particular attention to those for which exposure is ubiquitous. Consider as an example warnings about the possible carcinogenicity of electromagnetic fields (from electric power production, distribution, and use) *per se* rather than through electric or mechanical effects they produce. If these electromagnetic fields are carcinogenic and increase cancer rates by amounts just too small to detect in any epidemiological study, 1,000 people per year in the U.S. could get cancer (Wilson, 1996). However, experts in electromagnetism and thermodynamics have emphasized that it is impossible for any structures in the body to detect these fields at the typical intensities observed in everyday life. No part of the body can therefore have any response—beneficial or adverse—at the low field intensity of the power lines under consideration (APS 1995, NAS 1996, Hafemeister, 1996). Then the risk would be zero. The question arises: "how seriously should one take such warnings?; what is the risk of the impossible?" It is particularly important that we consider very carefully whether or not a risk belongs in the "impossible" category. If we do not, the pressure for a draconian application of the "Precautionary Principle" (decision framework 11 of Chapter 6) will increase. Such a draconian application will, by indirect effects, produce its own risks, which may be considerable. This issue is discussed by Kammen, Shlyakter and Wilson (1994). They discuss several cases where scientists have suggested a risk which is probably not there, and other cases where a risk has been denied which probably exists. There should be no shame in making a suggestion that a risk exists. It is usual for a non-scientist to attribute to a substance he does not understand all the problems that he does not understand. A scientist may make some such conjecture and then explore the consequences of his conjecture. Some persons, inexpert in electromagnetic fields, find no problem in attributing to them unusual properties. But once the logical problems have been demonstrated, a good scientist will abandon his initial conjecture. Meanwhile, a risk analyst must be wary.

Large and Immeasurable Risks

There is a small class of potentially catastrophic but presently immeasurable risks; we discuss two; the risk of an all-out nuclear war and the risk of a major epidemic (perhaps an airborne AIDS or Ebola virus) that is worse than the Black Death of the 13th century A.D.

The risk of nuclear war is particularly troubling. While there still exist in the world over 5,000 nuclear weapons, most of them more powerful than the one used on Hiroshima, there is a possibility that someone, inadvertently or deliberately, may set off one that starts a war where all are used. While many persons think of the radiation danger (as suggested for example by the book "On the Beach" by Neville Shute), it must be remembered that at Hiroshima and Nagasaki the effects of blast exceeded, by 1000-fold, the effects of radiation, and that the much discussed "nuclear winter" would be caused by soot from fires. Although the effects of nuclear war could be exceeded by a meteorite impact of a size expected every 100 million years, nuclear war seems more probable and subject to man's control. In a manner similar to that used above in giving an *upper limit* to the probability of a nuclear reactor accident, Pauling (1970) noted that we have had no nuclear war since it became possible in 1945. Then he made an upper bound estimate of P, which (updated) comes to 0.01 per year. This risk would apply to everyone in the world and is *larger* than most of all the risks listed in Chapter 7 (only the probability of US or Egyptian presidential assassination is greater). These observations suggest that *any* action that increases the risk of nuclear war even by a small amount must be avoided, and any action that decreases it must be taken. It is widely assumed (without proof) that use of nuclear fission for production of electricity increases that risk because of the increased availability of fissile material. However one of us (Wilson, 1999b) has argued that the existence of a group of active professionals in nuclear matters can reduce it. Important though it is, the possibility of reducing this large risk has not been discussed explicitly by risk analysts.

Similarly, the risk of a virus as infectious and contagious in humans as foot-and-mouth disease is in hoofed animals, but as deadly and as difficult to treat as AIDS, has not been fully faced. Such a development could wipe out the human race, or at least a large part of it. Again mankind must be alert to anything that might increase this risk. For such a risk, there is a conflict in risk management between the demands of individuals and the demand of society as a whole. Individuals want to maximize the time between the time of infection with HIV (the AIDS virus) and death. At the same time society wants to ensure that HIV does not spread, and has the smallest chance of mutating to a more dangerous form. Quarantine is one approach that can satisfy both desires, but may conflict with other values.

The Chimera of Zero Risk—Predictable but Irrelevant

As a final class of risks, and as an amusing example of the fact that zero risk is unattainable, we may consider certain risks that are predictable by very well verified physical theories, but that involve events which have never been observed and probably never will be observed. These are due to the inherent probabilistic nature of certain phenomena. It may be recalled that the air, which we breathe, is composed of molecules in constant motion, motion that is essentially random in nature. There is thus a finite, but very small probability that all the air in a room may spontaneously move to one end of that room resulting in decompression of any occupant of the other end.

On an even more fundamental level, it appears that all matter obeys the laws of quantum mechanics, which are inherently probabilistic. One of the consequences of this is that there is always a finite chance (albeit very small for macroscopic bodies) of any object spontaneously converting into a lower energy state even if there is a substantial energy barrier to be overcome. Since there apparently exist lower energy states for such bodies as the sun or earth, in the form of black holes, there is a theoretical possibility that the sun or earth might spontaneously convert to a black hole. Such an event has such a small probability that it is practically meaningless, but it is nevertheless finite, and of no consequence to a man who would not then exist.

Notes

1   Some agencies and risk assessors define a Virtually Safe Dose (VSD), which is the dose at which the risk calculated by the formula above, is one-in-a-million. Thus VSD = $1/(1,000,000 \, \beta)$.

2   One of the world's great dam designers, the late professor Arthur Casagrande, designed many of the earth-filled dams in North America, none of which has failed. However when asked (in the 1960s) by a Parliamentary Committee in Canada whether his design was absolutely safe, he impatiently responded: 'Perhaps the Right Honorable gentleman would prefer not to have been born into this risky world." (stated to one of the authors by Professor Casagrande)

3

Uncertainty and Variability

"Round Numbers are always false."
    —*Samuel Johnson 03/30/1778 in: Boswell "Life of Johnson" 3:226*

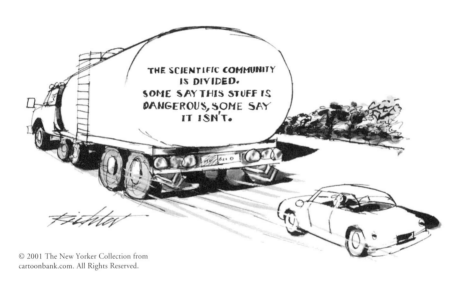

© 2001 The New Yorker Collection from cartoonbank.com. All Rights Reserved.

Risk Implies Uncertainty

The very word risk implies uncertainty. Conversely if there is an uncertainty whether a hazard exists, there remains a probability that it does, and therefore a risk. It might be argued that we should ignore "uncertain risks," but further thought suggests that such an approach would be paradoxical and contradictory. Simply because the existence of a hazard has not been convincingly proven does not make it small. The risk due to such a hazard may be called an "uncertain risk," but a study of risks shows that if we only attempt to reduce those risks with well-defined magnitude ("certain risks") we will miss most of the present opportunities to improve public health.

Common sense can guide us when scientific evidence is inconclusive. When sanitary engineers insisted on main drainage (connecting everyone to a sewer system) a century and a half ago, they did so upon general principles, not upon the basis of reliable data showing that failure to remove raw sewage or provide pure water caused bad health; the rule was to provide the best drainage and the purest water reasonably possible. Sir Edwin Chadwick's famous report on sanitary conditions of the laboring population was presented to the British Government in 1842. It preceded the demonstration in 1849 by Dr John Snow of the role of fecal pollution of drinking water in epidemicity of cholera, and by many more years the discoveries of Louis Pasteur (Fair and Geyer, 1954). There is now no question that this action was correct even though the benefits at the time must have seemed very uncertain.

Quantitative analysis of uncertainty and variability is receiving growing acceptance in risk assessment. It is an important step forward from multiplying simple point estimates of the individual risk factors as it provides a decision-maker with more information about the reliability of the results.

In this chapter we contrast several different types of uncertainty: stochastic uncertainties vs. uncertainties of fact and objective vs. subjective uncertainties. We also discuss relationship between uncertainty and variability. (Wilson, Crouch and Zeise, 1985).

The concept of risk and the notion of uncertainty are closely related. We may say that the lifetime risk of death by cancer is approximately 25%, meaning that approximately 25% of all people both develop cancer in their lifetimes and die from it (Of course, not everyone who develops cancer will die from it). Once an individual develops a terminal cancer, we can no longer talk about risks, but instead we talk about near certainties (for even the most deadly cancers, there is usually a small chance of survival). Similarly, if a man lies dying after a car accident, the risk of his dying of cancer clearly drops to nearly zero. Thus estimates of risks, insofar as they are expressions of uncertainty, will change as knowledge improves.

In most risk estimates, the measure of risk estimated is not a definite quantity but summarizes in some way a set of probabilities. Often a useful summary quantity is an expected value, or means value, of the risk measure. We can illustrate with a hypothetical example: suppose every year every member of some population played Russian Roulette just once (one bullet, six chambers in the gun). Then we would say that the annual risk of death from Russian Roulette in that population is ⅙, i.e. on average ⅙ of the population would be killed each year. But we would not expect exactly ⅙ of the population to die each year—the actual number in any year could be from none to all — and we certainly cannot tell in advance which members of the population would die in any given year. The expected value is ⅙, but in any given year there would almost certainly be some deviation from ⅙. Now suppose that we do not know that the population all plays Russian Roulette with a six-shooter, but simply observe that every year approximately ⅙ of the population ends up dead of a gunshot wound, with year-to-year variations. We would hypothesize some sort of process occurring that had a probability of about ⅙, but we would not know that it was exactly ⅙ without knowing about the Russian Roulette. The best we could do would be to average the death rate over several years, and find that the risk was ⅙ per year, plus or minus a bit. The "plus or minus a bit" would then represent a statistical uncertainty in our estimate. We chose a model with which to analyze the observations (here, a constant risk of death each year, with the annual fluctuations corresponding to the nature of risk), then estimated the parameters of that model (the constant annual risk of death). The fluctuations caused by the nature of risk ensured that there was some uncertainty in our estimate. This process, in more complex form, is how we usually analyze risks — we choose some model that explains the risk, and that incorporates an explanation of any fluctuations in observations either as dependent on parameters of the model, or as random fluctuations. Then the model is fitted to the observations by selecting the parameter values to minimize the difference between predictions and observations; but that selection is always uncertain. Unfortunately, all too often the risk analyst fails to state the uncertainty.

Different Types of Uncertainty

Different uncertainties appear in risk estimation in different ways. Here we emphasize two distinct types of uncertainty according to the way they appear which we here call "stochastic uncertainty" and "systematic uncertainty." There is clearly a risk that an individual will be killed by a car if he or she walks blindfold (and with earplugs) across a busy street. One part of this risk is stochastic; it depends upon whether the individual steps off the curb at the precise moment that a car arrives. Another part of the risk might be systematic; it will depend upon the density of traffic and nature of the fenders and other features of the car. Similarly, if two people are both heavy cigarette smokers, one may die of cancer and the other not; we cannot tell in advance. However, there is a systematic difference in this respect between being a heavy and a light smoker, or between a heavy smoker and a gluttonous eater of peanut butter with its aflatoxin content. Although aflatoxin is known to cause cancer (quite likely even in humans), the cancer risk of eating peanut butter is much lower than that of smoking cigarettes. Exactly how much lower is uncertain, but it is possible to make estimates of how much lower, and also to make estimates of how uncertain we are about the difference (to reassure peanut-butter eaters, it is certainly much, much, lower).

Some estimates of uncertainties are subjective, with differences of opinion arising because there is disagreement among those assessing the risks. Suppose one wishes to assess the risk (to humans) of some new chemical being introduced into the environment, or of a new technology. Without any further information, all we can say about any measure of the risk is that it lies between zero and unity. Extreme opinions might be voiced: one person might say that one should initially assume a risk of unity, because we do not know that the chemical or technology is safe; another might take the opposite extreme, and argue that one should initially assume that there is zero risk, because nothing has been proven dangerous. Here and elsewhere, we argue that it is the task of the risk assessor to use whatever information is available to obtain a risk estimate, with as much precision as possible, together with an estimate of the imprecision. In this context, the statement "we do not know" can be viewed only as procrastination, and not responsive to the request for a risk estimate (although this is not to condemn procrastination in all circumstances.)

The second extreme mentioned above is surprisingly common, even in some government agencies that are supposed to take risks into account in their promulgation of regulations. It arises in hidden form whenever there is a propensity to ignore anything, which is not a proven hazard, or when potential or proven hazards outside the authority of some agency are induced by the agency's attempts to deal with hazards within its authority. Such an attitude is usually logically inconsistent, and users of risk assessments should beware of this danger. Fortunately, if risk assessors have been diligent in searching out hazards to assess, few hazards posing large risks will be missed in this way, so that there may be little direct danger to human health from a continuation of the attitude. The attitude may also lead to economic inefficiencies, however, and can easily lead to unnecessary aggravations.

As Risk Changes with Time, So Does Uncertainty

Risk and uncertainty, have different qualitative meanings at different times. I may say that I have a risk of dying of cancer, meaning that it is uncertain whether or not I will develop cancer and die. If I should develop cancer, the magnitude of the risk would at once be changed. It is still not a certainty that I would die of cancer, since (some) cancers can be cured and there is the chance of spontaneous remission. But once all attempts at cure have failed, the risk of death becomes a certainty. Numerically the risk (R) of death has become unity.

Stochastic Uncertainties

The first type of uncertainty to consider is the stochastic uncertainty of some processes. We consider, for example, the process of developing cancer. Some persons exposed to a large dose of carcinogens, for example, lifetime cigarette smoking, will develop lung cancer; others will not. Whether any particular smoker will develop lung cancer appears to be largely random: there is a stochastic component of uncertainty. Similarly some persons crossing a crowded road blindfolded will be run down and killed, whereas others will not. Weather predictions are uncertain, and probably stochastic; climate predictions cover a longer time and would not normally be considered stochastic.

It is easy to see that it does not really matter in this example whether the onset of cancer is actually a stochastic process or not in the sense of quantum physics. Scientists consider radioactive decay a stochastic process but the Oxford English Dictionary goes further and traces "stochastic" from the Greek "to aim at a mark, guess." In aiming at a mark, we can specify a general distribution of hits but not whether a particular point may be hit. Similarly the details of why a cancer occurs in a particular individual at a particular time is unknown and, with our present and foreseeable knowledge, largely unknowable. Thus arguments about whether the cancer is "really" started by a hit on an individual molecule are irrelevant.

We can list other examples of stochastic uncertainties. A typical risk assessment may estimate the probability that a person will be killed next year. For automobile accidents this may be done on the basis of historical experience: of the U.S. population of 281 million persons. Approximately 44,000 die in auto accidents each year, giving a (population) average risk of 180 per million per year. This estimate is fairly precise—it has been declining a few percent from year to year—so the probability of any one individual (randomly chosen from the population) being killed is also precise; but the individual cannot calculate his own time of death or whether he will in fact die from this cause. This uncertainty, inherent in the word "risk," is purely stochastic—provided the way we have analyzed the historical data is correct. People with different functions and responsibilities will see the uncertainties in different ways. A hospital administrator whose responsibility is to provide emergency services will only be interested in the total number of automobile accidents in his region in any one day because he needs to know the number of injured people for whom he must plan. Although this will fluctuate around the mean the uncertainty in his planning caused by this variability will not be as great as that seen by an individual who sees it as a large uncertainty. It therefore requires careful scrutiny of the problem at issue to evaluate whether measurements are being correctly used.

Variability vs. Uncertainty

Uncertainty and Variability: What they Are

It is often useful to distinguish between "variability" and "uncertainty" in risk assessments. McKone (1994) calls these Type A and Type B uncertainties. Variability is the variation (in some quantity) between different members of a population. For example, everybody's weight is different, and the variation among members of the population, or among some sub-group of the population, represents variability for that population. Similarly, people live all over the United States, and enjoy (or suffer) different climates. The differences in various aspects of the climate (such as rainfall, or average annual temperature), may be considered a variability among the population of the United States. It should be realized that the variation being discussed here is immutable—it is not an artifact of the measurement process used to estimate the values. People's weights really are different, and the annual average rainfall really is different for different areas of the country. No amount of measurement will reduce these differences.

Uncertainty, on the other hand, is the result of not having sufficient information. In the simplest circumstances, it is the result of imprecise methods of measurement—and almost all methods of measurement are imprecise to some degree. For example, we may go out and measure some quantity several times and find different answers, even though we are certain that the quantity in question does not change between measurements. The scatter in our measurements is a measurement uncertainty, and we can usually get a better estimate of the true value of the quantity by taking multiple measurements and averaging the results. Indeed, if the measurements have no bias, we can reduce the uncertainty to any desired degree by taking enough measurements (although with rapidly diminishing returns on our efforts).

These two descriptions convey the essence of the difference between variability and uncertainty. The first is an essential component of the description of the quantity, and the second represents an unwanted limit on how accurately we know about the quantity.

This distinction is useful because for human risk assessment we are sometimes interested in the risk to particular individuals, or to particular small sub-groups of the population, as opposed to the risk to the whole population in aggregate or to random members of the population. Where we are so concerned, the variation in risk among the members of a population is of interest, so we need to separate, as best as possible, the variability in risks among the population from the uncertainty in risks for the whole population. Many of the risk estimates given in this book do not make any such distinction—we are concerned with the risk to a randomly selected member of the population, and we know nothing special about the characteristics of any such randomly selected member. However, it is obvious that for some risks there are large differences between particular sub-groups of the population, or among individuals.

To take a concrete example, the risk of cirrhosis of the liver is given as 2.9 in 100,000 people in Chapter 7, and that is indeed the population average, or a best estimate for a randomly chosen member of the (U.S.) population. However, the risk of cirrhosis of the liver to an individual is largely (although not entirely) driven by the quantities of alcohol that the individual consumes. The risk to a randomly chosen inhabitant of Utah would be considerably lower than the national average given, because of the lower average alcohol consumption in Utah. Similarly, if we know about the alcohol consumption of a particular individual, we can make a much better estimate of that person's risk of cirrhosis of the liver. In some circumstances, we might want to evaluate the variability in the risk of cirrhosis, and distinguish it from our estimate of the uncertainty in that risk. Even though the average risk of cirrhosis is not large, it is plausible that the variability could be huge, with the risk ranging from 100% in genetically pre-disposed alcoholics down to practically zero in certain teetotalers.

As mentioned above, the distinction between uncertainty and variability becomes of importance when examining sub-groups of populations. The U.S. EPA and FDA have become interested in examining such sub-groups, out of a desire to be protective for every member of a population. The FDA, for example, has suggested that one should examine the 99th percentile highest eater of any particular food (e.g., potatoes, apples, prunes, and less obvious foods like lemon rind) in order to ensure that all individuals in a population are adequately protected. The FDA use the descriptive phrase "gluttonous consumer" to describe a person at the 99th percentile. The U.S. EPA also regulates under some statutes that demand the protection of every member of a population—for example, the Clean Air Act calls for such protection of every member of the population with an adequate margin of safety. And in other cases, the U.S. EPA typically demands that its risk assessments apply to the upper end of any variability distribution.

Uncertainty and Variability: It Depends upon the Question

When a set of measurements have been made on some quantity that is going to be used in a risk assessment, do the variations between those measurements represent a variability or an uncertainty? As often occurs in a risk assessment, the answer may depend on what question is being asked.

Some quantities are obviously not variable for different members of any population, so that the variations in measurements always represent uncertainties. Many physical quantities fall into this category—for example, measurements of the octanol-water partition coefficient of a chemical at a particular temperature and pressure are independent of location or individuals. Similarly for most physical and chemical properties measured under fixed conditions.

Other quantities vary from place to place, time to time, and among members of the population. People's body weights vary, so that if the problem involves body weight, and variability is of interest, the distribution of body weights will be a variability distribution for that problem. Of course, the variation may be small relative to other variabilities, and might be ignorable. On the other hand, if the problem involves a random individual from a population, then the variation in body weight may be irrelevant, or may affect the uncertainty distribution. For example, if the properties of the population are measured by measuring a sample, then the uncertainty in the average body weight estimate for that population is directly related to the variability distribution across the population.

Which is which is different when viewed from different perspectives. One might ask what is the risk of exposure to a pollutant in a major city. Since the exposure obviously varies across the city, so also will the risk. If the person asking the question knows where he will live, and the exposure at that location, he can calculate his risk, which will vary depending upon the location. But if the person asking the question does not know where he will live but merely that he will live in a "typical" or average location, the variability becomes an uncertainty to be folded in with other uncertainties of the risk calculation (Hoffman and Hammonds, 1994).

Similarly in calculations of reactor safety one must include a knowledge of how often crucial components are likely to fail. No one knows exactly whether a particular pump will fail, but an estimate of probability with its uncertainty, can be gained from the historical record of the variability of pump failure rates. Therefore a general study of reactor safety will consider the variation to be an uncertainty. But a more detailed study might separate pumps from different manufacturers, or different designs, and determine the failure rates of each. This might then suggest a safety improvement by switching manufacturers.

Whether a given parameter distribution contributes to variability or whether it contributes to uncertainty is may depend, therefore, on a distinction between slightly different questions being addressed by the risk analysts (Hattis and Burmeister, 1994).

Uncertainty vs. Error

The mathematical theory of measurement error is nearly two centuries old, and is called "the theory of error." For example the famous scientist Gauss, when describing his measurements of geographical locations of German mountains invented the method of "least squares" and modestly suggested that no previous geographer has been as thorough. In his theory each measurement is assumed to be statistically independent of every other. Then errors of the measurements can be "added in quadrature" (the square of the combined error is the sum of the squares of the component errors).

The word "error" that is used in formal statistical theory has another connotation when used in discussions of public health and medicine and can mean "mistake" for which the perpetrator might be legally and economically liable.[1] Therefore in public health risk analysis the words "uncertainty analysis" replace "theory of error." But that does not mean that mistakes are not considered by risk analysts. In reactor safety analyses for example, the postulated initiating event is often someone's mistake or error. An analysis of the frequency and distribution of these mistakes is an important input to any full probabilistic risk analysis (PRA).

Independence of Uncertainties

In reactor and other technology assessment it is vital to discover whether or not two factors in a risk equation are statistically independent and to take account of any dependence. If they are independent, uncertainties can be combined in quadrature. For a technological system, oil refinery, space shuttle or nuclear power plant, ensuring that failures of different components are independent may be a crucial part of system design. For a purely observational analysis, such as the analysis of chemical carcinogens, or a study of global warming, the skill of the analyst is to choose those parts of the system which are approximately independent of each other both for ease of calculation and for ease of understanding. In technical terms this can be called "diagonalizing the error matrix."

For example, a reactor safety system is designed so that if a coolant pipe breaks (frequency P_A in the risk equation of Chapter 2) an Emergency Core Cooling System (ECCS) re-injects water into the system. The ECCS itself has a failure probability P_C. If that fails, the reactor containment should hold any radioactive fission products. But the containment might fail with probability P_D for an overall probability of accident $P = P_A P_B P_C$ if these systems are independent. If each of the factors is small, perhaps 1/100 per year might be practical, then P is much smaller at 1/1,000,000 per year, which is often considered acceptable. A correlation between these terms is called in reactor accident analysis a "common cause failure" or a "common mode failure." If there is a complete correlation between two factors, P immediately increases to 10^{-4} per year, a value that is usually considered unacceptable.

Typical examples of common cause failures in reactor safety calculations are fire that destroys all control cables that are (stupidly) installed in the same cable tray (as happened at Browns Ferry in 1976), and intentional sabotage by someone who understands the weak points of the system. An example of a "common mode" failure is the common use of a defective component from a single manufacturer. One must pay special attention to those cases because then the factors are not statistically independent and we must calculate the risk separately either "by hand" or by careful inclusion of correlations in a Monte Carlo program (Rasmussen et al., 1975).

Uncertainty in Cancer Risk Assessment

In Chapter 2, equation 4, we described the risk of cancer caused by chemical carcinogens with four factors:

$$R = \beta_a \times K_{ah} \times d \times E(d) \qquad (3\text{-}1)$$

These factors are approximately independent of each other. Gauss' procedure for combining uncertainties is especially simple if each factor can be described by a lognormal distribution (the logarithm of each factor described by a normal distribution). Then the risk itself is a lognormal distribution with variance equal to the sum of the variances of the individual distributions. Thus we can understand the way in which uncertainties propagate by assuming that each term in the fundamental equation can be approximated, or bounded, by a lognormal distribution and taking the logarithm of both sides:

$$\ln R = + \ln \beta + \ln K + \ln d + \ln E \qquad (3\text{-}2)$$

Each term in the logarithmic form of the equation is approximated by a normal distribution, and then $\ln R$ is also approximated by a normal.

$$\ln R = (1/\sigma_R)(1/2\pi)^{0.5} \exp - [(\ln R - \ln R_m)^2/2\sigma_R^2] \qquad (3\text{-}3)$$

where $\ln R_m$ is the peak of the distribution of $\ln R$, and σ_R is the standard deviation. If the distributions are not exactly normal, approximations that successfully reproduce the mean and the variance are (The mean IS the first moment about zero. The variance is the second moment about the mean) often adequate. If the process described by each term is independent of the others, then the distribution of $\ln R$ is also normal (distribution of R is lognormal), with a variance given by (Crouch and Wilson, 1991).

$$\sigma_R^2 = \sigma^2_\beta + \sigma_K^2 + \sigma_d^2 + \sigma_E^2 \qquad (3\text{-}4)$$

Of course, if the distributions are not lognormal, but are known, the "risk distribution" (the distribution of the function R) can still be evaluated on a computer by a Monte Carlo program and many programs are commercially available for this purpose. But the simple analytic calculations with an approximate lognormal fit can be readily performed, and are always worthwhile to perform, to ensure that no simple human errors are made.

Although in the above we have considered the extrapolation factor E(d) in the same way as the other three, it has many different features. As noted in Chapter 2, it is usually not derivable directly from data and depends upon indirect evidence. It would not normally be considered to have a lognormal distribution, but might simply have one of two values, zero or unity. In that case, a better way of proceeding is to leave out this factor, and calculate with two separate models; one with a threshold (E(d) = 0) at low doses and the other with linearity (E(d) = 1). Then the two results would be presented separately to the decision maker with some estimate for the likelihood of each. This is discussed further under Model Uncertainty.

Often overlooked is that while the median of the distribution of R is the product of the medians of the distributions for each factor, this does not apply to any other parameter of the distribution. In particular, any upper percentile of R is *less than* the product of the same upper percentiles of the individual distributions(for example, the upper 95th percentile of R is less than the product of 95th percentiles of each of the terms). A failure to realize this has resulted in many overestimates of risk. This fact is particularly important because of the tendency of regulatory agencies to quote only an upper percentile of the distributions of these 4 separate factors; of cancer potency in the bioassay; of exposure; and so forth. All too often the product of what are stated to be upper 95th percentiles is erroneously quoted by persons with positions of authority as the upper 95th percentile of the risk. The error although widespread is extremely simple. In a game of throwing dice the probability of throwing a double 6 is $\frac{1}{36}$ or 0.028. But the probability of throwing a double 6 four times in a row is *not* $\frac{1}{36}$, but much less than that.

The 4 parameter equation for risks of cancer from exposure to chemicals is sometimes used, but more often the extrapolation parameter is set equal to 1 and linearity is assumed, leading to three parameters. However it assumes that the *dose* is known. In some situations that is true; the concentration in the blood of phenoxy chemicals or of lead can be, or is measured. But in regulation of chemical exposure it is more common to use a calculation to estimate the dose. The calculation of dose then depends on a large number of factors, (for example, 4 factors m, n, o, and p) (d = mnop) some of which are poorly known, others of which vary extensively over a population. Many of these factors might be approximately independent, so that we can express the distribution of dose in turn by lognormal distributions with appropriate geometric means and geometric standard deviations and write:

$$\sigma_d^2 = \sigma_m^2 + \sigma_n^2 + \sigma_o^2 + \sigma_p^2 \qquad (3\text{-}5)$$

Monte Carlo Models

The combination of uncertainties that we espoused above assumes that the uncertainty distribution of each term in the equation can be fit by a lognormal curve. The important feature of course is to fit the geometric mean and the geometric standard deviation—which are the first two moments of the distribution. Then if the terms are independent, the resultant risk distribution will also be lognormal and the geometric mean and the geometric standard deviation will be correctly given. We recommend this procedure for a rapid-back-of-the-envelope calculation. But when the distribution of one of the terms is far from Gaussian this may not be adequate. For these purposes a Monte Carlo calculation can be performed.

The Monte Carlo procedure has been used for combining results for 50 years. It was used by Rasmussen (1975) for evaluating uncertainties in the reactor safety calculations. It was used by Wilson et al. (1983) for obtaining a distribution of risks when risks from different pollutants are added (a problem that is not analytically tractable). But the major use in chemical risk assessment came with fast PCs and commercial software packages. The U.S. EPA (EPA, 1999a) has written a guidance document on the topic. The flexibility of a Monte Carlo analysis enables any distribution to be incorporated, and correlations to be taken into account. A number of authors have written extensively on this topic, and produced calculational procedures that, for example, distinguish the effect of variability and uncertainty on the final answer (McKone and Ryan, 1989; Green et al., 1993; McKone and Bogen, 1991; McKone, 1994; Bogen, 1995).

The accuracy of the calculational technique (Cox, 1996) is much greater than the reliability of the assumptions that go into it so that these assumptions must constantly be challenged.

In the calculation of risk from chemical carcinogens it is far from obvious that all the relevant variables are independent of each other. However, Smith et al. (1992) argue that the residual correlation is small and that assuming independence gives little error.

Model Uncertainty

Unfortunately, life is not quite as simple as the foregoing discussion makes it appear. In Chapter 2 we emphasized that any risk estimate involves a model—even if it is a simple one such as "next year will be like last year." Because of the randomness of real life, the data used to construct the model will contain some deviations from the expected values, so that in fitting the model to such data, we will almost invariably get it slightly wrong, so that the values predicted by the model will also be wrong (both in expected value and uncertainty estimate). This effect is, however, relatively straightforward to allow for using statistical techniques, the result being an increase in the size of the uncertainty.

The more difficult problem is to try and estimate the uncertainty due to the possible choice of an erroneous model (Bouville et al, 1994). The likelihood that any estimates suffer from this type of error depends on the case being considered, and the theories being used—on how well tested they have been and their applicability In engineering systems it is common to describe phenomena by a model, hopefully based on sound physical theory, and derive the parameters of the model, with their uncertainties or variations, by fits to data. This procedure is usually adequate for summarizing a quantity of data and enables the data to be described by an analytic expression. But often the model is used to predict the behavior of a system beyond the region where data exist. If the model is well founded scientifically this extrapolation is reliable; otherwise it may be complete nonsense. The model may fit very well to any existing data, and give extrapolated estimates with small statistical error estimates. But those extrapolated estimates may nevertheless be which are nevertheless many times further from the real world values than would be expected from such statistical error estimates.

There is no general technique for estimating this sort of error, although there are some methods, which may be, used that sometimes may give an idea of their magnitude, although quantitative statements are difficult to make.

These methods can be summarized as "choosing worst (or best) cases." Different models are tried, adjusted to fit the available data as well as possible, and then examined to assess what they predict in the required situation. The different models may be variations on a single theme (obtained, for example, by varying some parameters within the original model) that cannot be adequately selected by available data or may be widely disparate in underlying philosophy. The only requirement is plausibility and consistency with available data (this consistency should be extended to include relevant other cases where data is available), but the test of plausibility is necessarily dependent on opinion. If any consensus can be reached on best and worst estimates, then these represent some measure of uncertainty, but it must be recognized that no quantitative statements can be made about such estimates—they are statements of belief.

One example where uncertainty could be grossly underestimated by slavish use of a model is in the event tree calculations. Rasmussen (1975) in his first report estimated the uncertainty by assuming independence of all the terms in the overall risk of reactor accident, and combining the uncertainties. But, as we noted above, independence is only an approximation (footnote 1). One procedure used is to consider an initiating event where the different terms are coupled as the start of a separate event tree, to work out the overall probability for that tree and then to add the probabilities for the two trees together at the end.

Another particular case of a major model uncertainty appears in the estimated of risks from chemical substances where there is uncertainty whether or not there is a dose-response relationship at low doses. As noted above, the procedure we espouse is the one usually adopted: we calculate with and without a threshold and present the results separately with a brief commentary. This is what we do in the tables of Chapter 7.

Uncertainty in Expert Elicitation

In Chapter 2 we noted that "expert elication" may be used to estimate the risk when there seems to be no good objective way of estimating the risk otherwise. Of course the uncertainty in such a procedure is considerable. One can both ask the experts their estimate of the risk and their estimate of the uncertainty, and it seems reasonable for the analyst to assign an uncertainty, which includes the bounds from all experts. However these bounds may not be great enough and must be used with caution because experts are often as over-confident as members of the public. The experts will probably be using a variety of models to extrapolate to the situation of interest, and fitting their models to a wide array of data. The variation between experts may therefore be considered one example of the previously mentioned model uncertainties. Estimates of the non-statistical errors are notoriously difficult to make, and it is a natural trait to be confident in one opinion and therefore overconfident about the accuracy of one's estimate.

A particular example might be to elicit opinions on the risk of cancer due to low doses of a particular chemical, a problem in which the extrapolation factor E above is important. Webler et al. (1991) propose a novel group Delphi to reduce uncertainty. However this procedure has not achieved general acceptance. Some toxicologists may tend to assume a threshold, by analogy with many toxic effects, whereas modelers may well assume linearity. This might lead to a bimodal distribution with weights depending critically on the choice of experts, a classic fable describes the problem. A group was asked their opinion about the height of the Emperor of China. Being an intelligent, if uninformed, group, they reasoned that Chinese are often shorter than Caucasians, and suggested heights varying from 5 feet 2 inches to 5 feet 8 inches. The mean was 5 feet 5 inches and the uncertainty of the mean about one half an inch. The principal problem with the answer is that there *is* no

Emperor of China! The question asked of the "experts" in this case had an implicit assumption: "assuming that there is an Emperor of China." The assumption was not included in the statement of the answer. If the group had assumed that the question applied before 1912, then there was an emperor of China (but if in 1912, a better estimate of his height would have been about 3.5 ft, since he was only 5 years old. In Chapter 2 we recommended that all data that any of the experts considered to be relevant to the problem should be available to the whole group of experts. The, hopefully, there will be no implicit assumptions that lead to errors of this sort.

Overconfidence in Uncertainty Estimates

Lawyers in particular have often pointed out that as research continues, the uncertainty increases. Of course it is only the perception of uncertainty that increases—the actual uncertainty (whatever it is) stays the same or goes down. (Hammitt, 1995). Two studies have shown that this change in perception applies to the experts as well as to the public. Morgan et al. (1984) asked a group of experts about the risk of premature mortality posed by air pollution at present levels. The spread of opinions was wide. After five years of research into air pollution the same group was questioned again; the opinion spread was even wider! Morgan and Keith (1995) asked a group of experts their opinions on the temperature rise caused by increased greenhouse gas emissions. Then they asked the same group to develop a research program. Finally their opinions about the temperature rise were elicited again. The stated uncertainty had increased!

This is part of a general phenomenon noted by Tversky that probability judgments are attached not to the events but to description of events (Tversky and Koehler, 1994). As the description of events become more specific and detailed (the phenomenon is "unpacked") the perceived probability of the sum of the descriptions becomes greater. This will be discussed further in Chapter 4.

Various authors have parametrized the overconfidence in estimates. Perhaps surprisingly, the same sort of overconfidence is found in uncertainty estimates for both direct measurements as well as for extrapolations. The uncertainties in the most rigorous measurements, of basic physical quantities, are found to have been underestimated. And, less surprisingly, uncertainty estimates of extreme extrapolations, like projections of energy use, or economic growth rate, are also found to be substantially underestimated. The degree of overconfidence in these estimates can be quantified by examining how they have changed over time; and it is possible to fit an empirical distribution to the degree of overconfidence. Although the absolute error in measurements usually decreases with time the estimated uncertainty is also smaller so that the probability of "large" deviations relative to the estimated uncertainty is roughly the same (Morgan and Henrion, 1989; Shlyakhter, 1994). There are two ways of contemplating and using the empirical distribution of overconfidence. The first is purely empirical; one can assume that if practitioners in a given field have understated the uncertainties in a particular way and by a particular amount, then other practitioners in the same field are likely to underestimate errors in the same way.

One may also approach the problem more theoretically. The standard uncertainty analysis can be supplemented with an analysis of "uncertainty of uncertainty." If this uncertainty of uncertainty is itself expected to have a Gaussian distribution, the distribution of risk can be shown to have a long tail similar to that seen in the historical comparisons.

Standard uncertainty analysis provides an estimate of the width of the probability distribution around a simple point estimate. However, the commonly used 95 percent confidence intervals are determined by the tails of the distribution that are very sensitive to such underestimation of the uncertainties. In particular, the commonly used 95 percent upper bounds for normal and lognormal distributions are very sensitive to the underestimation of the true uncertainty. For example, the width of the 95% CI is 1.19 times the width of the 90% CI ($Z_{0.95}/Z_{0.90}=1.96/1.64=1.19$) for a Gaussian (normal) distribution. This implies that an underestimation of the standard deviation (uncertainty) of such a distribution by 20 percent will underestimate by a factor of two the probability of the true value being outside the confidence interval (10 percent instead of the estimated 5 percent). This increase becomes even more important when it is realized that the underestimation of uncertainties particularly affects the tails of the distribution as noted in the previous paragraphs.

Notes

1 Rasmussen's procedure was clearly incorrect in his analysis of the Anticipated Transient Without Scram (ATWS) in a Boiling Water Reactor (BWR), although the final answer may well have been about right. Recent reactor safety calculations avoid this error.

4

Perception of Risks

"Any politician would prefer a dead body to a frightened voter"
—J.Dunster, UK Health and Safety Executive

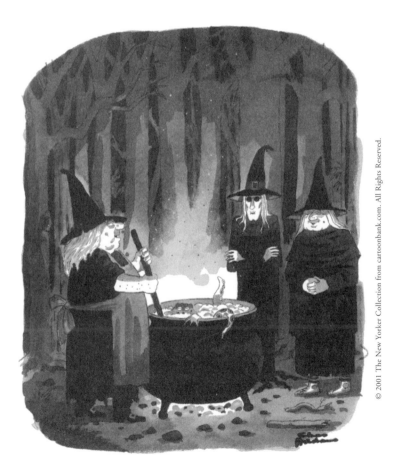

© 2001 The New Yorker Collection from cartoonbank.com. All Rights Reserved.

"It's going to be great! All natural ingredients."

The estimation of risks discussed in Chapter 2, with their uncertainties discussed in Chapter 3, is moderately objective. Benefits of any action, or lack of action, are harder to analyze, vary from person to person and depend upon the decision at issue. However in particular cases benefits can be written down. Once this has been done many people would say that the role of the professional risk analyst is complete. But a decision has yet to be made, and in any given case the way in which risks and benefits are weighed will depend upon how decision makers perceive risks, or believe their constituencies perceive risks, and how they decide which risks to accept. In this chapter we will start by considering various fundamental studies of the way in which people perceive risks, proceed to a review of the surveys of how people actually perceive several risks of topical interest, and conclude with a check list of items that influence perception that must be seriously considered by an analyst. The more the analyst can address these items, and any concerns that they raise, in advance, the better the chance of the analysis being accepted and used.

We assume in this book that "real" numerical values for a risk and its associated uncertainty exist, but all that any analyst can describe is his estimate of those values based upon his perceptions. A fundamental assumption is then made by risk analysts that the perception of an "expert," and therefore the risk estimate based upon this perception, is better than the perception of a "common man" or lay person. Whether or not this is true, a risk *manager* ignores the perceptions and risk estimates of the "common man" at his peril. This influences him in at least two distinct ways. If the common man has an "incorrect" estimate (meaning an estimate that appreciably differs from that of the expert), this is susceptible to correction and change. But some attributes of a risk, such as whether lives are lost one at a time or many at a time in a large accident, are likely to lead to perceptions that persist almost independent of any risk estimate. Such perceptions contribute to "value judgements" which the decision maker must take into account.

Tversky's Analyses

Some of the most perceptive analyses of the way in which people perceive risks are by the late Amos Tversky and collaborators (Tversky and Kahneman, 1971; Tversky, 1975; Tversky et al., 1982). Tversky and Kahneman (1981) show that the way people perceive risks, at least when asked about them, depends very critically upon the way the question is framed or posed. When discussing risks, they attempted to raise as few emotions as possible by careful selection of format. They asked a class in psychology at Stanford University a set of carefully worded questions. Assuming that the U.S. is preparing for an outbreak of a disease imported from Asia two alternative programs, A and B, have been suggested. If program A is adopted 200 people would be saved but if program B is adopted there is a 1 in 3 chance that 600 will be saved and 2 in 3 chance that no one will be saved. 72% of students chose A and 28% chose B. That more students chose the definite result, rather than a risky prospect with the same expectation, is surprising to few people. Another group of respondents was given a different formulation of the alternative programs. If program C is adopted 400 people will die. If program D is adopted there is a ⅓ probability that no one will die and a ⅔ probability that 600 would die. A moment's arithmetic tells us that C and D are the same as A and B, the choice being expressed as people dying rather than people being saved. Yet the students' choice inverted. 78% of the students chose program D.

In the first presentation the problem was presented as a choice between gains. Then the students were risk averse. In the second it appeared as a choice between losses and the students were risk takers. An interesting facet is the *stability* of the responses at different times and places. One of the present authors has found an almost identical distribution of responses among students in his risk analysis classes.

Tversky and Kahneman showed another example of such irrational behavior. Imagine that you are about to purchase a jacket for $125. You then find out that it can be purchased at the other end of town for $120, a saving of $5. When asked whether they would make an extra trip to save $5 on a $15 calculator, 68% of students were willing to travel for 20 minutes to save $5. But the same students would *not* be willing to travel for 20 minutes to save $5 on a $125 jacket!

Risk aversion obviously depends upon context. Many persons are risk takers when buying on the stock exchange but risk averse as they insure their houses. A similar issue arises with risk reduction. Most people would be willing to spend as much on reducing risk from one in ten thousand to one in a million, as to reduce a (larger) risk from 2% to 1%. Another discussion in the same vein as Tversky and Kahneman has been presented in a very readable paper by Piatelli-Palmarini (1991).

In another paper by Tversky and Koehler (1994) the authors show that a risk that might be acceptable when looked at in aggregate can become unacceptable when broken down into its individual parts. In buying an old car there is a risk that it might break down. Many people would accept that risk. But the same people might be overwhelmed when a long list is presented of the ways it might break down! In financial affairs this often can appear as an increase in an estimate for work to be done when that estimate must be itemized.

A very important result, associated with the paper by Tversky and Koehler is that when people try to understand risks, and assign an uncertainty to the numerical value that they attach, the quoted uncertainty *increases*. This applies even for experts. For example Morgan and Keith (1995) assembled a group of climate experts to discuss the uncertainties attached to a single parameter—the prediction of temperature rise if the carbon dioxide (CO_2) levels in the atmosphere doubled. The experts were first asked their opinion on the uncertainty range. Then they were asked to lay out a research program with the intention of narrowing those uncertainties. Finally they were asked what they believed the uncertainty range would be at the end of the research program. Instead of decreasing, the uncertainty range would increase! This result (which is well known in many other less well documented examples) appears illogical until it is realized that it is only the *perception* of the uncertainty that increases. Trial lawyers know this very well. If they want definite statements from a witness he should not be encumbered too much with facts. The opposing lawyer's job is of course to increase the perception of uncertainty.

Other Attributes and Dimensions

In addition to Tversky's papers there is a large literature related to perception of risk and methods for decision-making relating to risks. The authors include: Arkes and Hammond (1986), Clark and Van Horn (1976), Ebbin and Kaspar (1974), Fischoff et al. (1977, 1980), Jasonoff (1986, 1993, 1996), Kimsky and Plough (1988), Kasperson et al. (1988), Nelkin (1971), Renn et al. (1992), Shrader-Frechette (1980, 1991, 1993), Slovic et al. (1974, 1976, 1977), Van Horn and Wilson (1976) and Ziman (1968). In addition there are a number of case studies of public protests over technological risks (Lawless (1976), Mazur (1975), Van Horn (1976), Wilson and Crouch (1982, Chapter 6). Slovic (2000) is an excellent recent book on the subject.

The seminal papers of Tversky and collaborators addressed various types of risks, often of a relatively trivial financial nature (as in the example above). The conclusions of these papers applicable to the type of risks discussed in this book, but there are additional cognitive factors that can have a substantial effect on how such risks are perceived and interpreted. Tversky and Kahneman (1974) discussed three distinct ways in which information is processed that result in a persistent bias in interpretation.

■ *Representativeness.* Similarities between events are used to infer that one class of events, usually small in size, is representative of a large class of events. Often small samples may erroneously be viewed as reliable. Associated events may also be considered as representative of another class of events. As an hypothetical extreme case, a person might view a particular automobile as representative of the manufacturer's entire line or assume that limited data characterize the entire fleet. Such stereotyping may result in judgments that correspond to the stereotype rather than actual cases.

■ *Anchoring* is a judgmental process that occurs when a first approximation or estimate is progressively adjusted to account for subsequent occurrences. Where anchoring occurs the adjustment is inaccurate. For example, the Boeing jumbo jets (747, 757, 767) are now regarded to be quite safe, but had the accident in the Canary Islands (in which two Boeing 747 aircraft collided on the ground) occurred shortly after their introduction into service, they would probably be regarded as risky airplanes, even if the cumulative accident record (1 death per billion passenger miles) were identical over time. Thus, first estimates of a probability or of any numerical value seem to define a psychological range into which subsequent estimates will fall. "Anchored" estimates depend more heavily on the initial estimate than a statistical assessment of experience indicates, so that this phenomenon results in an inaccurate revision of probabilities. This will particularly occur for those cases where the risk is delayed, such as cigarette smoking, where individual initial adverse reactions are small, leading to perceptions of low risk.

■ *Availability* is another cognitive factor resulting in mis-estimates of risk (Tversky and Kahneman, 1973). It arises from the ease of recollection of events; the paradigm is given in the Tversky and Koehler (1994) paper— "If I can conceive of a number of ways for something to fail, the probability of failure must be high." The ease in which occurrences are brought to mind will therefore bias risk perception.

Although risk perceptions vary from country to country and from one community to another (Savage 1993), the above three factors remain remarkably stable. Others have suggested other risk attributes that we add to this list.

■ *Voluntariness* of the risk was suggested in a seminal paper by Starr (1972). Risk acceptability depends on the extent to which we choose to be exposed to the risk situation; i.e. "we are loath to let others do unto us what we happily do unto ourselves." Natural hazards are usually considered to be voluntary in this sense and therefore more acceptable (Slovic et al., 1974).

■ *Availability of alternatives.* Closely related to the voluntariness of the risk is the ability to choose among alternatives. This is largely related to the belief, which in occupational safety is well founded, that if the person who is enduring the risk has a choice he is likely to be able to reduce the risk at little or no cost. Therefore if a choice is available, acceptance may become easier even if the choosing person or public picks an alternative with higher calculated risk. (e.g., many people choose automobile travel over airplane travel).

■ *Necessity.* The question of necessity is also related to voluntariness. But here again, one man's meat is another man's poison. The authors feel no need to dye their hair; others may feel that such a need outweighs the (slight) risks from hair dye use. However, it is neither our desire, nor our duty, to influence such decisions as long as these others are fully informed about the risks.

■ *Immediacy* is stressed by Lowrance (1976) and Fischhoff (1977, 1980). Are the consequences immediate or delayed? Is there a latency period and how does it affect the perception of the risk situation? Lowrance and Fischhoff imply that if the threat is immediate it is perceived as worse than if it is delayed. A latent period puts a risk out of mind. But in contrast to this view, the risk of cancer fills some people with a horror which far exceeds any objectively assessed risk. This leads to the next item:

■ *Dread* is a concept stressed by Kasperson (Kasperson et al., 1988). Does the nature of the risk have a connotation that is dreaded by people? Many people fear developing a cancer more than they fear death itself. In part, but certainly not entirely, this is because it can be a lingering disease. But other lingering diseases are often dreaded less. Radiation cancers are particularly dreaded. "Dread" clearly varies with the person. Nobel Laureate Marie Curie said "There is nothing in the world to be feared—only to be understood." But those who have not yet understood may well fear.

■ *Rare yet catastrophic* —apparently closely related to dread. It seems that many people are more concerned about risks that are catastrophic (with many fatalities) and rare than those which involve fewer fatalities but are more frequent, even when the average risk is the same. Some refer to this by saying that "it is not the odds that matter but the stakes." Many of us (including the present authors) are much more concerned about a risk that would wipe out the whole human race (4 billion people) with a probability of once in 3,000,000 years (approximately the calculated risk for a meteor or comet impact) than the numerically similar individual risk of 1 in 3 million per year incurred regularly. But others clearly do not agree. The U.S. is doing nothing much about the former risk but is trying to regulate many risks of the latter type which are 1 in a million per lifetime—20 times smaller than one in 3 million per year.

- *Knowledge about risk.* How well is it perceived that the risk analyst can determine the risk and how large are the uncertainties? How well do persons exposed to the risks understand the risk, its probability, consequences, and uncertainties? If many people are skeptical about the calculations and if there is disagreement among "experts" the risk is usually perceived to be larger, and even a small risk can become unacceptable.

- *Familiarity.* Old and familiar risks, such as automobile accidents, are accepted more readily than new and strange ones, particularly those (such as those due to radiation or low-level chemical poisons) that cannot be seen. There is a close relationship to Tversky's "anchoring."

- *Distribution of risk.* Is the risk situation widespread; does it affect average persons or especially sensitive persons?

- *Potential for misuse or abuse.* If there is an increased risk if and when the technology is misused, there is often a perception that the risk is high even when properly used. An example is nuclear electric power where there can be very serious consequences if there is misuse—particularly if the separated fissile fuel is used to make an atomic bomb.

- *Trust.* Slovic (1999), in particular, has emphasized the need for trust in the risk assessor. Trust is created slowly but can be destroyed quickly. Figure 4-1 shows his ranking of actions and events that increase or decrease trust. This is another example of the asymmetry in perception of risk suggested by Tversky and Kahneman (1991). As Abraham Lincoln observed in a letter to Alexander McClure (and a modern president might well take note), "If you once forfeit the confidence of your fellow citizens, you can never regain their respect and esteem." However, the ways in which trust is

FIGURE 4-1

Differential Impact of Trust-Increasing and Trust-Decreasing Events

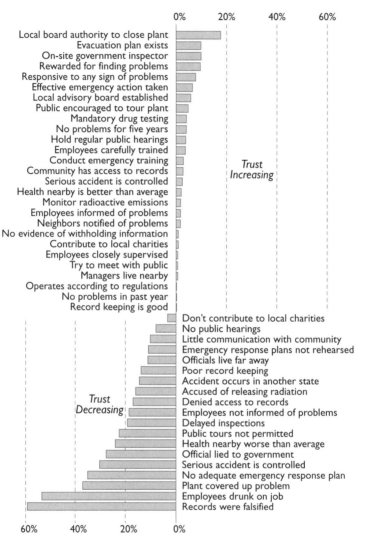

Percent Very Powerful Impact

Note: Only percentages of Category 7 ratings (very powerful impact) are shown here.
Source: Slovic (1993)

lost does not seem to be similar across technologies. Trust in air travel has remained in spite of continuing accidents, the most recent (in 2001) large accidents (more than 100 fatalities) in the US being the 1996 TWA crash, Moriches, NY (212 killed), and the Miami, FL, Valujet crash of 1996 (105 killed). At the same time, an accident that caused *no* deaths (Three Mile Island) caused considerable loss of trust. This suggests that other factors, such as *anchoring*, are also very important. Most peoples' first knowledge of nuclear and radiation issues was the atomic bomb. Most peoples' knowledge of dioxin was its use as Agent Orange in Vietnam.

Managers and Decision Makers Consider Public Perception

We do not suggest that any of these considerations be explicitly introduced into a calculation of a risk, and indeed we suggest that they should *not* be so introduced because that would introduce an excessive degree of subjectivity on the part of the analyst. But the analyst must present his results in a form to be useful to the decision maker who acts on behalf of the public, so that some consideration of them is essential. This is part of a general rule; if a risk analysis cannot be understood, it cannot be used.

At all stages in presentation it becomes useful to compare the risk calculation with other risks with which the reader may be more familiar from everyday life. We will in Chapter 7 calculate and list some of these risks just for this reason. But comparisons should not necessarily imply judgments. Cigarette smoke and air pollution both probably cause lung cancer, and the former probably causes (in the U.S.) 20 times as much as the latter. Yet cigarettes are smoked voluntarily and air pollution is involuntary, so even individuals who understand the numbers well can rationally oppose other sources of air pollution while smoking like chimneys themselves.[1]

To the extent that a risk manager must address the risk as perceived by the public, he must discover what the perceptions really are. In any survey about risks the answer given will depend upon the detailed question and may not even be an honest answer. Therefore analysts have developed several approaches to measure perceived risk. These may be categorized as the "revealed preference" method, the "expressed preference" method, and the "implied preference" method. The revealed preference method examines the historical behavior of society using statistical risk and benefit data. It presumes that society has adjusted to an acceptable balance between risk and benefit. Starr (1969) was one of the original advocates of this approach. However, several shortcomings of the revealed preference method can easily be seen. For example, the methodology finds out what existed, independent of desirability or other preferences. A use of this method must be careful not to imply that any results it finds are necessarily desirable or undesirable (such terms are value judgements that do not enter the methodology). Moreover, the method assumes that past relationships are still relevant—that the surveys on which the methodology is based can keep up with society as it changes. In rapidly changing times, this may not be true. It is plausible that reason or choice might have led to different preferences if the risks and benefits had been analyzed in advance. Finally, the methodology requires that risks and benefits can be accurately determined. Some of the measurement difficulties have been pointed out by Otway and Cohen (1975), Fischhoff et. al. (1977), and Slovic (1998).

Although the revealed preference method is usually more reliable, neither the revealed preference method or the expressed preference method will us whether the preference is held after careful thought or because of some outside influence. We therefore suggest a further category, which we call the "imposed preference" method, in which an activist or a politician manages to convince sufficient people of their preference.

In order to determine the revealed preferences of society, one study (Baldweicz et al., 1974) determined baseline historical trends of risk levels for natural hazards such as floods, tornadoes, and lightning; man-made hazards such as commercial aviation, rail transportation, and rail grade crossings; and occupational hazards such as fire fighting, steel working, coal mining, and railroading. However, this study did not attempt to assess the benefits of the technologies associated with these hazards. Examination of existing data and historical trends in risk levels, such as are provided in the National Safety Council's "Accident Facts," can provide useful comparisons with public perception of risk levels determined by other methods.

Cohen (1980) went further. He reviewed a number of decisions where money has been or was about to be spent to save lives. For each decision he estimated how much money society was willing to spend to save one life. This analysis could be thought of as a measurement of the constant g in the formal risk benefit equation of Chapter 5. There is a huge variation in these amounts of money (see Table 7-6 on pages 214–217). We cannot tell whether this variation is due to intrinsic differences in society's valuation, or due to the fact that in most cases, a detailed risk benefit comparison was only made after the decision. Tengs et al. (1995) calculated in detail some 500 such "life saving actions" and also found a very large spread. Both are certainly lists of what society *has been* willing to pay; an optimist could say it is what society *will be* willing to pay to reduce similar risks, or even what society *should be* willing to pay. We do not go this far, but suggest that a well executed assessment, well presented, might reduce the tendency for decision makers to pay much more or much less than the mean for risk reduction and to this extent, improve decision making. To aid the decision maker the analyst must, inter alia, make clear the relationship between public perception, myth and objective reality. Whether or not this view is correct, we believe that a risk analyst does well to separate clearly where assessment is based on fact, clearly separating those assumptions where the judgement of the decision maker comes into play.

In the "expressed preference" method, samples of the public are asked directly to express their preferences. Although the method accounts for current preferences, it is fraught with sampling difficulties. Not only is it difficult to obtain a large sample of individuals with the time and willingness to state their preferences, but the representativeness of any sample group can be challenged. Some individuals may be atypically uninformed, or others may attempt to deliberately bias results. However, if carefully designed questions are used, these drawbacks may be less severe than those of the revealed preference method which is retrospective in outlook. The expressed preference method of evaluating risk perception has been used by Fischhoff et al. (1977) and Lichtenstein et al. (1978) to assess the importance of various characteristics of risks and to rate subjects' perceptions of the total risks and benefits accruing to society from each of thirty activities and technologies. The risk measure used was the total expected annual number of deaths in the U.S. The results showed that subjects believed that activities which (at least in the eyes of the respondent) benefit society in other ways could have higher levels of risk, and that double standards of risk acceptance existed for certain characteristics of the risk including voluntariness, controllability, familiarity, immediacy, and dread. The implication of this work is that any method for assessing the "magnitude" and "acceptability" of risks should consider all of these factors in concert, as well as benefits. Moreover, care must be exercised in defining terms such as "magnitude of perceived risks" and "acceptability of risks" since these terms have different meanings to various individuals and may be interpreted differently for different measures of risk. The relative rankings (see Figure 4-2) of hazards obtained using this method differ from those based strictly on objective measures (actual annual U.S. deaths).

F I G U R E   4 - 2

Relationship Between Judged Frequency and Actual Number of Fatalities per Year for 41 Causes of Death[a]

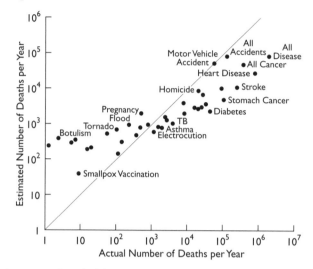

a. Respondents were informed of the actual number of motor vehicle accidents.
Source: Lichtenstein et al. (1978).

In the third method for assessing public perceptions of risks, the "implied preferences" approach, one examines the societal institutions which have been developed to cope with risk benefit tradeoffs in the past. Legislative, judicial, and industrial standards reflect current balances achieved by society as a whole. Concepts such as "reasonableness," "best prevailing professional practice," and "lowest practicable exposure," imply tradeoffs among costs, risks and benefits.

Various researchers have used the methods just described to extensively study people's perceptions of risks. In Table 4-1, we show a compendium assembled by Slovic (1988) of the rank ordering of several hazards (determined by the expressed preference method). In this plot the authors do not label the axes, indicating the scale. This, we presume, was an intentional indication of considerable arbitrariness in the quantitative magnitude. As we note several times in this book, the differences in perception between experts and others is greater for risks posed by nuclear power than for any other.

T A B L E   4 - 1

Ordering of Perceived Risk for 30 Activities and Technologies (ordering by different, non-overlapping, groups)

Activity or Technology	League of Women Voters	College Students	Active Club Members	Experts
Nuclear power	1	1	8	20
Motor vehicles	2	5	3	1
Handguns	3	2	1	4
Smoking	4	3	4	2
Motorcycles	5	6	2	6
Alcoholic beverages	6	7	5	3
General (private) aviation	7	15	11	12
Police work	8	8	7	17
Pesticides	9	4	15	8
Surgery	10	11	9	5
Fire fighting	11	10	6	18
Large construction	12	14	13	13
Hunting	13	18	10	23
Spray cans	14	13	23	26
Mountain climbing	15	22	12	29
Bicycles	16	24	14	15
Commercial aviation	17	16	18	16
Electric power (non-nuclear)	18	19	19	9
Swimming	19	30	17	10
Contraceptives	20	9	22	11
Skiing	21	25	16	30
X-rays	22	17	24	7
High school and college football	23	26	21	27
Railroads	24	23	29	19
Food preservatives	25	12	28	14
Food coloring	26	20	30	21
Power mowers	27	28	25	28
Prescription antibiotics	28	21	26	24
Home appliances	29	27	27	22
Vaccinations	30	29	29	25

Note: The ordering is based on the geometric mean risk ratings within each group. Arbitrarily placed in the order assigned by sample from the League of Women Voters. Rank 1 represents the most risky activity or technology. (From Slovic)

In Figure 4-3 we reproduce from Slovic (1987) a two dimensional chart showing the location of 31 hazards based upon the attributes of *dread* and *unknown risk*, two of the attributes listed above. Kasperson et al. (1988) and Renn et al. (1992) introduced the concept of "social amplification of risk" whereby the experts' risk numbers are amplified for risks possessing one or more of the attributes previously listed. It also appears that strong regulation can lead to amplification. "If NRC thinks it is dangerous then it must be *very* dangerous." It is easy to see that where the extent of regulation on risk perception such amplification provides positive feedback, perhaps leading to instability. Some observers think that this may be the situation with nuclear power.

In Figure 4-4 we show Slovic's (1998) view of levels of risk that are acceptable as a function of their voluntary nature, with the relevant accepted

---

FIGURE   4 - 3

Location of 31 Hazards on a Two-Dimensional Plot from 15 Risk Characteristics

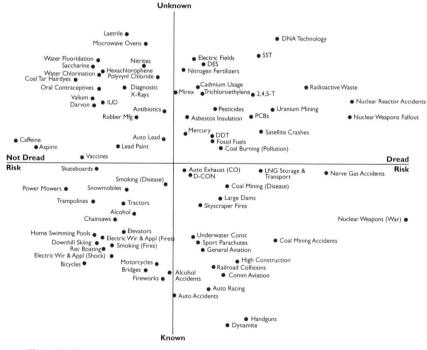

Source: Slovic (1987).

---

risks in railroad transportation superimposed. Finally we show in Figure 4-5 an overall matrix summary, prepared by Dr. Ortwin Renn, of the various factors influencing perception of risks. Dr. Renn did not supply a detailed explanation of this matrix, and we present it here as an example of the complexity that social scientists tend to introduce, which complexity we admit that we do not understand.

Of course, standards and factors influencing public response may change. People's stated attitudes and their actual behavior often differ, people and governments may not be adequately informed, and they may desire unattainable risk levels. In addition, different approaches to determining public preferences, including alternate formulations of questions, can elicit different responses. Thus, estimates of risk perception are not definitive and will usually be representative of only a section of the population. Nevertheless, with a full appreciation of the difficulties in our efforts to understand and quantify the public's perception of risks, this work should improve our capability to assess and deal with future risks.

FIGURE   4 - 4

Maximum Individual Risk as a Function of Risk Categories

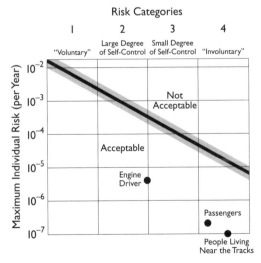

Note: The three specific values refer to the transportation of hazardous materials.
Source: Slovic 1998.

FIGURE   4-5

Matrix of Approaches in Perception of Risk

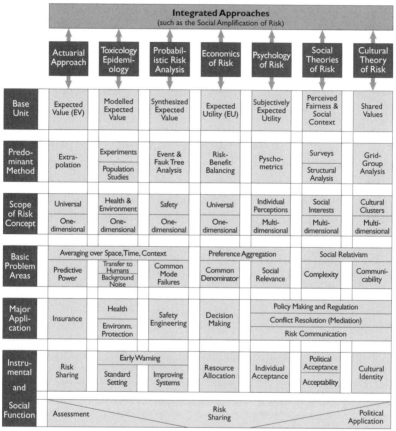

Source: Renn 1998.

Comparing Risks (Risk-Risk Comparisons)

"That's how I judge pain Lucille…. Will it hurt more than a punch in the nose or less than a punch in the nose?" —*From a Charles Schulz "Peanuts" cartoon*

There are several reasons for comparing risks with each other. Perhaps the most important reason is to gain understanding and improve our perception. None of us are born with a concept of what one in a million means, although we have learned that some risks are small and others large. We find it helpful to compare risks that are calculated in a similar way and we presume that others will find it helpful also. Then some of the familiarity and understanding of the older risk can be transferred to the new one. For example, in Chapter 1 we contrasted the risk of automobile travel with that of traveling by horse, for both of which the risks could be calculated from historical experience.

Another common procedure is to compare exposures only. Table 4-2 shows a list of radiation exposures in typical situations (Wilson and Jones, 1974). The dose response relationship for radiations with similar dE/dx [rate of loss, with additions, of energy by the charged particle as it slows down in matter, sometimes called the linear energy transfer (LET)], will be similar, although there may be some correction required for dose rate effects. Thus, ordering by

TABLE 4-2

Comparison of Several Common Radiation Risks

Action	Dose (mr/yr)	Cancers/yr if all U.S. pop. exposed (assuming linearity)
Medical X rays (annual U.S. 2000)	40	3,000
Single Chest X ray annual (2000)	7	600
Single Chest X ray annual (1945)	900	70,000
Radon gas at 1.24 pCi /l (equivalent dose)	175–225	15,000–22,000
Potassium 40 naturally in own body	30	2,500
Cosmic radiation at sea level, U.S.	40	3,000
Cosmic radiation at Denver	65	5,500
Total exposure at sea level (Vermont)	100	*
Total exposure at sea level (Kerala, India)	1,000	*
Exposure at Grand Central Station NY	500	*
Weapons test fall out	2	150
One transcontinental round trip by air	5	400
Air crew exposure at 60 hours per month	400	*
Av. within 20 miles of U.S. nuclear plant	0.002	0.2*
Dose to average resident near Chornobyl	5,000 1st yr**	NA
Dose to highest exposed area (in Bryansk oblast) of Russian Federation	8,000 1st yr**	NA
Cumulative dose to highest exposed area in Bryansk oblast	16,700	NA

* It is not possible for all the U.S. population to live at Grand Central station or be within 20 miles of a nuclear power plant, and so forth, so that these totals are not possible.

** Dose in mrem.
NA Not applicable — not an exposure for the US population.

exposure should be similar to ordering by risk, and the relative risk should be similar to the relative dose. In estimating the number of lethal cancers using a linear dose response hypothesis, we have here assumed approximately 3,000 manrems per cancer (at low doses)—based upon the most recent analyses of the Hiroshima and Nagasaki data (Pierce and Preston, 2000), with a correction factor of 2 for a lower dose rate. This correction factor may not apply to medical X-ray exposures. The estimate is uncertain by 30% or more even if a linear dose response is assumed. If there is a threshold dose below which risk is not increased (or is even reduced), all of these numbers could be zero.

Doses from exposure to radon gas cannot be directly compared to whole body external exposure. For Table 4-2 the risk value comes from a study of uranium miners, and the comparison is on the basis of an equal number of cancers. This comparison has an uncertainty of at least a factor of 3. The risk to smokers is greater than the risk to non-smokers and indeed if there is a threshold below which there is no effect, that threshold may only apply to non-smokers. The concentration of 1.24 pCi/liter is approximately the current US population average exposure to radon (NAS, 1999; the cancer numbers come from the same source). The effect of this exposure appears to be larger than many risks that are currently regulated by U.S. EPA and other government agencies at this time, although no agencies are specifically charged with regulating indoor air in homes, which is where the majority of the exposure occurs. While it is uncertain whether the risk applies at all to smokers, it is curious that this risk, which can be mitigated with relatively low-cost measures, has been largely ignored, particularly when contrasted with the many other smaller risks that have been addressed.

The total background radiation exposure varies from place to place even at sea level, primarily because of the variation of external natural radiation. Even though this table suggests that radiation (in normal operation) from a nuclear power plant could well be ignored in comparison with the medical X-rays or background radioactivity, there is a common public perception that the reverse is the case. This has been repeatedly shown by surveys. For example in a survey of 1,000 college students from Harvard, MIT, and Princeton, most of the students at each institution had the order reversed (Red, 1973). This illustrates very clearly that other factors, such as dread of man-made ionizing radiation, strongly influence perception.

When exposures are not to the same agent but are nevertheless similar, another slightly more complex comparison can be made. An example of such a comparison of risks that are similarly calculated is the comparison of risks of various chlorinated hydrocarbons in drinking water (Table 4-3) (toxicity data from NTP Chemical Health & Safety database, available on the NTP website (see Chapter 8). The animal carcinogenic potency is the potency at the most sensitive site from a book by Gold and Zeiger (1997), which is also available in a paper and supplements (Gold et al., 1984, 1986, 1987, 1990, 1993, 1995, 1999) and on a website: http://potency.berkeley.edu/cpdb.html.

The risks to humans have to be estimated from carcinogen bioassays in rats and mice. Since these are similar materials one might initially expect that the dose response relationships to have the same shape. In setting standards for carcinogens the US EPA first ask whether it is expected that the dose response is linear at low doses, and if so, set a Maximum Contaminant Level Goal (MCLG) of zero, a procedure which supplies little information. Then they decide on a Maximum Contaminant Level based on other criteria. The MCLGs for all of these three chemicals was originally set at zero in 1998. (But see the further comment two paragraphs down). Since zero cannot be met, EPA choose an Maximum Contaminant Level (MCL) based upon other considerations. A comparison such as Table 4-3 suggests suggests that chloro-

T A B L E   4 - 3
A Comparison of Some Hydrocarbons

	Chloroform	Bromoform	TCE
Chemical abstract No.	67-66-3	75-25-2	79-01-6
Acute Toxicity (LD50) in mg/(kg body weight) (smaller numbers more toxic)			
in mice oral	36	1,400	2,402
in mice sc	704	1,820	16,000
in rats oral	908	1,147	N/D
in rats ip	894	414	1,282
in people n(LDLO)	143	7,000	N/D
Carcinogenic potency (oral) in $[mg/(kg\text{-}b.w \times day)]^{-1}$			
in mice (gavage)	0.015	0.009	0.0017
in mice (other)	0.0013 (wat)	N/D	0.0003 (inhl)
in rats (gavage)	0.01	0.009	0.0001
in rats (other)	0.0008 (wat)	N/D	0.0001 (inhl)
in people	N/D	N/D	N/D
Mutagenic *in vitro*	No	No	No
Regulatory level in water	100ppb	5 ppb	5ppb

ip = interperitoneal; sc = subcutaneous; inhl = inhalation; wat = in water;
N/D = No Data

form is more toxic than trichloroethylene (TCE). Then it might seem logical that standards for chloroform, bromoform, and trichloroethylene in drinking water ought to be more stringent for chloroform than for TCE with bromoform in the middle. Moreover, although neither is known to cause cancer in people, we might expect from the gavage data that chloroform would do so 20 or more times as readily as TCE. Yet the U.S. EPA set regulatory levels in the opposite order (EPA, 1979)! This poses a major paradox. Why did not the U.S. EPA set the levels in the same order as the calculated hazard? The public deserved, and did not get, an explanation of what other considerations influenced the order of the MCLs. One explanation we suggest is that Chloroform in drinking water is produced by the action of chlorine on organic material during the chlorination process used to kill bacteria. This process is almost universal for surface water supplies and common for public supplies of groundwater. Bromoform occurs naturally in some ground waters. They are hard to avoid, and reduction invloves public expense. TCE is an industrial solvent that is occasionally found in well waters as a result of accidental pollution which is, in principle avoidable, and the expense is mostly paid by private industry.

In Figure 4-6, from Condran and Cheney (1982), we show the incidence of typhoid in Philadelphia, from 1870–1930, showing the marked reduction when sewage separation, filtration and chlorination of water were instituted around 1900–1915. Although separation of the effects of the three is not possible since the three measures were instituted about the same time, no scientist wanted to return to the "bad old days" where water was not chlorinated. Leaving a slight excess of free chlorine in the water enables bacteria to be destroyed even after the filtration plant. Clearly any good decision maker will try to avoid regulating chloroform to the extent of recreating the higher risk of the nineteenth century. But the EPA failed in what we believe was its duty, to explain the apparent paradox to the public and, even worse, failed to explain it to its own regional and district offices. In 1980, there was a perception among many members of the public that TCE was unusually dangerous and there was strong public pressure to regulate it. Indeed, a major film, "A Civil Action," has been made about a court case involving adverse effects claimed to have occurred as a result of exposure to TCE. In 1979, the director of the office of drinking water standards explained to one of the authors (RW) in an elitist remark that "the public would not understand" (even such a simple graph as Figure 4-6)! As a result, many public health officials gave incorrect advice to the public. There are many cases where a

Deaths from Typhoid Fever: Philadelphia, 1870–1930

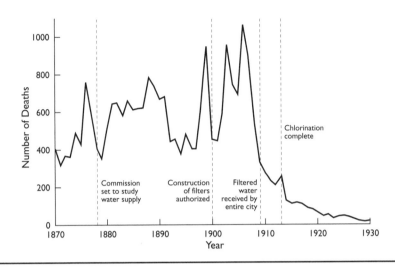

person, or a community, receives their water from a deep well. In a few, there has been industrial pollution so that the TCE level just exceeds the EPA guideline, but there was no chloroform. In some cases, EPA officials have recommended transfer to the city water which comes from the treated surface waters, and therefore has an amount of chloroform substantially higher (in ppb) than the TCE that was avoided. By this switch, the risk was increased a hundredfold, and considerable expense was incurred. In an inverse situation, it appears that regulators in Peru, following U.S. concerns about chloroform, allowed chlorination to be reduced (Anderson et al., 1991) thereby allowing a cholera epidemic (Ries et al., 1992).

EPA has improved its public communication since then. It is possible, and many scientists now believe, that the comparison shown in Table 4-3 may be entirely irrelevant for cancer effects. Animal toxicologists claim that they understand the mechanism by which chloroform causes cancer in animals and that at low concentrations in water it does not cause cancer in animals, and probably in people, at all. Following this argument the EPA in 1998 proposed an MCLG (Maximum Contaminant Level Goal) of 300 ppb for chloroform in drinking water. However, this did not receive universal acceptance (perhaps because they failed to directly address the argument of Crump et al. (1976) discussed in Chapter 2) and later, in 1998, the EPA instead promulgated a rule that set the MCLG of chloroform to zero (EPA's policy default value for carcinogens). This MCLG was vacated by court order in 2000 because of EPA's "failure to regulate in accordance with the scientific evidence." EPA subsequently removed the MCLG for chloroform from its National Primary Drinking Water Regulations. The same toxicologists do not believe that they can make a similar argument for TCE (but see Rhomberg et al. 1997).

This is very relevant to, and calls into question, the way in which human cancer potencies data are inferred from animal potencies that we described in Chapter 2. Because the toxicologists failed to address the Crump et al. argument, the scientific jury is still out as to whether chloroform, TCE or for that matter other non-genotoxic carcinogens can cause human cancer at low doses.

More usually such a direct comparison as Table 4-3 is impossible and calculated risks must be compared. Objections have been raised to comparisons of risks on the ground that such comparisons are misleading. The same charge could be leveled at any approach to examination of risks; but comparison of risks is just one way of presenting information, it does not force actions. It would be naive to insist that risks of the same magnitude must be treated similarly; that would be an optimal approach only in the most circumscribed of circumstances, and it is not how people behave. In general, we must consider, along with the risk, not only the benefit, but also some features of risk perception. There are circumstances, however, where side-by-side comparison of risks that are of a similar magnitude can be enlightening. In Table 4-4 we give an example by comparing and *contrasting* the carcinogenic effects of aflatoxin B1 and dioxin—both among the most carcinogenic chemicals known (toxicity data from the National Toxicology Program (NTP) Chemical Health & Safety database, available on the NTP website (see Chapter 8). Animal carcinogenic potencies are the highest in any site from the book by Gold and Zeiger (1997), and human carcinogenic potencies from Wu-Williams et al., 1992).

Aflatoxin has about $1/_{100}$ of the toxicity of dioxin. (LD50 about 100 times as great). The carcinogenic potency in rats and mice is also about $1/_{10}$ to $1/_{100}$ of the potency of dioxin. Both vary substantially with species tested. Yet regulatory agencies take dioxin more than 100 times as seriously! It is worth examining this carefully. What is the evidence for carcinogenicity at low doses? Since we first made this comparison (Crouch and Wilson, 1987) the evidence has changed.

TABLE 4-4

Comparison of Two Very Toxic Chemicals

	Aflatoxin B1	Dioxin
Chemical Abstract number	1162-65-8	1746-01-6
Acute toxicity in mg/kg (smaller number more toxic)		
In mice	9	0.1
In rats	5	0.02
Carcinogenic potency (in $[mg/kg \cdot day]^{-1}$)		
In people with hepatitis B1*	150	unknown
In people w/o hepatitis B1*	6	unknown
In mice (gavage)	N/D	8,020
In mice (in diet)	256	N/D
In rats (gavage)	N/D	6,900
In rats (in diet)	511	104,000**
Mutagenic in vitro	Yes	No
Certainty of information on human carcinogenicity	High	Medium
Activity (initiator/promotor)	Initiator	Promoter?
Possibility of threshold dose-response	Low	High
Source	Molds (Natural)	Combustion
Common knowledge	little known	agent orange
Regulatory level in peanuts (FDA)	20 ppb	N/R
Level of concern in soil (CDC)	N/R	0.1ppb***

* Wu-Williams et al. (1992).

** this is calculated from the response at high doses. In this study (Kociba, 1978), the tumor rate goes DOWN at an intermediate dose. If taken seriously, this shows that dioxin is anti-carcinogenic at environmental doses.

*** quoted by Dr Kimbrough in public talks in the 1980s; also Kimbough et al. (1984).

N/D = No data N/R = Not Relevant

Early epidemiological studies (Peers and Linsell, 1973; Shank et al., 1972; Van Rensberg et al., 1974) showed that aflatoxin causes liver cancer in people But the data comes from regions of the world where hepatitis B is endemic. Hepatatis B is a major risk factor for liver cancer. When the synergistic effect is factored out, the potency of aflatoxin B1 in humans is lower than previously believed. Aflatoxin is more potent in animals than in people (Butler and Barnes, 1968; Butler, Greenblatt and Lijinsky, 1969; Wogan, Papliolunga and Newbreme, 1974) but the potencies are consistent with the "ordinary" interspecies comparison discussed in Chapter 2. The ratios between the animal and human potencies is at the top end of the range expected if experimental mice and rats (chosen to be sensitive to liver carcinogens) are considered more equivalent to humans with hepatitis B than to humans without hepatitis B.

Nonetheless, aflatoxin is a mutagen *in vitro* and dioxin is not. Dioxin may be a promoter and pose a minuscule risk at low doses, whereas aflatoxin is almost certainly also an initiator. When it was thought that mutagens are likely to show a linear dose response at low doses, and non-mutagens might show a threshold, this suggested that dioxin at low doses should be taken *less* seriously than aflatoxin. But as noted in Chapters 2 and 3, low dose linearity can be a result of other reasons.

The contrast between the behavior of regulatory agencies to these two chemicals cannot be explained solely by a comparison of the risk numbers. We suggest that public perceptions of risk have affected the way they are treated. Aflatoxin is a constituent of molds that naturally grow on nut and corn products. Dioxin is mostly produced by human activities, and was a trace component of a chemical mixture, agent orange, that was used in warfare. We have never failed to stimulate thought by this table especially when we ask this question after discussion of the last three rows in the table: "Which one do you eat?"

Although naturally occurring, the growth of molds that grow on foods may be controlled and so the concentration of aflatoxin in foods may be controlled by society. Careful storage of grain, and elimination of peanuts with cracked shells serves to reduce concentrations. Nonetheless regulatory agencies have refused to regulate these naturally growing molds as rigorously as they regulate dioxin.

Comparing Risks for the Same Benefit (Cost Effectiveness)

Comparisons of risks for different activities that provide the same benefit are relatively easy to assimilate. An example is the comparisons of risks for electricity generation. An early very brief comparison was by Wilson (1972). A full volume was devoted to the risks of different energy sources in 1980. (SFEN, 1980). The most recent of these studies (ExternE) has been funded by the European Commission (European Commission, 1999). Clearly, a guiding principle of any comparative risk analysis process should be a consistent approach in terms of its scope and execution for each energy option. The system boundaries of the assessment, including the time-period examined, should be the same for all compared fuel sources. Differences may arise legitimately where it is apparent that a particular aspect of the fuel cycle is important for one option but is unimportant and can reasonably be neglected in another. However, it is essential that such distinctions and approximations be clearly stated and justified in any comparative study.

While striving for consistency is an important principle it must be acknowledged that the current state of knowledge on key aspects of comparative assessment is not identical for all fuel chains. A clear definition of the assessment, and explanations of the data utilized and of the assumptions, will enhance the utility of, and users' confidence in, the results. This can also help to ensure that the results will be used in an appropriate way. Some of the important features of the ExternE study have been summarized by Krewitt et al. (1998) and by Rabl and Spadaro (2000). ExternE expressed the results in monetary terms (see Chapter 6). In the first ExternE reports this was done by expressing the amount to pay to save a "calculated" or "statistical" life of $4,000,000 per life, but in the more recent work the amount is expressed in Euros per years of life lost (YOLL). Some ExternE results are reproduced in Table 4-5.

Although these calculations are the "state of the art," various authors (IAEA 1996, 1999; Wilson 1999) pointed out that the comparison is still critically dependent on assumptions. The risk estimate for coal is from air pollution at low levels (and whether such pollution causes a risk is still controversial) and from numerous small accidents and events which occur every day. The risk of nuclear power is primarily the small risk of a severe

TABLE   4 - 5
Typical Monetary Damage Costs in milliEuro per kWh of Electricity Generation, Numbers from ExternE (European Commission 1999)*

Type of Fuel	Coal	Oil	Gas	Nuclear	Hydro	Wind
Toxic pollutants	45	26	11	0	0	0
Greenhouse gases	27	18	12	0	0***	0
Radiation cancers (inc. accident)**	0	0	0	<2	0	0
Amenity & ecological	0	0	0	0	0–6	0–1

* At the time of the study the value of the dollar and the Euro were approximately equal (1 milliEuro ≈ ¹⁄₁₀ cent U.S.).

** The number for radiation cancers is almost all due to a hypothetical accident for which the probability is uncertain. The upper limit here is from A PRA for a European power plant in an unfavorable location. No aqccount is taken of especial aversion to rare accidents with large consequences.

*** But note a recent UN report that suggests that hydroelectric plants emit greenhouse gases.

Note: Numbers are rounded off to the nearest integer. Therefore the radiation cancers produced by emissions of natural radionuclides in burning coal, are small enough to be rounded to zero, as are cancers caused by storage of nuclear waste.

accident, with emission of radioactivity and subsequent cancer increase. The risks from the "renewable" technologies are smaller, and largely due to construction and maintenance of the facility, but since they are technologies diffuse in space and time the amenity costs can be appreciable and very site dependent.

Expression of Risks

Just as a comparison of risks is an aid to their understanding, so is a careful selection of the methods of expression. It is hard to comprehend the statistical (stochastic) nature of risk. There are ways to mitigate this difficulty in comprehension. We are almost all used to one such statistical concept—the expectation of life. When we talk about the expectation of life being 79 years (for a U.S. nonsmoking male—Figure 1-2) we all know that some die young, and that many live to be over 80. Thus the expression of a risk as the reduction of life expectancy caused by the risky action conveys some of the statistical concept essential to its understanding. One particular calculation of this type can be used as an anchor for many people, because it is easy to remember. The reduction of life expectancy by smoking cigarettes can be calculated from the risk, from cancer or heart disease, nearly one in a million, of smoking one cigarette, multiplied by the difference of the average life span of a nonsmoker and a smoking victim. This turns out to be 5 minutes, or the time it takes to smoke the one cigarette! But this comparison must not be overdone. Even though he/she may understand that regular cigarette smoking is very high on the list of risks, a cigarette smoker may still wish to reduce other, smaller risks. For him or her the "benefit" of smoking outweighs the risk.

It is important to realize that risks appear to be very different when expressed in different ways. One example of this can be seen if we consider the cancer risk to those persons exposed to radionuclides after the Chornobyl disaster. According to Russian estimates (reduced from the early 1986 estimates), the 24 thousand persons between 3 km and 15 km from the plant, but excluding the town of Pripyat, received and are expected to receive, 330 thousand person-rems total integrated dose, or about 14 rems average dose. Even if we assume a linear dose response relationship, with 3,000 person-rems per cancer, the risk may be expressed in different ways. Dividing 330,000 million manrems by 3,000 gives 110 cancers expected in the lifetimes of that population. This is larger than, and for some people more alarming than, the 31 people within the power plant itself who died of acute radiation sickness, combined with burns, within 60 days of the accident. Dividing the 110 again by the approximately 5,000 cancer deaths expected in this small group from other causes, the accident caused "only" a 2% increase in cancer. This seems small compared to the 30% of risk of cancer or heart disease caused by cigarette smoking. The difference is even more striking if we consider the 75 million people in Belarus and the Ukraine who received, and will receive, 28 million person-rems over their lifetimes. On the linear dose response relationship this leads to 9,000 "extra cancers"—surely a large number for one accident. But dividing by the 15,000,000 cancers expected in the whole Ukranian population leads to an increase of only 0.062 (6.2×10^{-4}) which might be considered insignificant in some contexts.

Of course, none of the methods of expressing the risk can be considered "right" in an absolute sense. Indeed, it is our belief that a full understanding of the risk involves expressing it in as many different ways as possible. We therefore urge that any responsible authority presenting a risk assessment to the public or to a decision maker do so in a variety of ways. Of course it is possible to misuse the whole process, by deliberately choosing a form of expression that either appears to make a risk appear large, or on the other side, to choose a form of expression that makes the same risk appear small. This happens very often, both by accident, and on occasion intentionally. In either case the remedy for some person or group who does not wish the public to be misled is simple. He can explain that there are several ways of expressing the same facts and he can then represent the same risk in a format more favorable to his own cause[2].

Public Misconceptions

General

It is important to attempt to discover, and to distinguish between, the various reasons for any difference in an expert and a lay perception of a risk. In some cases, for example, the difference may be a value judgement—a legitimate difference of opinion on what to do about a risk of a known quantitative value. But in others it may be due to a public misconception of the size of a risk. The first would be a legitimate issue to be brought to the attention of a decision maker. The second might be improved by improved education and understanding. Sometimes, moreover, a person may deliberately confuse the discussion and exaggerate a risk in order to attain another objective. An English physician, Anthony Daniels, writing about British misconceptions in the *Wall Street Journal*, shows that the problem is not restricted to the USA.

"Our, British, perception of the risks we face is grossly inaccurate, affected by dramatic scare stories, blown out of all proportion by the media, and by our daily experience of the incompetence of public services.

In fact, the British are half as likely to die in accidents, whether domestic, industrial, or during travel as they were in 1970. Half as many people die on our roads as died in 1925 when there were 1/20 the number of vehicles. Like other Western peoples we live longer than ever before. Our infant mortality rate is among the lowest ever experienced in human history. The idea that we live in hazardous times could not be more mistaken.

But our sense that things are falling apart is not based on the statistics that prove that we are the most fortunate people in our country's history. Statistics on our growth rate do not make up for the fact that it is impossible to ride the London Underground without finding escalators and elevators that don't work, unconscionable delays before a train arrives, entire routes closed down for repairs that never seem to affect anything..."

In the next paragraphs we discuss three situations where there have been clear misunderstandings about the numerical value of a risk. These are NOT value judgements although they may influence value judgements. These situations try the patience of scientists and risk assessors but without such patience improved communication is impossible.

Common Public Misconceptions

Cancer Clusters

Among the most important misconceptions that is common in the lay public is that many cancer clusters exist that are evidence of environmental pollution. These misconceptions occur in legal liability cases mentioned in Chapter 6. Of course cancer clusters exist, as do clusters of every kind of disease. They are certain to occur, simply because of randomness. Even unlikely ones will occur, with the expected low frequency. The common misconception is the mis-identification of a "cluster" as being non-random, the attribution of a real cluster to environmental pollution, or, most commonly, both. In what follows, we mean "non-random cluster" when we use the term "cluster." There are clusters of infectious disease, and occupational clusters of non-infectious disease, but very few purely environmental clusters of non-infectious diseases, such as cance rcaused by environmental agents (that is, something present in the environment, to which everyone is exposed). The problem has been discussed, for example, by Rothman (1990), Neutra (1990) and Gawande (1999). It has been said that the science of epidemiology started when Dr. Snow marked cases of cholera upon a map and found that they clustered around a particular (water) pump. Since then looking for clusters is clearly in the public mind. Clusters of *infectious* diseases are often found—such as the cluster of legionnaire's disease at a hotel in Philadelphia, and another cluster of the same disease in 2000 at a zoological park in Sydney, Australia. But not of cancer. Indeed, if cancer clusters existed in the environment they would be evidence for the infectious nature of cancer. One of the main reasons that we know that cancer is not usually an infectious disease is that clusters in the environment are not found.

To have a cancer cluster one needs to have a high exposure localized to the group containing the people who get the cancer. This can occur in occupational settings but is rare in the environment where exposures are more diffuse. The clusters that have been claimed to exist are usually due to chance or to some common lifestyle factor. Neutra (1990) suggested 8 characteristics that might enable one to distinguish real clusters from false ones (Neutra, remembering Cervantes' *Don Quixote*, calls the procedure distinguishing giants from windmills). The more of these characteristics a cluster shows, the more likely it would be that a multicommunity investigation would be fruitful.

1. There are at least 5 cases and the relative risk is very high (e.g. 20 or more).

2. The disease is one, like mesothelioma, for which an (almost) unique and detectable class of agents has been responsible in the past, or for which the pathophysiological mechanism is well understood.

3. The agent is persistent in the environment and can be measured there (there are relatively few such agents).

4. The agent is persistent in, or leaves a physiological response in, the bodies of those who have been exposed, and (the response) is rare in the normal population, so that it can be used as an index of exposure.

5. There is heterogeneity of exposure within the neighborhood so that the effect of exposure can be assessed.

6. The plausible route of exposure is such that subjects would be able to assess their own relevant exposure on a questionnaire or it could be reconstructed from records.

7. It would be feasible to carry out a multicommunity study consisting of several similarly exposed and some unexposed communities.

8. The cluster represents an as-yet-uninvestigated, endemic space-time cluster. This suggests a stable, persistent problem and perhaps a persistent agent to be found in the environment.

There are various examples of cancer clusters, although few can be explained by exposure to environmental agents; the others have not been explained. Outcroppings of erionite in a Turkish village of Karain led to a cluster of mesotheliomas in the village. The relative risk was over 1,000! The cluster had most of these characteristics. However, the erionite was used for many purposes, some domestic, which led to considerable exposure(Baris et al., 1978, 1987). A semi-occupational cluster of leukemias appeared near Sellafield in N.W. England among children of workers at the local nuclear processing plant. Yet the (measured) exposures of the parents were too small to attribute causation. The finding of a cluster of leukemias in Glenrothes new town with no nuclear facilities (Kinlen, 1988) led to the strong suggestion that the cause was that these leukemias are infectious.

In the above paragraphs the word "cluster" was used to describe a small group of people closely related by something—usually geography. This is distinct from a group of people with the same ailment in a larger region. In Taiwan, for example, those drinking from wells in a certain area developed skin cancer and various internal cancers (Chen et al. 1986). But the number of people "at risk" was large, perhaps 20,000, although the Risk Ratio was moderate in the first studies (about 3), the statistical accuracy was adequate and the attribution of the risk was generally accepted and subsequently confirmed.

Environmentally Caused Does Not Mean Caused by Industry

The development of cancer registries throughout the world, and achievement of consistency in the definitions of disease, enabled rates to be compared across countries. When that was done, variations in cancer rates could be attributed to differences in lifestyle including diet. This led the WHO in 1964, and many distinguished scientists before and since, to consider that "90% of cancers are environmentally caused" (Higginson and Muir, 1976). This has been misinterpreted as a statement that "90% of all cancers are caused by environmental pollution." But epidemiologists use the word "environment" in its broadest sense—including substances and agents naturally present in foods, sunlight, cigarette smoking, alcoholic beverages, and chemicals or radiations to which people are exposed in the course of their occupation or their daily lives (Eisenbud, 1978). As is shown in Chapter 7 (Figure 7-5) the trend of most age specific (or age adjusted) cancer rates is flat or declining. The main exception, a marked 10-fold increase in lung cancer from 1930 to 1970 and still increasing, is usually attributed to cigarette smoking. But there is little or no increase in cancers known to be caused by chemical pollution. In a major "gaffe," the U.S. Secretary of Labor stated that between 15 and 40% of all cancers were occupationally related (Califano, 1978). This was based upon a report, never published and usually discreetly forgotten, (but alas never formally repudiated) with appallingly bad arithmetic. The authoritative report by Doll and Peto (1981) attributes only 4% of cancers to occupational causes, based on past cases; in the intervening years since the dates that the environmental exposures occurred, the combined actions by employers, regulators and unions have probably reduced this proportion by a factor of two. Their estimates of cancer causes are presented here as Table 4-6 compared with those of Higginson and Muir (1976) and Wynder and Gori (1977). Nonetheless the Califano report was

TABLE 4-6

Proportion (%) of Cancer Deaths Attributed to Various Different Factors

	Doll & Peto, 1981		Higginson & Muir, 1976		Wynder & Gori, 1977	
	Best	Range	Male	Female	Male	Female
Tobacco	30	25–40	30	7	28	8
Alcohol	3	2–4	5	3	4	1
Diet	35	10–70	—	—	40	57
Food additives	<1	−5 - +2	—	—	—	—
Life style	—	—	30	63	—	—
Reproductive and sexual behavior	7	1–13	—	—	—	—
Occupation*	4	2–8	6	2	4	2
Pollution	2	<1–5	—	—	—	—
Industrial Products	<1	<1–2	—	—	—	—
Medicine & medical procedures	1	0.5–3	1	1	—	—
Geophysical factors**	3	2–4	11	11	8	8
Infection	10	1	—	—	—	—
Congenital	—	—	2	2	—	—
Unknown	?	?	15	11	16	20

* These figures are based on pre 1960 data and diminishing. The figure of Califano (1978) was over 50%.

** Includes sunlight and ionizing radiation. Only a few percent could be called "avoidable."

used by politicians 2 years after it was scientifically discredited, and claims continue to be made that industrial pollution is the cause of a large fraction of cancers. For example in an influential book about the decline of the USSR, Feshbach and Friendly (1992) attributes the declining life expectancy to chemical pollution—a claim that cannot be substantiated by any calculation of the product of concentrations (and therefore doses) and the potencies. Cancer rates have not increased and an examination of the age distribution of the death rate in Russia suggests that the major problems are increases in deaths from avoidable behavior (drinking, workplace accidents, suicides) and declining medical care (Leon et al., 1997).

Radiation Hazards Are Often Grossly Overstated

Whereas radiation (from radium sources for example) was thought 100 years ago to be medically beneficial, and people attended (and many still attend) spas (such as radium hot springs), radiation is now widely regarded as an anathema; and there are widespread misstatements. The Minister of Health of Ukraine reported in 1999 that 300,000 people are ill with "radiation sickness" from Chornobyl—yet the doses to the general public were all insufficient to cause acute radiation sickness. People in Utah, when members of their families died of cancer within a few years of the Atomic Bomb tests, steadfastly insisted that the tests were the cause of the cancers in spite of the well established long latency for cancers. The misconceptions of radiation hazards persist in spite of the fact that radiation doses are often the easiest of environmental exposures to determine, and the consequences are probably the best understood of all exposures. Pessimistically assuming the linear no-threshold (LNT) dose response leads various experts to suggest that 20,000 people worldwide *may* develop cancer from Chornobyl. Yet hundreds of thousands of Russians, Ukrainians and Byelorussians still claim that they have ailments that are caused by radiation from Chornobyl. The records of the 600,000 clean up workers (liquidators) many of whom got moderately high doses, show death rates that are less than people of comparable ages in Russia. This is the "healthy worker" effect that is well known in all studies within an occupation. There is no question that there are many illnesses in Russia, the Ukraine, and Byelorussia; and illnesses are probably occurring at higher rates. A few such illnesses may be due to Chornobyl. However, general societal disruption (which certainly occurred as the Soviet Union collapsed) is a much more likely the root cause of the great majority of the increased rate of illness (Leon et al., 1997).

In the U.S. there have been repeated reports by a small number of persons who claim large effects of radiation on people. Such claims have been repeatedly repudiated, for example, by Shihab-Eldin et al. (1992). These claims of large effects have been mostly concerned with nuclear bombs or nuclear power. Nuclear power is widely regarded as a potentially hazardous technology, so it is rigorously regulated. Curiously, there is an enormous difference between risk estimates by the professional experts and by many lay persons or experts in different fields (Wilson 1999, IAEA 1999, Nelkin 1974). In particular, both accident probabilities and accident consequences are often estimated 1000-fold higher than by professionals. Cohen (1989) reports that there are many more incorrect reports in the media on effects of radiation than correct ones. Whether such "biased" reporting is the major influence on public opinion (as Cohen suggests), or vice versa, is an open question. A perception that nuclear power production might be a contributor to the risk of nuclear war might be a principal cause of the adverse reactions to nuclear electric power. This involves all three of the effects of anchoring, availability and dread.

Do people really believe these statements that differ so widely from the estimates of the experts? If so, can their belief be changed by discussion and education (as is the general view of nuclear and radiation experts)? Or is the belief so deeply held that no argument can dissuade them? If so, is there some way to ensure that major societal decisions are not affected? Can technologists make changes in the technology to render moot the complaints of irate citizens (Shlyakhter, Stadie and Wilson, 1995)? Do some influential persons state these beliefs without holding them (as some cynics suggest) to achieve another desired end or to gain popularity and votes?[2] Do people deliberately state exaggerated risk estimates in an attempt to more strongly influence the decision maker? We do not pretend to answer these questions; our view is that society is best served by the most objective quantitative assessment possible, honestly presented with all its caveats.

Recipe for Communication

In this chapter we have examined some aspects of risk perception and summarized aspects of some risks we have examined. The examples are all taken from our experience in the U.S. Some may not apply in other circumstances, for example, in another country, but we hope that we have conveyed enough of the ideas that the reader may apply them to other situations. In the last 20 years there has developed a subfield on "risk communication," or how to communicate risks. However many authors in this field have addressed a somewhat different question: how to communicate acceptability. Often the two are barely compatible. The operator of a coal-fired power plant may well gain acceptability by showing that (with his scrubbers) the emissions are half what they were last year. But the risk may still be much larger for the existing facility than a different facility—gas fired or nuclear powered—replacing coal powered, as suggested in Table 4-5.

We recommend a careful comparison of risks to increase understanding of them. We have found that this has been helpful to many people ranging from students to juries in toxic tort cases. But such comparisons, even with improved understanding, may not improve acceptability of particular situations, as a simple historical example shows. An EPA official went to the Stringfellow dump site around 1990, and explained that the risk of living near the site was comparable to smoking one pack of cigarettes in a lifetime or eating several peanut butter sandwiches. He was physically attacked and commented that the attempt at risk communication had failed. But we believe that an alternative explanation is more likely. His communication probably succeeded but was unwelcome. It was unwelcome because if indeed the risks are small, the residents would have a hard time having the dump site removed or obtaining monetary compensation. This view is bolstered by the unpopularity of risk comparisons among lawyers trying to obtain damage awards for toxic chemical exposure believed by experts to be inconsequential, and the popularity of such comparisons among lawyers defending such cases. The former try to prevent explicit risk comparisons being made as irrelevant (and often succeed in so doing), while the latter find from experience that they are an effective way of communicating to a jury.

We propose a few general recommendations for risk communication. The first is to know the risk that you are talking about, in all its aspects. All too often risk communication is left to persons who do not themselves fully understand the risk and have never gone through the intellectual process of calculating risk estimates. It is all too easy to communicate the wrong message through failure to grasp some aspect of the problem. This is well illustrated by an EPA document (EPA 1992b) on "seven cardinal rules of risk communication," which leaves out our first rule: "understand the risk." Secondly, know your audience: what do they want to know? what are their preconceptions? are they really interested in your message or are they trying to tell *you* something? If the last, it is much better if you can listen rather than talk. The third is never to talk down to the audience. Everyone is capable of understanding risk to some extent. If the audience gets the feeling that you are talking down to them, they will also tend to feel that you are hiding something. The fourth is to try to explain, in so far as you can, why you are estimating risks. If the audience feels that you are trying to belittle their concerns, or are "putting profits ahead of people," the details of the message are likely to be ignored. A fifth is to be clear what you know, what you do not know and the uncertainties in your risk assessment. Your listener must not get the feeling that you are hiding something important. A sixth is to be clear that you as a risk assessor are *not* making a recommendation for action, but are only giving the facts so that the reader or audience may decide for themselves. The sixth particularly applies, of course, to giving expert testimony in a courtroom. It is the jury who must decide: not the expert witness. Most of these recommendations also apply when briefing a decision maker.

Fischoff's (1995) view of the issues is shown in Table 4-7 and many of these issues are discussed in Hammitt (2000).

T A B L E   4 - 7

Developmental Stages in Risk Management (Ontogeny Recapitulates Phylogeny)

- All we have to do is get the numbers right
- All we have to do is tell them the numbers
- All we have to do is explain what we mean by the numbers
- All we have to do is show them that they've accepted similar risks in the past
- All we have to do is show them that it's a good deal for them
- All we have to do is treat them nice
- All we have to do is make them partners
- All of the above

Source: Fischhoff (1995)

Notes

1 Anybody is entitled to act inconsistently, irrationally, illogically, unreasonably, and contrary to their own interest at any time. There is no law to prevent them doing so. Nobody has to justify their opinions or actions, providing they are legal.

2 One of us knows personally three persons who have each been part of a group opposing an overhead power line near their residences. To achieve their ends the group made a claim that the power lines would increase cancer. None of the three believed this, but two went along with the group to achieve the desired end of blocking the power line. The third, to his credit, left the group.

5

Formal Comparison of Risk and Benefit

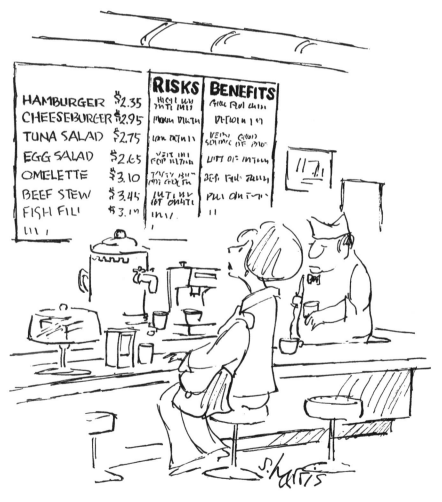

© 2001 The New Yorker Collection from cartoonbank.com. All Rights Reserved.

There are many reasons for evaluating risks. These include academic interest, analyzing risks in order to find ways of reducing them, and providing inputs into decision processes about taking various actions. This last reason is the concern of this chapter. The question to be answered is: are the risks of the action big enough to outweigh any of its benefits? The answer may then be used as one (but of course only one) input to a decision process.

In many cases the comparison is easy, and the subsequent decision a foregone conclusion. The risk may be so large that once it is perceived, something is done about it almost independent of other concerns, like cost (e.g. evacuation of the populace around spilled toxic chemicals). In other cases the risk may be obviously so small that it is not worth the trouble to think about it (e.g. occupational risk to a waitress sweeping up spilled saccharin powder).

Such cases are barely worth calling to attention since there is no controversy. Still other risks may in fact belong to one or other of these two categories but are not perceived to be so either because the calculation has not been done, or because the risk is complex enough or badly enough perceived that it is not understood when such calculations are done (occasional hair dye use is not very dangerous; the smoking habit is). Most of the use made of risk analysis so far lies in taking risks in a third category (unknown) and putting them into the first (large) or second category (negligible). For this purpose a great deal of precision in calculation is not necessary; in the first (large) case it is obvious that the risk exceeds the benefit and in the second (negligible) case it is obvious that the benefit exceeds the risk. For these cases little more need to be written. What follows is a discussion of a procedure for assessing risks and aiding decisions in more marginal cases.

A primary problem in setting up a formal structure is the time lapse between action and risk, cost, or benefit. The risks of any action may not all accrue at one time. Accidents may occur at the time of the action, but cancer and disease caused by air pollution, among others, can occur many years later. Moreover, there are even later effects of environmental pollution. Toxic chemical wastes or radioactive substances can enter the biosphere hundreds of years or more after the actions causing them. The risk, therefore, of mortality (for example) is not a simple quantity but is a function of time, $R(t)$ say, and similarly other measures of risk will vary with time. Benefits do not all occur at once either. The risks of coal mining start when the coal is mined; but the benefits come later, when it is burned. There is a stream of benefits, $B(t)$, and of costs $C(t)$. These risks and benefits are usually incommensurate quantities, although of course monetary costs and benefits are both measured in monetary units (dollars). For decision making it is usual to try to put them on a common basis by, for example, estimating society's willingness to pay to reduce a risk, or to forgo a benefit. In order to do this, we may introduce factors $\alpha(B,t)$, $\beta(C,t)$ and $\gamma(R,t)$, discussed more fully below, which, at some time, t, reduce respectively benefits, costs, and risks to a common scale, so that, on this scale, the part of net worth of the action attributable to time t is:

$$\text{Net worth} = W(t) = \alpha(B,t)B(t) - \beta(C,t)\,C(t) - \gamma(R,t)R(t) \qquad (5\text{-}1)$$

(We consider benefits to be positive and subtract costs and risks.) There is now the problem of adding such valuations at different times, t, in order to obtain the total effect, so we introduce a time factor $D(t)$ which discounts the value at time t to time zero (at the moment the decision is made) and hence obtain a net present value (NPV) of

$$\text{NPV} = \int_{t=0}^{t=T} D(t)\, W(t)dt \qquad (5\text{-}2)$$

where the integral is taken from $t = 0$ to $t = T$, the time horizon for the analysis, the distance into the future which will be taken into account in making any decision. In making business decisions using similar methodology, T is usually small (1 to 10 years) but for a full risk-cost-benefit analysis T may be very large. The usual choice for a discounting function $D(t)$ is the standard economist's choice:

$$D(t) = \frac{1}{(1 + r)^t} \qquad (5\text{-}3)$$

where r is a discount rate. This has the merit of simplicity and of consistency; if the ratio of income and benefit streams were the same at future times, one would still make the same decision at any arbitrary future time, and the decision will still appear correct at any time after making it, provided the results are evaluated using the same discount rate. The simple prescription for decisions is that the action should proceed if NPV is positive, and should not proceed if NPV is negative.

Distributional Inequity

But the above discussion is overly simplified for a real decision. The costs, risks and benefits do not necessarily accrue to the same individuals or populations. There can arise what is called a *distributional inequity*. For example the benefits derived from electricity production are shared among a population extending many miles from a coal-fired power station, but the amenity costs (loss of visual amenity, excess traffic for fuel transport, higher pollution, etc.) are largely borne by a local group living close to the station.

Distributional inequity is extremely common. To avoid it society has developed compensation mechanisms. Society might compensate the population around a power station through reduced property taxes (since the power station usually pays substantial property taxes which subsidize the local neighborhood) but often there remains inequity in distribution of the benefits, costs and risks. Distributional inequity may arise from any decision process—it is not unique to risk-cost-benefit analysis—and exists because of the imperfections of these compensation mechanisms. If the choices discussed above are correctly made, the net present value obtained will be correct for the whole population (and will take into account individuals at high risk, for example), and the formalism may be used to find values of the NPV for subpopulations. Thus for each risk, cost, benefit of type i and individual j to be included, we should evaluate the NPV as follows:

Note here the integral sign has the same limits as the limits as the sign for equation 5-2; t = 0 lower limit; t = T upper limit

$$\text{NPV} = \int_{t=0}^{t=T} \Sigma_{ij} \, D_j(t) \, \{\alpha_j(B_{ij},t)B_{ij}(t) - \beta_j(C_{ij},t)\,C_{ij}(t) - \gamma_j(R_{ij},t)R_{ij}(t)\}dt \quad (5\text{-}4)$$

By restricting the summations over the population (index j) we could obtain the NPV for subpopulations. Theoretically, but not practically, this would allow the design of compensating mechanisms (such as taxes and subsidies) which could ensure that every individual had a net benefit (all NPV are positive, assuming that the whole sum is positive). In practice, this is the field of political compromises—adjusting the actions so that some groups benefit, while others might suffer a loss that is not too large. With proper choice of α, β and γ, the effect of placing large burdens of cost or risk on individuals or small groups should already be accounted for in the NPV sum,—for example, if the NPV is expressed in monetary terms, γ will be the value obtained when offering money in exchange for taking a risk, and will thus probably increase rapidly for large values of risk.

Deriving Suitable Value Functions

There are many practical problems with the formal approach outlined. An obvious one is the difficulty of deriving factors α, β and γ, which reduce benefits, costs and risks to common units, and the discount function $D(t)$ with the discount rate r. Much criticism of risk-benefit analysis can be traced to discussions about the validity of using such numbers (Baram, 1976), and even where the basic validity is not questioned the actual value to use is questioned. Another problem is that of deciding upon the boundary of the analysis; for example, is the Net Present Value to be calculated for an individual (in which case, which individual?), for a group (in which case, which group?), or for society as a whole?

Consider the value of γ; or, to reduce it to (oversimplified) basics: "How much should one pay to avert a (premature) death?"

"We are not prepared to go to limitless expense to save lives that could be saved on the basis of the technical knowledge we possess." —Editorial, *The Observer* (London), 14 January, 1968

"Anyone who tries to deal with health in economic terms, which is a necessary part of a system-analytic point of view, is exposing himself to the risk of misunderstanding and even of bodily harm from outraged citizens." —Nobel Laureate Joshua Lederberg

The coefficient $\gamma(R)$ for the equivalent of a monetary cost of a risk R inevitably raises arguments and indeed arouses passion. It is an approximation to the economists' idealized utility function. We are attempting to obtain a measure of the utility of a risk (measured by some risk measure with value R) by assigning a numerical value (γ) per unit of risk, and usually expressed in monetary terms.

The following points are often misunderstood about this approach. The coefficient need not be a constant, independent of the size, or nature, of the risk, and everyone recognizes limitations on its use. The last may be illustrated by an interchange that one of us had with an attorney in a court room.

Q: I understand that you put a value on human life.

A: No, I decline to do so. I recognize that a human life is priceless. Most religions accept this, and heroism awards, such as the Carnegie award, are given to someone who acts without regard to the risk to his own life.

Q: What, then, is this number you use, with units of dollars per life?

A: Ideally it could be how much society *should* pay to avert a death or save a life. But it is not for me to say that either.

Q: What is it then?

A: One objective measure one can use for the quantity is the amount society *has paid* in the past to save a life. This assumes that society wants to spend the same in the future—unless society has clearly expressed a reason for spending more or less. This is sometimes called society's "willingness to pay." Economists have tended to use the phrase "Value of a Statistical Life" (VSL), which we prefer not to use.

γ will not necessarily be a constant. If we are looking at a risk, R, to an individual, the value of γ may increase or decrease as R increases, depending on the circumstances, so we have to write $\gamma(R)$; γ may be a function of the risk. Such behavior is perfectly consistent, may be theoretically derived from certain utility models and models of perception discussed in Chapter 4, and is easy to understand heuristically. We illustrate two different types of behavior. In the first we consider an individual faced with a risk of death of negligibly small value, say one in a million (10^{-6}) probability of dying. That person would probably be prepared to pay a (very) small amount in order to avoid such a risk. Similarly, for a larger, but still small risk, say 10^{-4} probability of dying, he or she might still pay a proportionally larger amount, possibly 100 times as much, in exchange for avoidance. But if the risk presented gets

---

FIGURE 5-1

Amount Paid per Unit of Risk (γ) to Avoid a Risk

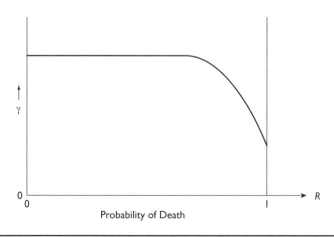

---

large enough, the limit of the ability of the individual to pay may be reached, so that the amount per unit of risk (γ) must thereafter decrease (Figure 5-1). An individual who makes decisions on this basis is displaying risk-prone behavior. An example of a different behavior occurs if an individual is invited to take a certain risk in exchange for money. For small enough risks the amount of money required in exchange for taking the risk may be proportional to the size of the risk, but for large enough risks (approaching certainty of death) it is plausible that no amount of money would provide sufficient inducement (Figure 5-2). This leads to a value of γ that increases as R increases. An individual who makes decisions on such a basis is displaying risk-averse behavior.

These examples indicate two different behaviors for γ that could be exhibited by the same individual, depending on the circumstances. It is quite possible, therefore, for γ to take on different values depending upon the way in which the risk occurs. In addition to those variations with the size and nature of the risk, the risk may also depend on time, t, so we write $\gamma = \gamma(R,t)$. If we are measuring the actual cost of repairing the damage caused when the risk is realized (if this is possible and if these actual costs are independent of

FIGURE 5 - 2

Amount Required per Unit of Risk (γ) to Take a Risk

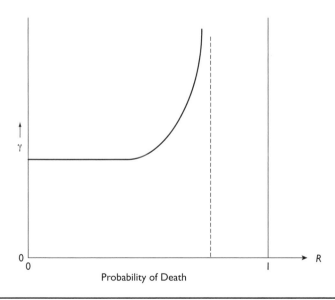

time—we are speaking of the economist's "real " costs here), then γ may be taken independent of time, since in such circumstances the discount rate fully takes account of the costs (see below). However, if it is necessary to use an individual's valuation of their life (for example), this may not be true, for such a valuation may vary with time. The simplest such case is if the valuation varies at the same rate as the (real) interest (discount) rate—e.g. a valuation which regards a life as being worth a fixed fraction of the total economic activity rather than the fixed amount of economic activity implied by the real cost case above. Here the applied discount rate in our NPV equation and the increasing value of exactly cancel, so that the present valuation of a life is identical for lives at any time in the future—or alternatively, that in the future greater absolute value is assigned to a life.

There is a lot of economic literature on the appropriate value of g to take in these calculations (Weisbrod, 1961; Starr, 1969; Rappaport, 1974; Thaler and Rosen, 1975; Zeckhauser, 1975; Zeckhauser and Shepard, 1976; Viscusi, 1992; Murray and Lopez, 1996; Rabl, 1996; EPA, 2000b). These are mostly based upon studies of the labor market and willingness to accept risk in exchange for additional money.

In one extensive set of risk analyses for energy systems (European Commission, 1999) a value of $4,000,000 per life has been used. U.S. EPA has recently used $6,100,000 for economic analyses (EPA, 2000b). However, the use of a single value must be treated with EXTREME caution. An interesting and instructive way of comparing risks is by comparing the amount people have paid in the past to reduce them. It might be thought that people would try to adjust their activities until the amount spent is roughly the same. Cohen (1980) has shown that the amounts spent vary by a factor of more than a million. Some of his figures will be presented in Table 7-6 (see also Table 7-8, by Tengs et al., 1995). For example, Cohen shows that it would be possible, even for an American, to save lives in Indonesia by aiding in immunization at $200 per life saved (1975 figures doubled to match a 2000 economy). People are willing to spend more on environmental protection to prevent cancer (over $2,000,000 per life) than they are willing to spend direct medical intervention (from less than $100,000 per life with the high value of $400,000 for kidney dialysis). This ratio is in rough accord with the maxim "an ounce of protection is better than a pound of cure." People willingly to spend $50 million per life for reducing the dangerous professions of mining—especially coal mining. They are willing to spend still more upon radiation protection at nuclear power plants and upon waste disposal (over a billion dollars per life saved undiscounted). We think it likely that people are aware in a general way of these differences, and of the general reasons for them. Economists and others often argue that efficiency depends upon society adjusting until the amounts spent to save lives in different situations are equalized. It seems that society does not work that way. We hear very little by way of calls by well-known activists for increased aid for medical help to Indonesia. We hear continued, and much more vocal, calls for increased efforts on reducing risks of toxic waste disposal and for radiation protection. Nevertheless, we believe that increased consistency is possible and would be desirable, particularly within similar groups of activities. We suggest that this information always be provided to a decision maker so that he can make an informed decision.

Similar calculations on the amounts paid to save lives have been performed by Schwing (1979), and a more recent study by Tengs et al. (1995) confirms the wide variation in costs to reduce a risk. Because of the wide variation, many early comparisons of health risk in energy systems (Bozzo et al., 1979; Hamilton et al., 1980) deliberately stopped short of making a monetary comparison.

Choice of Discounting Rates

The choice of the appropriate discount rate is controversial, especially for intergenerational costs. In a classic paper, Raiffa, Weinstein and Zeckhauser (1977) argued that lives should be discounted at the same rate as money. If the discounted cost of the future risk is invested at the ordinary market rate, then the return will be enough to yield the full cost at the time the risk is actually incurred. Cropper and Portney (1992) agree. Of course, the rate must be inflation corrected because this procedure implicitly assumes that the dollar value to be assigned to a risk is the same in the future as it is today. Explicitly it is the difference between the rate at which future costs will evolve and the uncorrected discount rate that matters. This difference ("effective discount rate") is likely to be positive but small. It is equivalent to saying, for example, that the discounted amount we are willing to pay now to save a life in the future decreases as the time of that life-saving gets more remote. This is reasonable if the amount discounted is an accurate reflection of the cost of saving that life, since economic use of the discounted amount from now until the future data will yield a return sufficient to bear the cost of saving the life. Indeed, few people worry (in the sense of taking action) about their great-grandchildren (50 years hence), which corresponds to discounting their lives at a rate greater than ~5%. If the amount used is an estimate of the value of a life (determined subjectively, for example), this argument may break down, but this can be taken care of in our formalism, as we show below.

The problems arise because the intergenerational risks of most public concern, for example, disposal of long lived nuclear waste and emission of CO_2 with its potential for global warming, become negligible unless the discount rate is very close to zero (no discounting) (Shlyakhter, Valverde and Wilson, 1996). The present furor over these particular issues suggests a trend toward low or even zero discount rates for some future risks. It has been suggested that no subsequent generation be exposed to a risk greater than that to which we are willing to expose ourselves. While this might be interpreted as a call for zero discount rate [$D(t)=1$], it is unclear whether this is a permanent public opinion, or a temporary fad. It is also unclear how to apply this concept to such issues as intergenerational resource allocation (Cairns and Dickson, 1995).

Some analysts have disagreed with the above conventional approach to intergenerational costs. They distinguish two main components of the discount rate: economic growth, and pure time preference (i.e. the premium people pay to be able to consume now rather than in the future). If one chooses as a criterion for evaluating risks the preference of future generations, the appropriate discount rate for intergenerational effects is significantly lower than the conventional social discount rate, because it should include only the growth of the economy. The pure time preference component of the discount rate involves only redistribution within the current generation and does not create wealth to compensate future generations, as shown by Rabl (1996). The key question is an ethical one: should the generation that makes a decision compensate future generations for all the damages imposed on them? To see why such compensation is not possible with the conventional discount rate, imagine that a special fund is set up to cover all future damages and reinvested permanently at the conventional discount rate; that is in fact the implicit assumption of a cost-benefit analysis. Assuming rates to remain constant, the money will indeed be there to pay for all damages. However, most of this money will have been paid by intervening generations (thanks to their time preference) and only the income generated by the growth component of the discount rate can be considered a contribution by the initial generation.

The uncertainties and controversies about intergenerational discounting are one of the reasons why it is advisable to keep long term impacts in a category apart, thereby allowing decision makers to see the consequence of applying different discount rates. A good analyst will therefore use a range of discount rates in the analysis to illuminate this factor in the decision process. For example, to get a simple upper bound of costs and to facilitate the conversion to impacts the "effective discount rate" can be set equal to 0.

Approximations and Simplified Schemes

Although the basic NPV equation may be useful for understanding details of the analysis, it is not usually useful for its presentation. Large approximations are usually made in the estimation of the benefits, the risks, and the costs. Large approximations may also be made in estimating the coefficients α, β and γ, without altering the outcomes. For example, if the cost and/or risk terms are included without discounting (or equivalently by making the terms β and γ increase with time at the discount rate), and the NPV is still positive, it is clear that the benefits outweigh risks and costs. If all the risks are small (i.e. the risk to all individuals is small enough), a constant value of γ is likely adequate (i.e. independent of the size of the risk). This is probably true for all probabilities of death below about 10^{-6} to 10^{-7} per year, as may be judged by consulting the tables of actual risks affecting individuals in the U.S. shown in Chapter 7.

If it is required to evaluate which is the better of two options providing similar benefits, rather than making decisions about a single scheme, some simplifications may be made. The simplest case is that in which both benefits and costs are identical, but the risks differ, in which case all that is required is the evaluation of the difference in (discounted) risks. In these cases, since all that is being evaluated are the effects of risks, the absolute values of the coefficients γ_j (see equation 5-4) does not affect the sign of the comparison, but only the relative value. Thus in this case only the relative value of different risk measures are required, but problems of discounting of the risks and distributional inequity remain—as represented by sums over possibly different risk types (subscript $_i$ in equation 5-4), possibly different populations (subscript $_j$ in equation 5-4) and the discount factor $D(t)$. Although even this simplified comparison looks a formidable task, practical cases suggest that it is possible to manage with fairly simple approximations. For example, in examining the option of using X-rays for screening whole populations or subgroups of populations for potentially fatal diseases, almost the only risk of concern is that of death—or disability—either from the disease or from a cancer induced by the X-rays. The benefit is the possibly early detection and cure of the disease (there may be side benefits, like the potential discovery of other conditions). Since benefit and risks are both in the same units (probabilities of dying or disability) there is no problem of assigning dollars to lives. To extend the analysis would require the introduction of the cost of the screening (assuming one finds that the risks are decreased by such screening). Even though an absolute evaluation of the value of such a screening program then requires a valuation of the risks, this problem may be avoided if only comparisons between different screening options are required, for then the cost effectiveness may be a suitable comparison measure. This situation is exactly that involved in the decision on whether or not to undergo X-ray exposure (a mammogram) to screen for possible breast cancer. Here the time situation enters. If radiation is given at a young age, and leads to a cancer, there is a greater loss of years of life than if the radiation and the cancer arrive later in life. On the other hand the average benefit of early detection increases markedly with age since it is weighted by an increased probability of a cancer. An analysis suggests that the largest net benefits accrue if regular screening mammograms are undertaken by a woman over about 45 years old[1].

In the ultimate analysis in which the aim is to maximize subjective utility, rather than an objective cost measure, the values of α, β and γ, depend upon individual perception of risk. They differ for different individuals and for different types of risk (as we suggest above by use of subscripts), although in many analyses representative values are sufficient for public policy purposes.

Often a decision maker will be able to use a scheme that is simplified from the full cost-benefit analysis. Thus if a decision can be made by a direct comparison of risks (Risk-Risk analysis), then one can avoid the discussion of the "value of a life." This was discussed in Chapter 4 and will be discussed again as one of the decision frameworks of Chapter 6.

Notes

1 Objective measures of gamma (γ) may be obtained from various measurements of what society does or individuals do; but they may miss people's desires and intent, or otherwise mis-measure true utility. It is quite plausible, and in some circumstances likely, that people are happier (higher utility) even though worse off by the objective measures discussed here (higher risks for the same cost, or higher costs for the same risk).

6

Risk Management: Managing and Reducing Risks

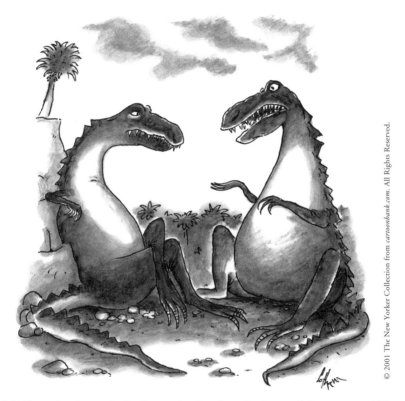

"All I'm saying is <u>now</u> is the time to develop the technology to deflect an asteroid."

© 2001 The New Yorker Collection from *cartoonbank.com*. All Rights Reserved.

"The consideration of [the] risk-benefit ratio is basic to any intelligent discussion of any problem involving technology and society, and is all too often ignored in the utterances of consumer advocates and industry spokesmen."

—Jean Meyer 1976. In the forward to Eaters Digest *by M.F. Jacobson, New York, Doubleday (Anchor Books).*

We Calculate Risks in Order to Reduce Them

As previously noted, one of the many reasons for evaluating risks is to find ways of reducing them, and to provide an input into decision processes about taking various actions. We have already mentioned in Chapter 1 that some risks are "obviously" too large to be acceptable, and others are too small to be worth discussing. As we said in Chapter 5 (page 136), large enough perceived risks are immediately dealt with, and small enough ones are ignored. For the middle ground, one can apply the cost-benefit procedures of Chapter 5 in more or less detail; but then one has to do something (or refrain from doing anything) — that is, make a decision on action.

It is important to realize that most decisions about risks are made every day by millions of ordinary individuals. We are the decision makers! In this book we argue that the method of managing risks by professional risk managers should not differ too much from the methods used by ordinary people in their decisions, lest the decision be harder to explain and be less acceptable. Therefore it is important to have a procedure, and a terminology, that are consistent with these "ordinary" methods.

As we also previously said in Chapter 5, some risks may in fact belong to one or the other of the two easy categories (obviously large or obviously small) but are not perceived to be so either because the calculation has not been done, or because the risk is complex enough or badly enough perceived that it is not understood when the calculations are done (occasional hair dye use is not very dangerous; the smoking habit is dangerous, yet these risks are not always perceived in this order).

Schemes for Analyzing Risk Management Options

There are a number of schemes for analyzing management options that discuss how risk management follows from risk assessment. Most of them stress that risk management (what society does about the risks) should be distinct from risk assessment (assigning a numerical value, with its attendant uncertainty, to the risk). In the first edition of this book we espoused the general scheme of Figure 6-1 that includes this distinction. The manager should not directly influence the assessment based upon his prejudices on how the risk is to be managed. The risk should first be assessed without regard for how it is managed, and then a decision made on how to manage it. The assessment and the management decision are different functions, although they may sometimes be performed by the same person.[1] We also made a more important distinction between data collection and risk assessment. The assessment inevitably adds to the data various assumptions to interpret the data and sometimes even to fill in gaps in the data. Another important feature of this scheme is its explicit recognition of the multiple pressures that are placed upon the decision maker, and the fact that the decision maker has multiple objectives. Although, for example, the Administrator of EPA has a duty to protect the environment and public health, he will also have a very strong incentive to "look good" in the eyes of the public and the President who appointed him, and to live within his budget. Decision analysts distinguish between good decisions and good outcomes. A single unpopular decision might cost the decision maker his job and reputation. Steady environmental improvement, particularly if only the indirect results of his decisions, might be ignored. Any subordinate bringing a risk analysis to a decision maker's attention must be aware of these constraints. A legislature intent on providing effective laws will frame the laws in such a way

FIGURE 6-1

Idealized Scheme for Risk Analysis, from Crouch and Wilson (1982)

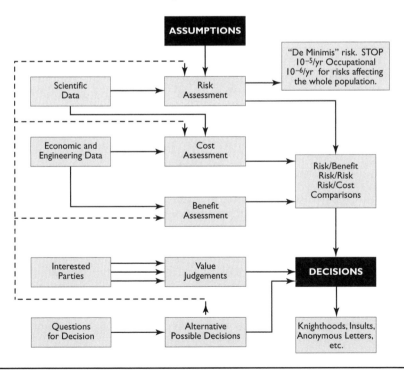

that the personal incentives to the decision maker coincide as far as possible with the needs and desires of society.

A committee of the National Academy of Sciences (chaired by Dr. Stallones) (NAS, 1982) proposed the scheme shown in Figure 6-2 (the committee report, with a red cover, is often called the "Red Book"). The two schemes of Figures 6-1 and 6-2 agree in separating the functions of risk assessment and risk management, which were becoming somewhat blurred during the 1970s. The NAS scheme is espoused by the regulatory authorities, in particular the U.S. Environmental Protection Agency, and was probably a codification of the best practice of the time. The NAS scheme of Figure 6-2 also makes a distinction between "Hazard Identification" and "Risk Assessment." This is a dangerous distinction. As used by the EPA, it has sometimes been an excuse for ignoring risks where a hazard has not been identified (which, as noted in Chapter 1, a colleague called "uncertain risks") — for example, the possibility that a particular chemical might cause cancer is ignored until there is specific evidence (like an animal bioassay) that it does. We believe that this is logically inconsistent. The NAS scheme, in separating risk management, also did not allow (as ours did) for the risk manager to "commission" a risk assessment on a subject upon which he must later make a decision. EPA later modified the

FIGURE   6-2

Elements of Risk Assessment and Risk Management (from the "Red Book," NAS 1982)

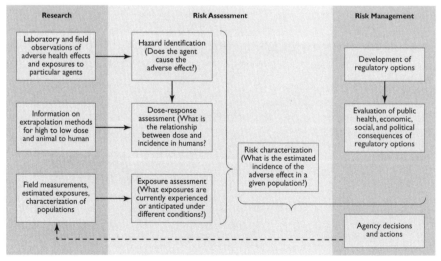

NAS procedure in 1987 by allowing that link (drawn as a dotted line at the bottom of Figure 6-2). But even more importantly, the NAS approach was designed for risk assessment for chemicals in the environment, and the steps in the process do not match (for example) the risk assessment for industrial accident risks. This has led to an undesirable separation of risk analysts into two groups: those assessing risks of an individual chemical in the diet or the environment, and those assessing the risk of an accident in a chemical or industrial facility, by a "Probabilistic Risk Assessment." Each of these two groups is then unable to learn from the insights gained by the other.

Although we cannot find a direct criticism of either Figure 6-1 or the NAS "Red Book" scheme of Figure 6-2, various social scientists (Jasonoff, 1993; Shrader-Frechette, 1985) and others have implicitly criticized such schemes. Firstly, some have argued that the distinction between risk assessment and risk management is artificial and should not be made. We believe that that criticism is more valid when addressed to the NAS scheme than to ours. We suggest that a risk assessor must be well aware of the question that the decision maker is attempting to answer. Indeed the risk assessment may be explicitly "commissioned." Moreover a good assessment, particularly one using an impact pathway approach, will often bring to light several places where intervention can reduce the risk (Kates et al., 1985). In discussing this distinction, Wilson and Clark (1991) suggest that the "separation should not mean divorce." The second and perhaps the most important criticism arose as some early risk managers asked the risk assessors for a single, simple number rather than a description. This, combined with the desire to be "on the safe side," leads to demands for risk estimates to be calculated with the highly biased estimates of all quantities. The same demands lead to a consistent use of a low dose linearity assumption for risk analysis of radiation or toxic chemicals. Scientists disagree (sometimes with extreme heat) on what happens at low doses (where epidemiological and experimental data are impossible to obtain), so this is a policy matter of which every decision maker should be aware. Such introduced biases are therefore sometimes called "risk assessment policy."

Thirdly, some social scientists have gone so far as to say that an assessment should be based upon "perception of risk" rather than one based, however poorly, upon facts. We, and others (Cross, 1992), are appalled by such suggestions. Uncertain though many risk assessments based upon facts are (as noted in Chapter 3), the uncertainty and variability (both from place to place and time to time) of public perceptions are far worse. Worse still, such a procedure is likely to be unstable, particularly if it were to be applied in regulation. Already public concern tends to be raised when a risk is mentioned by a regulatory agency. This increased perception is likely to lead to, in engineering parlance, a positive feedback. We suggest in Figure 6-1 that the demand for addressing public perceptions is best met when it is left to the decision maker to take societal values into account. Some proposals that perceptions of risk be used for risk estimates have gone so far as to suggest that risk comparisons should not be considered. We do not believe that risk comparisons should be the sole basis for decision-making, although we have been so misquoted previously (Wilson, 1990). But we *do* agree with Professor Jean Meyer, as quoted at the beginning of this chapter, that the risk-benefit ratio is basic and that the onus should be on the decision maker to explain the basis of his decision if it differs from what a technical analysis would suggest. Figure 6-3 shows a historical development of society's understanding of risk and its regulation. However, this figure omits any specific reference to the progress made in application of the scientific principles by engineers.

Criteria for Risk Management

Various criteria have been advanced as appropriate for deciding whether and how to manage risks. These include:

I. *Zero risk*—on this criterion any action which involves any risk at all should be rejected. The definiteness and simplicity of decision processes based on such a criterion is soon seen to be false, since although the criterion may be stated, it is not possible to achieve it. Every action (including inaction) has some risk associated with it, either directly or through indirect risks—e.g. to build thicker and thicker walls as protection leads (statistically) to deaths and injuries in cement production and in the building trade.

IIa. *As Low As Reasonably Achievable* (ALARA)—all risks should be made as low as reasonably achievable in any action dependent on the decision process. Such a criterion needs a decision rule which specifies what is "reasonable," a decision which will ultimately depend on physical limits — how thick a roof can be constructed — and the cost of implementation — how much more will it cost to brace the walls some more so we can build a thicker roof. Such decision rules may be made on an ad hoc basis, case by case, or may specify arbitrary cost figures. Although workable, they will lead to inconsistencies in effective valuation of various

FIGURE 6-3

Developments from Various Branches of Science that Contribute to
Risk Assessments of Nuclear Facilities and Hazardous Chemical Use and
Disposal, from Renn (1998)

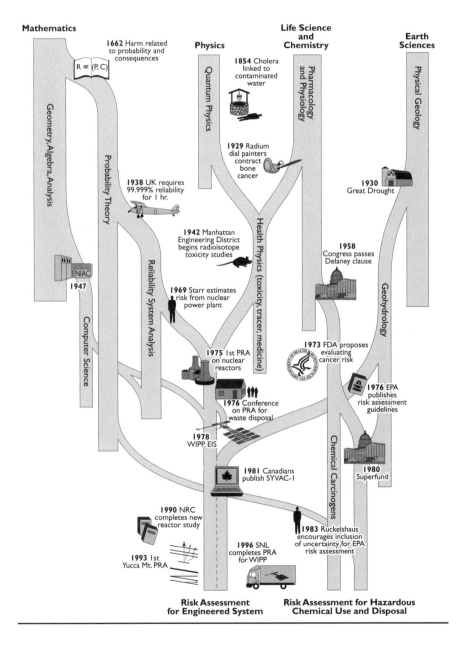

risks, and have inefficiencies in the sense that a more consistent criterion would be capable of saving more lives at the same cost, or the same number at lower cost.

IIb. *Best Available Control Technology* (BACT)—requires that risks be reduced using the best available technology for so doing. The problem here is in knowing what is the best available technology. Usually it is taken to mean a technology that is available commercially, in a tested design and at a cost which is not exorbitant. In the case of removal of sulfur oxides from power plant exhaust gases, it is possible to build equipment which would be more effective than that currently considered BACT, but the running costs would be impractically high, so such equipment has not been built on a large scale and is unlikely to be built. This was the method adopted by the U.S. Congress in enacting the Clean Air Acts of the 1970s. A similar approach was used by OSHA in requiring occupational exposures to be reduced to the Lowest Feasible Level.

III. *Cost-risk-benefit analysis*—requires that explicit account be taken of values to be assigned to various risks, so that they may be traded against the costs and benefits. This was discussed in Chapter 5.

Lave (1981) listed eight possible frameworks for decisions about risks. We approximately map the ones that we consider the most fundamental into the three categories above:

1. *Market regulation.* For efficient working, this requires that cost be assigned to the environmental and health items. Then it is a subset of our group III.

2. *No-risk.* This is clearly a ban: group I

3. *Technology-based standards.* This is a clear group II

4. *Risk-risk: direct*

5. *Risk-risk: indirect*

6. *Cost effectiveness*

We considered each of these three comparisons in Chapter 4 to aid in understanding the risks. They are all subsets of a full risk-cost-benefit analysis (our group III) that might, on occasion enable a decision maker to bypass psychologically difficult questions such as the "value of a life" (our constant γ).

7. *Regulatory budget.* Again, this is a subset of our group III

8. *Benefit-cost.* This is a simpler procedure where risk, the subject of this book, need not enter

The above alternative criteria all implicitly (or explicitly) assign a value to the risks they are designed to control, but some do so more consistently than others.

The Ban or Taboo

The first risk management approach—a ban—was used by many primitive societies. Many activities were subject to taboo. As societies developed, these taboos changed. There is, in this context, an important difference between the risks we are concerned about today and the risks of the last century. 100 years ago, many risks, e.g., from tuberculosis and contaminated water supplies, were sufficiently large that when the causes were recognized, the risks could be almost completely eliminated at modest cost (both financial and in the sense of introducing new risks), and in an obvious fashion by the use of a ban. Today we consider many smaller risks, which are expensive (possibly in both senses above) to eliminate completely.

In modern times we can consider the Delaney Amendment to the Federal Food, Drug and Cosmetic Acts of 1958 (U.S.C. 1958) a form of taboo. Contrary to a common belief of its detractors, it did *not* mandate zero risk. It mandated "that no additive shall be deemed to be safe if it is found to induce cancer when ingested by man or animal, or if it is found by tests appropriate for the evaluation of the safety of food additives to induce cancer in man or animals," (USC, 1958). At the time of its enactment, cancer was even less well understood than it is now, and few human carcinogens were recognized—such as cigarettes, beta-naphthylamine and radiation. Moreover the analytical methods for detecting small quantities of pollutants were not developed, and impurities could only be detected at a level of one part in a million or so. Any chemical known to be carcinogenic was, in the terminology we described in Chapter 2, a potent carcinogen. If it was detectable, it must have been present at levels of one part per million or more, so that the risk of cancer from frequent use worked out to be high (10^{-5} per year or more). It therefore seemed scientifically very sensible to ban all such chemicals, and if it became necessary to allow a carcinogen, to handle that on a case-by-case basis in Congress. (Such modifications were in fact made for aflatoxin B1 and saccharin). But it is typical of bans that they give inappropriate feedbacks and are unstable. How should a Macchiavellian industry executive respond? The incentive is to try to avoid testing a chemical, and if forced to test to use the least sensitive detection system he can get away with! Other procedures that provide incentives are discussed below.

"The best way to get a bad law repealed is to enforce it strictly"
— Abraham Lincoln

By 1980 animal carcinogen tests had become more sensitive and concentration measurements much more sensitive. Now we have more than 30 chemicals known to be carcinogens in humans (the International Agency for Research on Cancer, IARC, currently recognizes 87 agents or groups of agents, mixtures, or exposure circumstances that are known human carcinogens, IARC, 2001, but this list includes viruses, specific radionuclides, and other agents that we would not list as "chemicals" in this context). Several hundred chemicals (as well as quite a few other agents and exposure circumstances) are known to be carcinogenic in animals and, by implication, in humans, so that the Delaney clause, if strictly applied, would become a broad ban. In these circumstances FDA tried to use a "de minimis" level of one in million lifetime risk for chemical compounds given to animals (FDA, 1977). The U.S. National Academy of Sciences, at the request of the EPA, similarly recommended that the Delaney Clause be replaced by a "negligible risk" standard for both raw and processed foods (NAS, 1987). The Food and Drug Administration (FDA) and commissioned a review panel to study the question, and also recommended a 1 in a million "de minimis" risk with a sound scientific basis (Hart et al., 1986). But on a challenge by the National Resources Defense Council, Public Citizen, AFL-CIO and several individuals, the regulation formalizing this approach was turned down by the United States Ninth Circuit Court of Appeals in July 1992, who urged FDA to go to Congress.

The Delaney Clause in either the Food Additive regulations, or the Color Additive regulations of the FDA, while seemingly illogical in the present day and age, do not in themselves, pose great problems for society. But a potentially disastrous dilemma arose when the Delaney Clause was applied to the pesticide residues on food. Since many pesticides are slightly carcinogenic in animals, and even minute residues can be measured, all pesticide use would have to be banned. Food production would suffer. This was resolved by the

Food Quality Protection Act of 1996, EPA (1996b, 1996d) (Public Law 104-170), which allows EPA to apply a "negligible risk" standard if the incremental lifetime risk does not exceed one in a million in a lifetime of exposure. This law applies only to pesticide residues. The food additive and color additive provisions on the Delaney Clause are unchanged. The long time between Schneiderman and Mantel's paper in 1973 (Schneiderman and Mantel, 1973), and the 1996 law shows how long it takes to build up the support to change a law or regulation, and Abraham Lincoln's suggested procedure was only partially adopted.

Best Available Control Technology or As Low As Reasonably Achievable

The second type of hazard management, the demand to reduce a pollutant as much as possible subject to feasible economic demands, may also be useful in certain situations. The Occupational Health and Safety Administration (OSHA) wanted carcinogens in the work place to be reduced to the Lowest Feasible Level. The Clean Air Acts administered by the Environmental Protection Agency, demand that (in non-attainment areas) there be the Lowest Achievable Emission Rate (LEAR), and in all areas the Best Available Control Technology (BACT) must be used. We list in Chapter 7 a death rate and a risk due to living in urban polluted air — typical of the Eastern U.S. (Chicago, Boston, New York, Washington). There is substantial uncertainty in the risk of death, and particularly in the estimate of loss of life expectancy, not least because of uncertainty as to whether air pollution really causes these deaths (or whether the observed correlations are non-causal). The suggested death rate of 50,000/year is large. If we believe we should spend $6,100,000 to save a life (as has been suggested in another context, EPA, 2000), we should be prepared to spend as much as $305 billion per year to reduce air pollution—a huge amount of money, which might lead to large scale bankruptcies and other disruptions. In these circumstances, almost any amount short of bankruptcy might seem reasonable under an ALARA or BACT principle. Lave (1981) criticized such approaches and suggested that they tended to "impose costs arbitrarily among industries until all were at a minimum level of profit." However, actual implementation by the states has been better than Lave feared. This suggests a dual approach to risk management. The academic wants a logical structure that, if adopted and followed, will allow sensible regulation automatically with no contradictions. The best manager will recognize that no logical structure is perfect. He will examine the result of each analysis to see whether it violates "common sense" (which we all know is too uncommon) and make *ad hoc* adjustments as appropriate.

The principle of Best Available Control Technology has been applied, successfully and with common sense, for nearly a century to water pollution. Until recently legislation demanded pure water almost independent of cost—but the legislators never specified how pure or set a risk limit. In principle it would be possible to have much purer water than any existing public water supply by distilling it. But that would be expensive. In practice water supplies are merely chlorinated and perhaps filtered, and there has been no legal objection to stopping technology short at this point. In this case, the cost difference between the two technical mitigation methods, chlorination and distillation, was so great that no detailed risk-cost-benefit analysis was necessary to decide between them. However, several organic carcinogens appear in drinking water as a consequence of chlorination (we include chloroform in our catalogue of risks in Chapter 7), and it needs sophisticated analysis to decide whether and how much to remove (more accurately, prevent the formation of) chloroform. This more sophisticated analysis is now encouraged by the U.S. Congress in the 1996 amendments to the Safe Drinking Water Act.

Risk-Cost-Benefit Analysis

It is the last of these procedures—a thorough risk-cost-benefit analysis—that we espouse in this book, with a very strong emphasis on the word *thorough*. Many attempts to perform risk-benefit analysis have been inadequate. If time, knowledge and resources do not admit of a thorough analysis, sometimes one of the other approaches might be justifiable. When a risk is so large that the action or substance must obviously be banned or so small as obviously to be ignored a detailed analysis is unnecessary. It seems logical to use the less sophisticated management methods, a ban or best available technology until someone has done a risk-cost-benefit analysis. Who decides, and who should decide, when a risk analysis is good enough to replace the cruder approach? Presumably the legislature (with the courts acting, as usual, to prod along the administration when necessary). This can be a branch of "multiple criteria decision analysis" (Belton, 1994).

The Precautionary Principle

"Once harm has been done, even a fool understands it."
—Homer, The Iliad, Book XVII, 1.32

It is always difficult to decide upon a preventive approach when mankind has no experience of the particular situation or technology. In the 1990s it became popular to invoke a "Precautionary Principle": to refrain from an action the consequences of which are not understood, to ban a chemical on which there are no epidemiological data and a new technology with which there is no experience. As the quotation above illustrates, this is NOT a new idea.

The "Precautionary Principle" is not usually well defined. It has been indirectly invoked in a discussion of the exposure to Electromagnetic Fields at low intensity, where some scientists have advocated "Prudent Avoidance" of exposure to electromagnetic fields. However, that immediately leads to the quantitative question, "What is the quantitative meaning of prudence?" It is also similar to the ALARA concept (discussed above) for radiation exposure. But that has been quantitatively defined in terms of a dose and its roughly equivalent cost. Until a quantitative meaning has been assigned, which proponents of either the Precautionary Principle or Prudent Avoidance tend to reject, one is open to Lord Kelvin's famous comment that until it has been expressed in numbers it has not been understood.

For example, an ignoramus might invoke the precautionary principle on an action of society which more informed people might accept. When, and whether, to accept such invocation is an important role of any decision maker. We hope that this book will help to guide such decisions.

Regulation on Upper Limit of Risk

In a classic paper Schneiderman and Mantel (1973) proposed that regulation always be based upon the upper limit of a risk distribution. This idea was extended by Zeise et al. (1984). They argued that it would be sensible to have a decision framework that gives incentives to perform useful studies and research. They suggested that the prior information and the way that uncertainties diminish with research be explicitly recognized. Then if regulation were to always be based on the upper 95th percentile of the risk distribution, it would become more lenient if the uncertainty were reduced, even if the central estimate of risk did not change. Incentives for good research and honest reporting would then be automatically created without an onerous regulatory structure. However sensible this sounds scientifically, it seems politically difficult. There have been very few cases of regulation becoming more lenient in the last 25 years. In the case of chloroform the U.S. EPA (EPA, 1998) has accepted, albeit subsequent to court order, a risk *assessment* that estimates a much smaller risk than heretofore. But the U.S. EPA was already regulating chloroform more than 100 times *less* strictly than other chlorinated hydrocarbons, so this has led to little change in regulation. It is also interesting to speculate whether the EPA would have made this change if the chloroform in question had been a commercial product rather than an unintended by-product of a process (water chlorination) essential for public health.

As with any other approach, regulation on an upper percentile of a risk distribution would require careful analysis. For example, it might be considered prudent to base estimates on the most sensitive animal species; but care has to be taken not to simply choose the single experiment that gives the highest result (which is a completely different idea). Imagine, for example, two identical animal experiments, or two halves of a single experiment, with 50 rodents each. To evaluate the species response requires combining these experiments in an appropriate manner, and using the resulting combined result and its upper percentiles. One experiment will clearly have a higher result (by chance) than the other or the average, and the statistical uncertainty will be greater. Therefore, taking each experiment separately, and choosing the highest result, will automatically give a higher result than the scientifically proper way of combining them. By splitting an experiment into pieces arbitrarily one can always get a higher number. Fortunately, such unscientific extremes are rare. But other logical traps can easily go unnoticed. The uncertainty attached to extrapolations to humans from animal experiments is usually larger than when direct human data are available. This can then result in a paradox, because when both are available, the less reliable animal data might be chosen because of its more conservative upper limit.

A logical paradox also arises in consideration of cases when the evidence for carcinogenicity is not statistically significant—cases that IARC would place in Group 3 (next section). Statistical insignificance simply means that the uncertainty distribution for the risk includes quite a high probability for zero risk. The standard practice is to ignore such cases. But this is inconsistent with regulation on the 95th percentile of the risk distribution—which still exists.

The potential danger of ignoring chemicals for which there are few or no data can be readily appreciated when looking at a risk assessment for an incinerator to destroy nerve gases. Most of the chemicals found in trace amounts in the stack gas are NOT on the EPA list of possible or probable carcinogens—mainly because they do not appear in commerce. While common sense suggests that they might be very dangerous, a bit of thought suggests that the great majority of such trace gases are likely to be similar to trace gases produced in many combustion processes. This example is useful to jog awake one's appreciation of the potential, but it is not otherwise particularly unusual. The standard approach (followed, for example, for the incinerator at Tooele, Utah) accepted by federal and state regulatory authorities is to set the risk of these chemicals to zero. Yet the chemicals for which there are no data are likely, in this instance of burning nerve gases (with which the EPA is not usually concerned), to be more dangerous than the chemicals for which there are data and are listed in the EPA lists. A more logical and complete approach would be to follow a Bayesian procedure and assume that there is a "prior" information on the carcinogenic potency that is updated by each experiment or new observation. Even when considering a chemical for which there have been no formal measurements a risk analyst starts with *some* information—however imprecise. Firstly, one might assume that an untested chemical is representative of the class of all chemicals that have been tested. The uncertainty distribution for carcinogenic potency then spans 7 decades with a geometric standard deviation of 2 or 3 decades (and, of course, it may be zero—there are many other complications in practice). By measuring some parameter such as acute toxicity, and using a toxicity-to-carcinogenicity correlation, this estimate can be updated and the uncertainty reduced to a geometric standard deviation of a decade or so. Measurement of the carcinogenicity in animals can further reduce the uncertainty to a decade or less, while adequate epidemiological data might reduce the uncertainty even more.

Risk versus Certainty of Information

The above suggested procedure of regulating on the basis of the magnitude of a risk estimate (and particularly on the upper 95th percentile) contrasts with a procedure that is often used and that amounts to regulation on the certainty of information. It is often useful to distinguish between the numerical value of an estimated risk and the reliability (certainty) of the information from which the value is derived. A specific case in point is the risk of developing cancer calculated from human data or animal data. As noted in Chapter 2, the risk at low doses of a carcinogen (which are hopefully the doses that will concern society in the future) can sometimes be derived from the measured risk to humans at much higher doses that were experienced in the past. The uncertainty here is the uncertainty of extrapolation to low doses. But it has become usual to use animal data to estimate the risk to humans. This involves an *interspecies* extrapolation in addition.

Many analysts have insisted that risks estimated from human data are "certain" risks, in distinction to the risks calculated from animal data, which they call "uncertain" or speculative. The distinction has led to classification schemes primarily based on strength of evidence for carcinogenicity of the chemical or agent. This is the *hazard,* rather than the *risk.* This is a combination of the statistical significance for observed effects and the perceived relevance of the underlying data for humans. An example of distinguishing and hence the risks thereof, according to the degree of certainty with which they are known, is the classification scheme of the International Agency for Research on Cancer (IARC), part of the World Health Orgainization (WHO). The U.S. EPA has a similar scheme:

Group 1   "Carcinogenic to humans": there is sufficient evidence for carcinogenicity in humans and usually in animals also.

Group 2A "Probably carcinogenic to humans": there is limited evidence for carcinogenicity in humans and sufficient evidence for carcinogenicity in animals.

Group 2B "Possibly carcinogenic to humans": there is sufficient evidence for carcinogenicity in experimental animals but inadequate evidence for cancer in exposed humans.

Group 3   "Not classifiable as to carcinogenicity to humans."

The ideas that led to this scheme, and the ideas that the scheme engenders, carry over to the management and regulation of risks. Some scientists propose to ban all substances in the first group, but cannot consistently ban those in the second because there are so many animal carcinogens including many that occur naturally. The Delaney clause insists that FDA ban chemicals in both groups. Whether one accepts it, this management proposal is a "value judgement" in the sense of our scheme of Figure 6-1. There then is a big difference in regulation between Group 1 and Group 2A and often between Group 2A and Group 2B, independent of the numerical value of the risk estimate. For FDA the difference is between Group 2 and Group 3.

One historical example suffices to show the paradoxes that can arise from this treatment. Vinyl chloride (monomer) is a chemical that has been shown unequivocally to cause angiosarcoma (a rare liver tumor) both in persons occupationally exposed and in Sprague-Dawley rats. The information is certain. The Risk Ratio is much larger than the 400 which is highly statistically significant, while a consistent and significant value of 2 is usually accepted as adequate evidence. There were cries to eliminate all exposure to vinyl chloride in all circumstances. But the past high exposures were limited to occupations, and less than 300 angiosarcomas were so caused, world wide, over 40 years. Occupational exposures have been reduced by a factor of 1,000 to 10,000 since the "bad old days" of the 1960s, and risk presumably reduced at least as much. Lifetime occupational risk estimates are down to less than one in ten thousand. Environmental exposures and lifetime risk estimates are even smaller—one in a million in a lifetime. This reduction is a fantastic success due to combined concern and pressure by workers, trade unions, industry and government. But there remains residual pressure to do more, largely in our view, because the certainty of information of carcinogenicity is great (albeit at high doses).

In contrast, there are many risks which are calculated from animal data where the numerical value of the risk is larger and the number of people exposed much larger. Yet for them there is often less public concern. These include benzopyrene in cooked foods, saccharin and aflatoxin. A later section discusses two other substances, asbestos and dioxin, in which this contrast has played a major role.

The logical contrast between the two procedures, regulation on an upper limit of risk and regulating on certainty of information, can be seen by noting that for chemicals for which there are few data, the uncertainty is very high and the regulation on the upper limit of a distribution would be very severe. What should one do about a new chemical? What should one do about electromagnetic fields at low intensity (3 milliGauss) where some scientists still believe that there is a possibility of a risk? Regulation on certainty of information avoids this problem — but so also would regulation on a mean, or mode, value of the risk. Such substances are likely to be Group 2B, and according to WHO or EPA criteria have only limited regulation. Conversely the risk for a Group 1 carcinogen is likely to be more precisely known, and then regulation on an upper limit of risk would be much closer to the regulation on "best estimate" of risk.

The "De Minimis" Risk

There was a young lawyer called Rex
Who was very deficient in sex
When charged with exposure
He replied with composure
De minimis non curat lex
(The law does not concern itself with trifles)

If the law does not concern itself with trifles, why should anyone else? What is the numerical value of a risk that is too small to be bothered about? Few aspects of risk management have been more discussed. One in a million is a small value that has captured the imagination. In the UK the Royal Commission on the Environment (1977) suggested one in a million *per annum*. This is 70 to 80 times larger that the one in a million *per life* often used in the U.S. But a lifetime cancer risk of one in a million (10^{-6}) or an annual risk of 1.5 x 10^{-8} averaged over all 275 million Americans leads to 4 cancers per year in the U.S. In practice, these four cancers would probably appear among groups of people with higher than usual exposure who would be at a much larger risk than the average. If one knew the identity of the 4 people who would get cancers one would clearly take preventive measures. But one does not and cannot know that identity—although differences in exposure between defined populations may be knowable. A discussion of how the legislature deals with such cancer risks is given by Rosenthal, Gray and Graham (1992). A simple example of risks distributed differently among populations is given later in Chapter 7—the risk of being killed by a bear, and who should be concerned about it. When considering the risk of chronic chemical exposure it may be unnecessary to consider a "de minimis" risk if *a threshold* exists below which the risk is zero. The management procedure is usually then to reduce exposure to below the threshold. However, if a linear-no-threshold theory applies for the dose response, a risk exists at low doses, and the "de minimis" level becomes important. Stokinger (1972) somewhat loosely defined a (n *effective)* threshold as being a level below which the risk is insignificant. By this artifice he avoided the words acceptable and "de minimis" risk. We believe that this artificial approach is no longer necessary or useful.

Risk-related Decisions of the U.S. EPA

"Once the detailed risk and benefit analyses are available, I must consider the extent of the risk, the benefits conferred by the substance, the availability of substitutes and the costs of control of the substance. On the basis of careful review, I may determine that the risks are so small or the benefits so great that no action or only limited action is warranted. Conversely, I may decide that the risks of some or all uses exceed the benefits and that stronger action is essential."
—Russell Train (Administrator of U.S. EPA) Federal Register, 41FR41102, 25 May, 1976

In a similar vein to Russell Train's statement above, William Ruckelshaus (1983, 1984, 1985) wrote several papers expanding on risk-benefit tradeoffs. Nevertheless, most of the early EPA risk regulations, before 1980, were attempts to reduce the estimated upper bound cancer risk to anyone below one in a million (10^{-6}) *per life*. The one in a million arose because it is a round number, and for a risk to an individual seems small. But if everyone in the U.S. were exposed to such a risk, there would be 280 cancers in a lifetime or four per year.

The origin of the one in a million is unclear. The U.K. Royal Commission on the Environment had suggested one in a million *per year*, which is a risk 80 times larger. The Food and Drug Administration had used a non-linear extrapolation to low doses (the Mantel-Bryan formula) for many years, and the dose corresponding to a one in a million lifetime risk was, using that formula, very close to the one in a million annual risk, so there was no apparent strain on industrial processes to take the smaller risk. The one in a million lifetime risk was used before 1980 to regulate water pollutants, such as Trichlorethylene (TCE) in drinking water. Data on carcinogenicity in mice, led to the regulatory level of 5 ppb noted in Table 4-3 above. (Our calculations were less pessimistic: see Wilson, Crouch and Zeise,1983.)

Newer, and more pessimistic, calculations of the one in a million risk put the level at 2.7 ppb (EPA, 1980 see also the EPA website list IRIS). EPA proposed around 1980, and set in place in 1985 (EPA, 1985) a more complex procedure. An unenforceable Recommended Maximum Contaminant Level (RMCL) (now a Maximum Contaminant Level Goal or MCLG) was established, and equated to zero for carcinogens for which low dose linearity of the dose response relationship was assumed (this was in spite of our formal public comment on the proposal that setting the RMCL (or MCLG) to zero is a "cop-out" that provides no information). An enforceable Maximum

Contaminant Level (MCL) was set to be as close to the RMCL or MCLG as feasible, given cost and practicality. The MCL for TCE was left at the 5 ppb decided earlier (EPA, 1987).

Other actions of the agency to control pollution in other media, have different mandates. Unlike the carcinogenic water pollutants for which a linear dose response was assumed, the clean air act requires that:

"National primary ambient air quality standards, prescribed under subsection (a) shall be ambient air quality standards the attainment and maintenance of which in the judgment of the Administrator, based on such criteria and allowing an adequate margin of safety, are requisite to protect the public health. The Secondary standards, however, must protect the public welfare from any known or anticipated adverse effects associated with the presence of such air pollutant in the ambient air."

Thus, if "protecting the public health" doesn't necessarily require zero risk, neither do the primary standards. So the EPA may implicitly have defined "protecting the public health" as an (unspecified) non-zero risk, rather than implicitly using a cost-based approach. However, there is no way out for the secondary standards, which are supposed to protect against "any" adverse effects. If there exists a threshold below which the risk is zero, the legislative requirement is clear. But scientific data since 1980 suggest that a linear dose response cannot be ruled out (indeed, any dose response that does not include a threshold causes the same problem) the agency must establish a criterion. The obvious criteria are cost and practicality.

Even a cursory examination of the risks listed in Chapter 7 shows that a reduction to one in a million lifetime risk does not appear possible for all risks. Perhaps in response such observations, the stated views of both the legislature and the agency have changed over the years. In the 1990s the EPA have changed their view of what risk is acceptable—although Congress has discouraged them from reviewing earlier regulations—and EPA now officially consider a range 10^{-6} to 10^{-4} per person-lifetime to be acceptable in a variety of regulations (EPA 1989, 1990, 1994, 1996a, 1998, 2000). It is nowhere specified how to decide upon a number in this range, and little indication of the specific processes applied other than Russell Train's statement in the first paragraph of this section and several articles by William Ruckelshaus after he left office (Ruckelshaus, 1983, 1984, 1985).

Until recently EPA argued that to be responsive to the various legislative goals they had no authority to take cost into account, but this approach appears to have leaked into decision-making in areas where cost *must* be taken into account. For example, the Federal Insecticide Rodenticide and Fungicide Act (FIFRA) explicitly requires taking cost into account, yet in discussion in 1984 of ethylene dibromide the Administrator (William Ruckelshaus) explicitly told the press that he asked his staff *not* to inform him of the costs even though in this case FIFRA applied! In deciding upon an MCL for a drinking water contaminant the EPA already used considerations of economics and practicality and the 1995 amendments to the clean water act explicitly permitted and encouraged a cost-benefit analysis. On the other hand, in February 2001 the U.S. Supreme Court ruled that an explicit cost-benefit analysis is not permitted by the explicit wording of the Clean Air Act. We suggest that it would be much preferable to make the approach explicit, so that the assumptions can be adequately examined (although, of course, to do so would require a change in the law).

A specific calculation for hazardous waste is discussed in detail in Appendix 2.

Probability of Causation

As noted in Chapter 2 it is often possible to calculate the Probability of Causation (POC) that a cancer has been caused by a particular pollutant:

$$\text{POC} = \frac{\begin{array}{c}\text{(Risk calculated from the} \\ \text{estimated exposure to the pollutant)}\end{array}}{\text{(Risk from all causes)}} \qquad (6\text{-}1)$$

In this equation Risk is used in a restricted sense, because it is the risk of developing a cancer at a particular moment in time, from an alleged exposure at another particular moment in time, and not the risk of developing cancer at any time during life. Once the POC has been calculated the science itself ends. What one does with the information is a policy matter for which the public is ill prepared (Upton and Wilson 2000). Cases of legal liability tend to be governed by a rule that it must be "more likely than not" that the postulated cause is the correct one. "More likely than not" should presumably mean that POC is greater than 50%, although different interpretations have been advanced; and when legal liability accrues is ultimately a matter of public policy. No matter what the legal definition, society might well choose a different procedure for regulatory and administrative purposes.

There are many examples where legislatures have explicitly modified the usual legal rule. Workers' compensation is a case in point. Enough workers have been exploited that there is a common sentiment to compensate workers even when POC has not been calculated. For example, in Massachussets and several other states there used to be, and in many states still is, a "heart law." It was assumed that firemen and policemen are under sufficient stress that any heart attack was presumed to have been caused by the job, and so was compensable. Moreover, a high exposure to a chemical used in an occupational setting was not uncommon in the recent past, so such exposure has often been assumed except where there is evidence to the contrary. However, common sense prevails even in legislatures, and laws can be changed when the etiology of particular diseases becomes better elucidated. When it was realized that the major cause of heart attack in firefighters was cigarette smoking, pressure arose to abolish the heart law. The pressure was resisted and instead the trade unions concerned agreed that their members would be non-smokers.

A discussion of various heuristics for compensation in occupational situations has been made by Harber and Shusterman (1996). Several of these heuristics accept the idea that one should compensate when a large risk is observed even when POC has not been explicitly calculated and attribution is not certain.

Armstrong et al. (1988) discussed compensating cancer victims in aluminum plants in Canada. The Quebec Worker's Compensation Board (CSST) decided to compensate workers whose POC exceeded 50%. Wakeford et al. (1998) describe a procedure used in the U.K. whereby compensation is paid to exposed radiation workers if the calculated POC is greater than 20%. The choice of 20%, rather than 50% was chosen to be "generous" to the workers and to encourage arbitration (using this procedure) rather than court action.

In another situation the U.S. Congress responded to concern from veterans that they had developed cancer from being "downwind" of atomic bomb tests. Congress specifically requested the National Cancer Institute to prepare tables so that the POC could be evaluated for these veterans (Congress 1983). Subsequently, Congress directed the Veterans Administration to establish compensation standards for radiation exposure claims from these veterans (Congress 1984). The Veterans Administration chose to adapt the radioepidemiological Tables NCI had developed to provide an uncertainty distribution for the dose that gives POC = 50%, and to use the upper 99th percentile as a "screening dose" for compensation, with the actual compensation to vary with the actual POC. The POC calculated for these "down winders" was lower than 50% in almost all cases. Congress then passed a law awarding compensation regardless of dose to any veteran with a "radiogenic" cancer—a cancer of a type that is known to be increased by high radiation doses (Congress, 1988).

This presumptive legislation seems to have been a political decision based upon a deep public feeling that the atom bomb tests were wrong and society must make amends. Scientists and scientific societies were not consulted. The sentiment and procedure seems similar to that in the "heart law" referred to above. The attempts to put a scientific veneer onto the procedure suggests that radiation exposure is more dangerous than it is. Fortunately, when President Reagan signed the bill, compensating veterans regardless of dose or POC, in the law accepting the risk management procedure based upon other societal values, he made a small attempt to improve public perception by stating that neither the bill nor his signature should imply that radiation actually caused the cancers which were being compensated[2].

Later this presumptive compensation was extended by Congress to apply to certain eligible "downwinders," uranium miners and veterans (Congress, 1990). In September 2000, the U.S. Congress passed an amendment to the defense authorization bill (Congress, 2000); the amendment extended this concept, compensating former workers, mainly on defense projects, at the AEC or its major contractors, for exposures exceeding the lower 99th percentile of the distribution of dose for which POC = 50%. Although at the April 2000 press conference DOE officials stated that they intend to use scientific procedures, the interagency group recommending this step was not a committee of scientific experts on the issue, knowledgeable scientists and scientific scientists were not consulted, and some who enquired, by polite letter, by angry letter, or by Freedom of Information Act request, received no useful information and concluded that they were deliberately kept in the dark. It remains to be seen how DOE will be administer the law and explain it. President Clinton, when signing this bill or when issuing an executive order implementing it could have repeated President Reagan's cautionary words. The absence of scientific discussion, or explanation that a societal value judgement overrides the POC calculation, suggests that DOE used a risk analysis procedure to "justify" a decision already made rather than to illuminate a decision not yet made. Such an approach was explicitly decried at the end of Chapter 1. Interestingly, such charges are more usually leveled at EPA's superfund program.

The ramifications of diverging from a simple application of the rule that compensation applies only when the calculated POC is 50% or higher are numerous. At POC = 50% and above it is usually well determined from observational (epidemiological) data. When a lower 99th percentile is used, or equivalently a value of POC of 5% to 10% is chosen, the estimated POC depends critically on the uncertain theoretical extrapolation to low does. Problems particularly arise for the rarer cancers such as leukemia where the denominator (incidence) is small. For example, even 5 years of chest X-rays in the 1950s—with the doses, then usual, of 1 Rem per chest X ray—would in principle allow most leukemia victims to claim compensation.

Most of the cancers known to be caused by radiation are moderately common. In contrast, there are situations where there is a rare disease that is increased by an external agent. Mesothelioma, for example, is a rare disease that is known to be caused by exposure to asbestos, and other, fibers. Then the compensation procedures are much simpler. Almost any occupational exposure to asbestos would be enough to establish causation and compensability, although in this case the usual interpretation of the plots of mesothelioma incidence with time suggest that 70% of the mesothelioma incidence in males, and 20% in females, is caused by the high occupational exposures of 30 years ago (Price and Wilson, 2001).

But the same principle applied to medical end points other than cancer (Crawford and Wilson, 1996) raises even more societal issues. For example, the DOE in providing compensation could consider compensating those members of the public adversely affected by one of its major *suppliers*—the local electricity company—in addition to the employees of its direct *contractors*. At the AEC plants in Portsmouth and Paducah, in the Ohio valley, the large amount of electricity consumed was produced by coal burning power plants which in the relevant period of the 1960s had very inadequate pollution control. It is in the Ohio Valley, at Steubenville, that the largest increase in death rates from respiratory diseases was found by the Harvard Six Cities study of air pollution (Wilson and Spengler, 1996). Many scientists believe that this increase (of about 50%), compared to less polluted areas, is causally related to air pollution in the Ohio Valley. This increase leads to a POC (roughly averaged over the whole population of the area) of about 30%. Undoubtedly, it is higher for many individuals. The DOE workers already had some compensation for their exposures—their *salaries*—but the general public did not. Not mentioned in the discussion is the fact that the dose to many of the DOE workers cannot be obtained solely from the film badge they wore at work. At Hanford, for example, the dose from the medical diagnostic X rays exceeded the dose from the occupation and was not explicitly recorded (Shihab-Eldin, Shlyakhter and Wilson 1992). Should DOE pay the compensation, or some medical agency?

A cut-off at 50% or any particular figure seems arbitrary and hard to justify. How sure is society that someone whose POC is 50.1% should be compensated and someone whose POC is 49.9% should not? This paradox has led to proposals for compensation *on a sliding scale* (Bond, 1981; Upton and Wilson, 2000). Society (or a court) could decide on a compensatory value for the disease in question (perhaps $500,000) and pay a fraction of this equal to $500,000 x POC, with perhaps a *"de minimis"* cut-off at some value of POC or suitable sum of money. This would avoid a hiatus that would occur if an improvement in scientific understanding changed the POC from 50.1% to 49.9%. But the decision on what constitutes adequate compensation would have to be independent of the POC calculation. As noted above, this is the procedure used by Wakeford et al. (1998).

A proportionate use of POC would have the additional advantage of automatically allowing, in a simple way, assignments of compensation to multiple causes or situations where cumulative exposure to a single substance is the cause, but there are many contributors to the cumulative exposure. The courts are ahead of scientists, experts in public policy and politicians in considering such complex problems in compensation. In asbestos litigation it may well be possible to argue that POC is greater than 50% for asbestos as a cause, but the assignment of the blame to individual asbestos suppliers leads to individual POCs for individual asbestos suppliers less than 50%. In Rutherford (1997) the court held that "plaintiffs may prove causation in asbestos-related cancer cases by demonstrating that the plaintiff's exposure to defendant's asbestos-containing product in reasonable medical probability was a substantial factor in contributing to the aggregate dose of asbestos the plaintiff or decedent inhaled or ingested, and hence to the risk of developing asbestos-related cancer, without the need to demonstrate that fibers from the defendant's particular product were the ones, or among the ones, that actually produced the malignant growth." 941 P.2d at 1219 (footnote omitted).

Radiation exposure is comparatively easy to evaluate—even after an accident such as that at Chornobyl. Radiation workers usually carry personal monitors (dosimeters) and the radioactive materials leave their signature. But past exposure to most chemicals is much harder to measure.

Emerson once said that "foolish consistency is the hobgoblin of small minds." Nonetheless, we feel it is the duty of a risk analyst to point out inconsistencies so that if they are retained they are retained deliberately.

Management by Avoiding Precursors

The discussion above is on *when* or *whether* to manage a technology, not about *how* to manage it. The usual method for prevention of accidents is to determine the actions and events that have caused accidents in the past, and may cause accidents in the future, and endeavor to avoid them. Car accidents have been caused by inadequate brakes and tires; most states mandate brake and tire inspection. More importantly human error is a major contributor to car accidents and many industrial accidents. It was a major contributor to both the Three Mile Island and the Chornobyl nuclear reactor accidents. The same procedure is applied to the more complex and larger technologies such as nuclear power or travel by aircraft. Two hundred years ago the principle was to let a technology develop and only regulate it if there appeared to be problems. This was replaced by an approach to developing standards.

More recently "fault tree" analyses for failure probabilities and "event tree" analyses for failure scenarios (as discussed in Chapter 2) have been used within industrial and engineering companies for reliability assessment and improvement. Such analyses are then known as reliability analyses. The 1975 report on Nuclear Reactor Safety (Rasmussen et al., 1975) used "event tree analysis" which was discussed briefly in Chapter 2. This new approach originally had detractors, and indeed the failure of manufacturers, utility companies, regulators and critics alike to use it may have contributed to the occurrence of the Three Mile Island Accident. If the event tree procedure, origi-

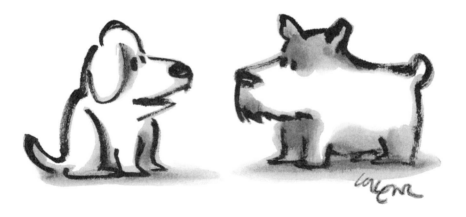

"I attribute it to human error. But then I attribute everything to human error."

© 2001 The New Yorker Collection from cartoonbank.com. All Rights Reserved.

nally applied to a single Westinghouse reactor and a single General Electric reactor, had been applied to other reactors, particularly those of a different manufacturer (Babcock & Wilcox), the different control system could have been noted, and probably the Three Mile Island accident could have been averted. Regulators quickly learned. An event tree analysis (called a Probabilistic Risk Analysis or PRA) is now demanded for every nuclear reactor made in the western world. The use of the analysis enables both the nuclear operator and the regulator to decide what are the biggest contributors to risk and then to take action to reduce them. In many cases the action is to reduce the frequency of precursors and enable the plant to stay on line more frequently. Such a reduction simultaneously improves safety and economic performance. The improvement in economic performance makes it accepted, and even popular, among nuclear operators.

Unfortunately, the authorities in the USSR and its remnants have been slow to understand. A full "event tree analysis" has recently been performed for the RBMK reactor at Ignalyina in Lithuania. Not only did this make apparent the design weakness responsible for the Chornobyl accident, but several other weaknesses were uncovered. The RBMK reactors are vulnerable to a hydraulic oscillation in the case of an Anticipated Transient Without Scram (ATWS). If not corrected these oscillations can lead with unknown but probably high probability to an accident with adverse health consequences comparable to Chornobyl.

The event tree procedure has also been applied to understanding risks of chemical plants and other industrial facilities. If such a study of the risk of each such technology were mandatory, it would hopefully locate opportunities for reducing risk. For example, a similar approach might have prevented the tragic accident at Bhopal (Kalelkar, 1998) where methyl isocyanate was accidentally released over a large, poor, residential area. Studies of the plant could have revealed that: (i) it was unnecessary to store as much methyl isocyanate in one location; (ii) the plant was designed so that sabotage was too easy; (iii) the personnel and the public were not aware of the simple and effective remediation steps in case of a release (spraying water at the plant to deposit the material and putting a damp cloth over the mouth to prevent inhalation of the vapor).

But the important issue of the present decade is when to stop reducing risk in a particular technology. A speed limit for automobiles of 10 miles per hour—which was the law in the UK in the year 1900—could reduce risk, but with a reduction in benefit. At what stage should one stop searching for small risks? This was addressed by the U.S. Nuclear Regulatory Commission in their *safety goals* promulgated after much open discussion (NRC, 1976).

It must be recognized that an event tree analysis can only tell us the risk of a group of plants built according to a set of standards. The plausible assumption is made that the risk calculated for the group, applies to an individual plant. But the event tree analysis cannot be the regulatory tool in itself. But it *can*, and in our opinion *should*, be used to tell whether a set of standards and regulations is adequate or overly restrictive.

A difficult issue in the issue of regulation is the extent to which a regulator should insist on a "clean house." A clean house rarely has a direct influence on risk, whether by accident frequency, or induction of disease, but it may have an indirect influence. A dirty house may mean a sloppy and careless owner. Likewise, there is often a belief that a clean nuclear power plant (for example) is run by people who have a high regard for safety. Although this belief is open to study (at least to the extent that precursors to accidents might be more frequent), this does not seem to have been done. Meanwhile the Nuclear Regulatory Commission in 1995 was insisting on a number of improvements even on power plants where the calculated accident probability was within its own guidelines (Wilson, 1997).

Asbestos and Dioxin

Asbestos and dioxin have been regulated in somewhat draconian ways that do not seem to be related to the real risks. It is therefore instructive to understand how and why this has occurred. It has been known for a century that asbestos at high exposures gives a toxic response called asbestosis, with an apparent threshold below which it does not occur. Starting about 1935 it was realized that asbestos exposure causes lung cancer and mesothelioma as well. Asbestos is not a mutagen (in standard assays), so that if one accepts the idea prevalent in the 1970s that only mutagens and initiators show linear behavior it should not have a linear dose response relationship. Before 1980 most scientists assumed that there was a threshold below which asbestos exposure did not cause cancer, but many scientists and the regulatory authorities now insist on considering a linear dose response. Some aspects of this were already discussed in Chapter 2.

But EPA regulation in the 1980s (encouraged by one group of scientists) was unrelated to dose or to any quantitative prediction of dose. Presence of asbestos was enough especially if it were in "friable" form. Moreover, EPA allowed inspectors of the asbestos, and those recommending action to be taken whenever it was found, to be also professionally involved in its removal. School systems all over the U.S. followed their advice, and this conflict of interest was a recipe for huge expense — an expense that many analysts believe to be out of proportion to the risks. Various business offices, state office buildings and school systems tried to recover the expense from the manufacturers of the asbestos. This led to the bankruptcy of Johns Manville (and other smaller companies). Moreover, it effectively led to the almost complete abrogation of authority and responsibility to the courts which were ill prepared to cope with the technical issues involved. Insurance companies were also heavily involved, and since insurance is "laid off" to the international market, the asbestos litigation was partially responsible for the financial debacle at Lloyds of London in the early 1990s.

The attitude of U.S. EPA changed. EPA officially recognize that concentrations of asbestos, and hence exposure and dose, are important in a risk calculation and subsequent management decision. But, even so, in 1989 a scare in New York City caused the shut down of schools for several weeks at the start of the school year. The health benefit of the extra asbestos removal was so small that it could not be measured, only calculated. The cost of asbestos removal worked out to be at least a billion dollars per calculated life saved (Wilson et al., 1994).

There seem to have been several factors involved in this failure to use the available tools of health risk analysis:

1. The scientists who urged a ban on EPA seem to have believed that the exposure from asbestos in place was likely to be very high, and the cost of asbestos removal modest. The opposite has been the case in the great majority of cases, although there were some horrendous exposure situations.

2. The asbestos manufacturers were careless in the past, slow to admit it, and reluctant to be more cautious in the future.

3. There was a belief that the available alternative insulation materials, such as fiberglass and cellulose fibers were "safe," although they had never been tested, since they had never been used as carelessly as asbestos has been in the past. Nonetheless, recent epidemiological data and models (Wilson, Nolan and Langer, 1999) do not suggest a large risk of the alternatives at present day exposures. But that applies also to asbestos which, carefully used, presents only a small risk (Wilson and Price, 2001).

4. All three of these items, but item 2 in particular, led to a lack of trust which is difficult to reverse (see Chapter 4), and it is not now possible to use asbestos in the U.S.

In the late 1990s the U.S.EPA proposed to ban asbestos completely, even for such uses with minuscule exposure such as packing for faucets and pipe fittings. This was considered a simpler regulatory strategy than deciding which exposures were adequately low. However, this was turned down by the courts (Corrosion Proof Fittings et al., 1991). Le Dou et al. (2001) called for an international ban, but there seems to be no new evidence since 1991 to justify one. In view of the 1991 court decision it seems unlikely that such a call can succeed without a comprehensive risk assessment presumably including risks of disposition as suggested by Camus (2001).

Dioxin (2,4,7,8 tetrachlorodibenzodioxin) is very toxic, as noted in Chapter 4. Only recently have enough data on effects of human exposure become available to allow it to be called a human carcinogen. But even now, the Risk Ratio in the epidemiological study is less than 2 and is only accepted because of conclusive animal data (IARC, 1997). However, dioxin is not mutagenic and is widely believed to display a threshold behavior. In fact the animal data of Kociba et al. (1978) show a *reduction* in tumors at moderate doses.

There seem to be three important issues that dominate the public discussion of the management of the dioxin risk. Firstly, dioxin is stored in fatty tissue, perhaps to a greater extent in man than in rodents. This may upset the "usual" animal/man comparison discussed in Chapter 2. Secondly, the amount of dioxin in the environment is large enough that the lifetime risk of eating ice cream daily, calculated from a linear dose response relationship is 1.9×10^{-4} (nineteen in ten thousand) (see Table 7-2B below). Thirdly, and probably most importantly, dioxin was an impurity in the defoliant 2-4-5T, which was used extensively as "agent orange" in the unpopular Vietnam war. All of these considerations lead to a regulation of dioxin on bases that are not fully scientific.

Reducing Risk by Technological Improvement

Even though we might, after a risk-benefit analysis, accept a technology, we want to make sure that technology is constantly improved to reduce risk. This procedure of technology improvement is often very slow and it seems worthwhile to find incentives and procedures to speed the improvement. We give three examples of this.

X-rays were discovered in 1897, and very soon thereafter their use for medical diagnosis began. Almost at once some serious adverse effects of ionizing radiation were discovered—skin erythema, radiation dermatitis and skin cancers were the first to be observed—but other cancers were discovered among radium dial painters in the 1920s. Although therefore the risk of using X-rays was well known, medical men stated their view, which is generally agreed to be correct, that the benefit of prompt diagnosis outweighed the possible risks. Yet the identical benefit can be obtained with less risk by reducing the X-ray exposure. It has long been known how to do this by using better X-ray film, intensifying screens, and shielding, including limiting the X-ray exposure to the region of the body being studied. But it took nearly 30 years for this risk reduction to be achieved even though it cost little. Even as late as 1950, the X-ray exposure for chest examinations was 1 Roentgen, 140 times greater than the 7 milliRoentgens commonly used today. In addition, as late as the 1950s, X-rays were used in applications (like shoe-fitting) for which the benefit to risk ratio was much lower than medical imaging. As a child of 7 years old, one of us, RW, clearly remembers repeatedly pressing the button on the radiography machine thereby ensuring a high radiation dose.

Pesticides and herbicides have enabled food production in the U.S. to increase considerably since 1940. The increase in well being, including reduction of risk of death from starvation and disease, is considerable, and is usually considered to outweigh the risks of the pesticides by a wide margin. But that is not the whole story. In "Silent Spring" Rachel Carson (1960) pointed out that there is a lot of unnecessary use of pesticides, and that the same benefit of improved crops can be obtained with less risk by using a little care, and that there were indirect effects (through effects on ecosystems) that had also to be incorporated in risk-benefit balancing.

Many scientists considered that the proposal of FDA to ban saccharin in prepared foods was foolish; they compared the risk of saccharin and the risk of sugar. Most Americans are overweight, and this brings many problems, including increased heart and blood pressure problems and perhaps an increased probability of cancer. If the choice were between more saccharin as a sweetener and more sugar as a sweetener, increased sugar poses a ten times greater risk. But those are not the only two possible choices. We can think at once of two more possible choices: not to use a sweetener at all, and to return to the use of cyclamates which may have been banned for incorrect reasons.

These examples have a common feature: the risk-benefit comparison was too narrowly posed. By posing the questions more broadly we can reduce the overall risk level in society. These examples must not be used to discredit the risk-benefit analyses that were actually performed. Diagnostic X-rays saved much misery and many lives, and pesticides increased agricultural production and our well being. The decisions to use them were (in our view) correctly taken. We do feel, however, that society must constantly look for new technological alternatives that can reduce risk.

There is, to our knowledge, no rigorous analytical procedure for finding new technological procedures. However, the very act of performing a risk assessment can often suggest ways of reducing risk. Indeed several practicing engineers have argued that the importance of such assessments is *not* in the numbers that they produce, which may be uncertain or otherwise unbelievable or unacceptable, but in the understanding of the system that the assessments provide. Since the understanding of the responsible plant manager and the plant workers is particularly important, it is vital that risk analyses be understood (and preferably performed) by the plant staff and not merely by an independent consultant or a regulator—however competent.

A method of reducing risk espoused by the U.S. Congress (in the automobile emission standards for example) is called "technology forcing." The Congress mandated a reduction of risk by a definite time. This is similar in its effect to the demanding Best Available Control Technology and is a less sensitive tool than demanding repeated risk-benefit analyses.

Radiation Protection

Radiation protection has been an important issue for many years. Moreover, since it was historically first, the procedures adopted tend to be adapted for regulation of other agents. In discussing the regulation of the burgeoning X-ray industry, the International Commission on Radiological Protection (ICRP) suggested in 1927 that a linear dose response relationship should be *assumed*. No dose should be received without expectation of some benefit. Doses should be reduced As Low As Practical [ALAP] (changed to As Low As Reasonably Achievable [ALARA]). The first Nuclear Regulatory Commission came to grips with what this might mean. After a two year hearing in which *inter alia* they asked participants what sum should be spent to reduce radiation doses they proposed (NRC, 1975) $1,000 per Man-Rem (now raised to $2,000 per Man-Rem (Kress, 1992)), which was a round figure larger than any "intervenor" in the hearing had proposed. NRCP (1993) propose a smaller number of about $20 per Man-Rem for occupational exposure. $2,000 per Man-Rem corresponds to a value of γ (Chapter 5). The value becomes about $6,000,000 per life saved in the dose response relationship on the basis of a linear dose response (infinity if there is a threshold) and seems in accord with the value suggested by economists (Chapter 5). But the effect of the standards and actions of NRC sometimes result in expenditure of sums 1,000 times greater than this (Tengs et al., 1995). This could be justified *if* (and only if) the dose reduction in question were a precursor to a major accident, or perhaps if were an indicator of sloppiness with its indirect effect upon accidents. This does not seem to be the claim. Although it has been slow in coming, the "Risk Informed Regulation" program of the Nuclear Regulatory Commission since 1995 begins to address the 1975 guideline. Many observers claim that this has been a major cause of an improvement of reliability, and has possibly also increased safety.

This is an example of the fact that society has only begun to decide how to cope with low doses and probabilities of adverse effects. Radiation protection experts had used the concept of an integrated population dose—measured in Man-Rems (now person-Sieverts). For a linear dose response, this integrated measure of dose is proportional to the total population effect of all exposures. When the whole world is exposed (as it is to Carbon 14 from a nuclear reprocessing plant unless an attempt is made to capture it) one can get big numbers for the integrated dose. But individual doses are small compared to natural background. In 1998 this regulatory problem has led to a demand in some quarters to *reject* the presumption of low dose linearity (in spite of the arguments in Chapter 2) and to regulate radiation exposure until it is below an assumed threshold.

Economic Incentives

Another risk reduction tool, particularly espoused by economists, is to provide incentives. In our capitalist society the obvious incentive is money, perhaps in the form of a risk fee (or pollution charge) on any risk that is imposed upon society. This might be at a level of $1–$10 million per life or $1–$10 for a risk of one in a million per lifetime encouraging an expenditure of $1–$10 million to save a life. Then there would be continuous financial incentive to reduce the fee by reducing the risk. Such financial incentives are not guarantees of the thought processes necessary to think of methods of risk reduction but may help. But these financial incentives, although attractive to most economists, are often unattractive politically. We do, however, suggest that a risk fee be calculated. This will be a useful guideline to the regulator to see whether his alternative regulation methods make sense or not.

An important variant of the economic incentive is the program of trading Emission Permits which have been successful for sulfur and ozone emissions. In a typical use of Emission Permits a company that has been emitting a substance for a long period of time, is given a permit to emit that amount but no more. If the company emits less than permitted, the permit may be traded on the open market to another company with wishes to emit more, to keep constant, or reduce, the total emissions in a geographical region.

It is important to choose the best place in an event tree for the emissions where it is easiest to regulate or control the permits. For sulfur and particle emissions from a power plant it will be the chimney stack of the plant, because the plant operator has the power to reduce emissions by stack gas scrubbers.

But for reducing carbon dioxide emissions to reduce the potential for global warming, it is simpler to regulate when carbon is taken out of the ground and put into the environment. Carbon is usually burned within a few years of being brought to the surface. For international rather than national control, where the carboniferous material is imported, regulation or a permit would be appropriate at the port of entry (Lackner et al., 2001).

Great care must be exercised to ensure that the permit procedure is not only applied at the best place from a materials flow standpoint, but also that it satisfies the ethical requirements of society. The cartoon (page 181) illustrates an application of tradable permits that most people consider undesirable.

The Multiple Uses of a Risk Assessment

In discussing the different regulations of the different agencies, and even of the different laws governing the actions of the same agency, it is useful to note that a well performed risk assessment can, with simple, small but necessary and appropriate modification illuminate more than one decision. For example, one can consider the risk caused by inhalation of benzene. The estimation of the risk can follow a similar path whether the risk is to an exposed worker or to the public. The assessments will differ because the exposure is much greater to the worker than the public. If there is a threshold, the risk to the former may be finite and to the latter can be zero. A discussion of the low dose behavior can be included to make the assessment applicable to both situations. It is in a consideration of the management options that the main difference comes. Society has always been willing to allow a worker (who is compensated by a salary) to have a somewhat higher risk from a few actions associated with his job than the general public, who are exposed to many actions in a smaller way. It must therefore be anticipated that the OSHA regulations will differ from those of the EPA, and NRC will have less strict rules for radiation workers than for the public.

Use of Comparisons to Guide a Manager

Although every government agency tends to insist that it makes a decision on the basis of the particular risk involved, there is in practice a great deal of comparison. Consider for example a set of decisions faced 20 years ago by the

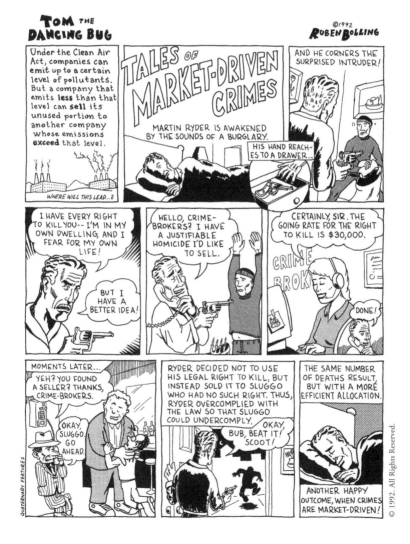

© 1992. All Rights Reserved.

TABLE 6-1

Substance	Annual Risk × Population	Reference
Aflatoxin B1	1,600	Chapter 7
Saccharin	500	FDA 1977
2-4 DAA (in hair dyes)	3	Wilson 1985

commissioner of the Food and Drug administration, Dr. Kennedy. In Table 6-1 the risk of three disparate substances is compared. All of these substances had been shown to cause cancer in animals, and aflatoxin B1 had been shown to cause cancer in people also. The table shows the annual number of persons who would die prematurely as a result of the exposures, according to risk assessors (using a linear dose response relation).

The public pressure by environmental groups was inversely proportional to the number of persons! The FDA could not act on the last of these (and still be intellectually honest) without acting on the first two. FDA side-stepped the aflatoxin issue (and declined to lower the "action level" for aflatoxin in peanut butter below 20 ppb) by calling it a "natural" additive. It is still present in the environment at about the same level.

Then FDA sent their 1977 risk analysis for saccharin to Congress (who promptly made an exception). Although 2-4 DAA was not subject to the same FDA rules (Clairol had obtained in the 1930s a "coal tar" exemption for use of chemical derivatives of coal tar), Clairol reformulated their hair dyes using chemicals not yet shown to be carcinogenic.

Scheuplein (1990) and other officials of the FDA have also publicly stated the problems with a law that requires regulation of man made chemicals to a *much* tougher standard than natural chemicals. This made the scientists in FDA "clean" and honest: but the effect was still a regulation that was not related to the risk.

A regulator might also look at the cost of reducing a risk as listed by Cohen (1980) or Tengs et al. (1995) (note that this is the quantity γ in the formal discussion of Chapter 5). Although (as noted in Chapter 5 and again in Chapter 7) costs for equal risks vary by a factor of a million there are groupings which might suggest the way in which a decision can be made in conformity with other decisions. For example, a risk manager in the U.S. would ignore risks in a foreign country if they cost more than $1,000 per life. An HMO would pay for cancer and other medical treatments that cost $100,000 per life, but few HMOs will pay more than this (kidney dialysis seems to be an exception). Agencies charged with cancer prevention will insist that those entities that they regulate pay $6,100,000 or more per calculated life (EPA, 2000b). Occupational hazards such as coal mining are more risky, but society seems willing to pay $30,000,000 or more to try to reduce them. But for the various nuclear power and radioactivity risks society seems to insist on upwards of $100,000,000 per calculated life saved—and of course if there is a threshold in the dose response relationship, an infinite amount per life saved.

Safety Culture and the Importance of Incentives

Many safety analysts have emphasized the importance of a safety culture in which all participants in an enterprise think about safety constantly. As the safety record improves, so does profitability in such different technologies as the railroad industry and the nuclear electric power industry. Establishment of incentives is an important aspect of such a culture. It then makes financial as well as human sense to use a good safety record as one of the criteria for year-end salary bonuses. There is a considerable variation in safety culture between countries, with the United States nearing the top of the list and Bangladesh near the bottom. But those of us who live in developed countries must recognize that the absence of a safety culture is among the least of the problems in Bangladesh.

Congress as the Filter for Societal Values

In the cases noted above, the executive branch of government has the primary responsibility for decisions about setting regulations and deciding upon other procedures for reducing or managing risks. In our diagram of Figure 6-1 we include three lines from interested parties conveying value judgements to the decision maker. Congress, however, sets the boundaries in which the agencies can make decisions. While the agencies have considerable latitude—some would say too much—Congress can and does override them. In discussion of the Probability of Causation above, we noted that it was Congress, not the Veterans Administration, that ordered compensation for veterans and other "downwinders." In superfund legislation Congress set out eight specific requirements that EPA had to take into account in its decisions:

1. Overall Protection of Human Health and the Environment
2. Compliance with ARARs (Applicable or Relevant and Appropriate Requirements)

These are clearly the requirements with which a risk assessor is principally concerned.

Balancing criteria:

3. Long-Term Effectiveness and Permanence

4. Reduction of Toxicity, Mobility, or Volume Through Treatment

4. Short-Term Effectiveness

5. Implementability

6. Cost

These allow the use of cost-benefit analysis but do not specify or suggest any discussion of the value of γ.

Modifying criteria:

7. State/Support Agency Acceptance

8. Community Acceptance

The acceptance criteria in numbers 7 and 8 clearly include both basic value judgements and value judgements based upon inadequate understanding (see discussion in Chapter 4).

The 1996 amendment to the safe drinking water acts, allowing the explicit use of cost-benefit analysis by EPA is a further step in defining the boundaries. Ultimately many observers think that Congress must specify the value of γ, the "cost of a statistical life." If so, it is our view that they should consider at the same time the appropriate "de minimis" risk and whether or not the linear-no-threshold theory should be used in the risk calculations. These are coupled together in discussion of risks in any actual decision.

The Dual Role of the Courts

"The responsibility of those who exercise power in a democratic society is not to reflect inflamed public feeling but to help form its understanding."
—Felix Frankfurter (former Supreme Court Justice) (1928), carved in stone on the wall of the Federal Court House, Boston

The law courts are the final arbiter of whether the risks are being managed according to the laws that society has set up for the purpose. There are two basically distinct ways in which the law courts in the United States influence the management of decisions. The first is in an oversight role of the regulatory agencies to see whether or not they are following the law and the constitution. The second is in a wide application of tort law to decisions involving risk.

In Industrial Union (1980) (the Benzene case) a plurality of the U.S. Supreme Court held that the Occupational Safety and Health Administration had erred in not performing a risk assessment for the risk of occupational exposure to benzene. OSHA had noted that benzene exposures have caused leukemia, but that causation could only be attributed at exposure levels above 10 ppm. Nonetheless OSHA claimed that lower concentrations pose a risk—albeit a hypothetical or theoretical one. OSHA proposed that the concentration limit in the work place be reduced from 10 ppm to the lowest feasible level, which they arbitrarily determined to be 1 ppm. The risk may be estimated from data at higher doses by assuming proportionality (a linear no-threshold dose response). Such an attempt leads to the risk esti-

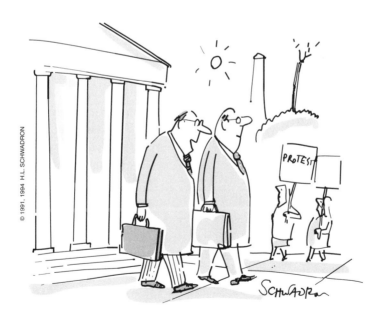

"Just for a change, wouldn't it be nice if Supreme Court justices had groupies and rock stars had dissenters?"

mates listed in the next chapter in Table 7-3. We see that this risk is comparable to other occupational risks and smaller than many; it could thus be considered insignificant. A majority of the U.S. Supreme Court held that the Secretary of Labor had not "found" that the risk was significant and by quoting the risk assessment implied that it might reasonably be used to discuss the significance. However, the Supreme Court fell short of deciding which risk level so calculated might be deemed acceptable—merely noting that 1 in 1,000 seems large and 1 in 1,000,000 seems small.

The principal agencies concerned, OSHA and EPA, seem to have interpreted the Court's decision in the following sense: management methods 1 and 2—bans and Best Available Control Technology, should be regarded as stopgap measures of risk management to be replaced whenever a good risk-benefit analysis is performed. In the case of benzene they have now performed this risk analysis, and although some analysts believe that the analysis is too conservative, OSHA has concluded that the level of 1 ppm is an appropriate one. This may not seem to be a gain since the level is the one originally proposed, but the process is now more open to view—the relevant assumptions have been laid out more thoroughly—and can therefore be considered more acceptable.

In contrast, the courts have declined to "second guess" the agencies that have a wide latitude in how to interpret the law and promulgate regulations. In Vermont Yankee Nuclear Power Co. (1978), the U.S. Supreme Court upheld the right of the Nuclear Regulatory Commission to establish reasonable rules.

Nor will the Court interfere with Congressional instructions on how an Agency promulgates regulations. In a recent decision (Whitman vs American Trucking Association, 2001), upheld the recent air pollution regulations, and rejected the idea that the U.S. EPA should perform a cost-benefit analysis in addressing how to achieve clean air. The court stated that the EPA had no authority to do this. Although the decision supported the regulation proposed by the EPA, the support leaves us with a logical impasse. Where a linear dose response relationship at low doses is likely, or even possible, as is true for air pollution, it is not possible to set a standard where there is no risk with an adequate margin of safety, as required by the Clean Air Act in this case. In practice the EPA has implicitly used cost as one of the criteria, and this may well be illegal.

It was probably the dilemmas of this sort that led William Ruckelshaus, when Administrator of the U.S. EPA in 1983, to state in a lecture at Harvard

University that "the statutes applicable to the EPA are inconsistent so that it is not possible to apply them all literally."

The effect of tort law is much more sweeping. The law (in the U.S.) is applied primarily by juries. These are picked by a process that is supposed to make them representative of the public, so that it can be said that "public perception" of a risk is the dominant factor in these decisions. If a product is widely available there is a potential for very damaging class action suits against a company with "deep pockets." A clear example of a dramatic effect is the bankruptcy of a company (Dow Corning) and the withdrawal of breast implants from the market (Angell, 1996). It seems that there is no reliable *direct* evidence that the harm claimed by the plaintiffs was caused by breast implants. However, direct evidence cannot rule out a small risk (a few percent in a lifetime) in this situation as in most others.

A problem that has been addressed by the courts in the last 10 years is that with enough financial incentive many honorable motives get perverted. Expert witnesses will exaggerate. Juries can be over responsive to this exaggeration. Judges are sometimes elected, search for campaign funds, and become susceptible to political influence. Juries can be over-responsive to this exaggeration. The process has been called a "random redistribution of wealth." Random or not, any manufacturer or distributor must pay attention to any potential health effect where risk perception is dominant.

In a dispute between two parties, judges and juries cannot be expected to know scientific details. For this reason, courts allow "expert witnesses" who can testify about the status of the science. Unlike other witnesses who can only testify to the facts in their personal knowledge, expert witnesses have a wider latitude. But in return they must be qualified as experts. The U.S. Supreme Court recently clarified the Federal Rules of Evidence that lay out what evidence may be properly brought before a federal court by an expert witness. This has been clarified in three important cases (Daubert, 1993; Joiner, 1997; Kumho Tire, 1999).

In Daubert, a lady took the drug Bendectin during pregnancy and blamed her child's birth defects on the drug. In the resultant law suit, an expert proffered an unpublished "reanalysis" of previously published human statistical studies (a "meta analysis") and purported to show that it was "more likely than not" that the Bendectin caused the problems. In remanding the case the Supreme Court mentioned (on their pages 593 and 594) several non-exclusive criteria by which such proffered testimony may be judged. None of the items in the list are absolutely necessary; nor is any individual item conclusive:

1. Has the theory been tested or can it be tested? In other words, is it falsifiable?

2. Has the theory been peer reviewed and published?

3. What is the known or potential risk of error?

4. Has the theory been generally accepted in the relevant scientific community?

5. Is the theory based on facts or data of a type reasonably relied upon by experts in the field?

6. Does the testimony have probative value that is greater than, or not outweighed by, a danger of unfair prejudice, confusion of issues, or misleading the jury?

Joiner was an engineer who had worked with transformer oil containing PCBs, and who alleged that the PCBs were the cause of his small-cell lung cancer. The testimony of two supposed "expert" witnesses were rejected by the district court, accepted by the appeal court, and finally rejected by the U.S. Supreme Court because it did not "rise above subjective belief or unsupported speculation." The Court held, inter alia, that the proffered testimony must be not only *relevant* but also *reliable.* In addition the Supreme Court emphasized that a lower court may "on its own motion or on the motion of any party" appoint an expert to serve on behalf of the court, and this expert may be selected as "agreed upon by the parties" or chosen by the court to aid in the gatekeeping role. This is sometimes arranged in a preliminary panel. Such a procedure has become known as a "Daubert Hearing."

In Kumho Tire, an automobile tire which everyone concerned agreed had a tread which was badly worn (nearly bald), exploded, and caused a crash in which a person was killed. An "expert" claimed that since he knew of no other obvious cause of the tire failure, the cause must be a manufacturing defect. His testimony was rejected by the circuit court and accepted by the court of appeals who argued that Daubert did not apply because "engineering is an art and not a science." The U.S. Supreme Court rejected this suggestion, and argued further that the less scientific the evidence, the more that the cautions that the Court had expressed in the Daubert judgement must apply.

Jasonoff (2000) has criticized these court decisions, implying that a person more influenced by "societal values" than by the standards of his expert field should be allowed to testify as to science of the issue before the courts. If a person was proffering testimony on "societal values," that might indeed be appropriate testimony to put before the jury. But in the above cases (Daubert, Joiner and Kumho Tire) the persons concerned did *not* proffer such testimony. Ideally in a toxic tort case a Probability of Causation would be calculated, but it is likely that one of Harber and Shusterman's (1996) lesser heuristics would also have a chance of success.

Notes

1 The problems of mixing assessment and decision functions might be illustrated by the following example. Two scientists A and B have both evaluated the risks of air pollution, and concluded that the risk of premature death (averaged over the population) lies somewhere in the range of 1 in a 100,000 to 1 in 10,000 per person per year. Both can agree that the problem is of such magnitude that $50 billion per year would be a reasonable sum to spend to reduce air pollution, given the general state of the economy. But if A is given decision-making authority, he is concerned this is too little, and so emphasizes the upper end of the uncertainty range, saying the risk "is" 1 in 10,000 per year (implying about 28,000 premature deaths per year, corresponding, at the EPA's figure of $6.1 million per life, to $171 billion). On the other hand, B is concerned that $171 billion is too much for society to pay, and so says that the risk "is" "only" 1 in 100,000 per year (corresponding to $17 billion). Both A and B may be making true statements from their point of view, but their statements are incomplete, having been colored by other considerations.

2 This was based, in part, on a suggestion by two nuclear scientists (E. Teller and R. Wilson) to the President.

7

Lists of Risks

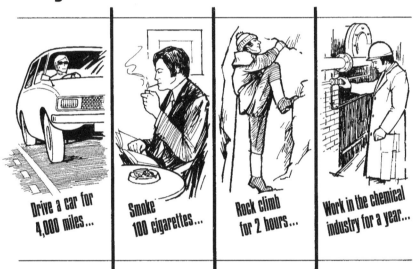

If you ...

Drive a car for 4,000 miles...

Smoke 100 cigarettes...

Rock climb for 2 hours...

Work in the chemical industry for a year...

... the risk to life is the same.

© 1980 T. Kletz.

"It is unquestionably true that [rail travel] is safer than traveling by coach or horseback...if one wants anything safer he must walk."
—H.G. Prout, (1892) The American Railway
New York, Charles Scribner and Son, p 191

The safety of technology-based systems improves with time. As will be seen below, most such systems have improved in the U.S. The first part of this quotation is still true in the year 2000. But expressed as deaths per mile traveled, train travel is now safer than walking.

Some Examples of Risk Calculations

As we said in the opening sentence of this book, life is a risky business. We went on to explain what this meant in qualitative terms, and then to describe how quantitative estimates may be made of the magnitudes of various measures of risk. The knowledge of such risk magnitudes from individual causes, however, may be of little use unless they can be related to the magnitudes of everyday risks. For otherwise one can obtain no sense of the importance of the risks, and how much notice should be taken of them.

This chapter is devoted to showing just how (quantitatively) risky are everyday life and actions by assigning numerical values to a collection of common actions which involve some element of risk. The object is to provide a background of values for familiar risks, against which the results of calculations of unfamiliar risks may be judged. Throughout the chapter we shall be specifically discussing risks of death, so that the risk measure used will be the probability of death—sometimes a population weighted average annual probability, at other times age specific annual average probabilities, and occasionally other averages. We do not claim, however, to present a complete list of risks. In order to present all the risks on as common a basis as possible, we have tried to arrange our examples so that we can specify some quantity or measure of activity which will give either a lifetime probability of 10^{-6} (one in a million) of dying from that activity, or an annual average probability of 10^{-6} of dying. Since the average expectation of life of a person in the U.S. is about 78 years (in the year 2000), for any given risk there will be a factor of about 78 difference between the numerical values of such measures. The annual average probability (that is, averaged over the lifetime of an individual) is about equal to the population average (that is, averaged over all ages according to the age structure of the population) provided the risks are small enough.

The Risk (of Death) in Living

The first risk (of death) to consider is that in living itself (i.e. the probability of dying). In case this sounds paradoxical, it must be realized that the sum total of all lifetime average risks (of death) must be one (absolute certainty) since everybody dies. From the risk analyst's point of view, we might say that the whole object of living is to die! Our efforts go into attempting to reduce annual risks, in order to make it more likely that the inevitable death will occur later, and longevity is increased. We look first at the probability of dying because it corresponds to the sum total of all the risks to which we are exposed. If we had a complete list of all activities undertaken by everybody, together with a list of the risks involved in such activities, and provided that we took care to avoid double counting, we could add all the risks together to obtain the total risk of dying. Evidently, for any individual or group, such a sum will vary from individual to individual or group to group, but if we average everything over the whole population we simply get the average risk

FIGURE 7-1

Time (in Hours) in Which Probability of Dying Is One in a Million, vs. Age (linear scale)

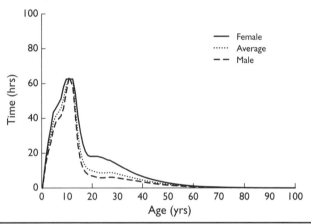

FIGURE 7-2

Time (in Hours) in Which Probability of Dying Is One in a Million, vs. Age (logarithmic scale)

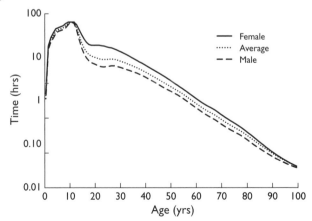

of dying for that population. Figures 7-1 and 7-2 show the time required to accumulate a probability of one in a million (10^{-6}) of dying at a given age for the U.S. population in 1998. This is a measure of the reciprocal of the total risk of living. Notice the linear scale in Figure 7-1 and the logarithmic scale in Figure 7-2.

The large range of times is better shown on the logarithmic scale of Figure 7-2, but Figure 7-1 may show the range more dramatically for those unfamiliar with logarithmic plots. The time required increases rapidly with age initially, reaching a maximum of 62 hours at age 10–11, and then falls rapidly. The dip in the curves near age 21–22, especially pronounced in males, is caused mainly by the risks of auto accidents. After age 30 the curves decrease steadily (this is especially obvious on Figure 7-2), reaching 7 minutes (males) to 11 minutes (females) at age 80. These curves are, of course, just the reciprocal of the age-specific death rate curves for the U.S. population, and convey the same information. If we know the number N of males aged 20 (for example) in the population, and the time to accumulate the one in a million ($10-6$) probability of dying for males aged 20 is 6.5 hours (from Figure 7-1), then in 1 year the probability of death is (8,760/6.5)/1,000,000 = 0.0013 (1.3×10^{-3}) and so 0.0013 N (1.3×10^{-3} N) males aged 20 die each year.

Life Expectancy

Figures 7-1 and 7-2 correspond to what occurred in the U.S. in 1997. From year to year the probabilities of dying change gradually as changes occur in our society, so they are not strictly applicable to other years, although the rate of change is small. If these probabilities were to remain constant, it is possible to calculate what the population age structure (represented, for example, by the fraction surviving to a given age) would be if the same number of children were born each year, and all grew up subject to the age specific risks of Figures 7-1 and 7-2 (and there was no immigration or emigration). The result is shown in Figure 7-3, where it was seen that most people would survive until their 60s, but there is a rapid drop off in survivors after age 75. The average age of the population shown in Figure 7-3 is known as the life expectancy or expectation of life (at birth) in 1998. It is not precisely the expected length of life of a child born in 1998. In actual fact, of course, such a child faces different risks—e.g., the actual risk for that child at age 5 is the 5-year-old's risk in 2004 (which is not yet measurable), not in 1998 (which *has* been measured). The expectation of life (at birth) is thus a form of

F I G U R E   7 - 3

Age Structure of Static Population in 1997

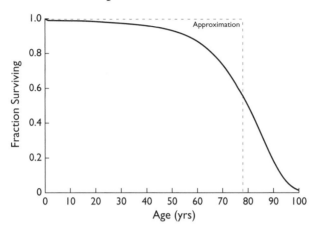

average measure of the risk of dying at all ages, since the risks at all ages are taken into account in computing it, and is thus a measure which may be used to compare between years to see if risks have been increasing or decreasing on average. The variation of expectation of life (at birth) with time was shown for the U.S. in Figure 1-2 and for various other countries in Figure 1-3. The expectation of life has been increasing, mostly steadily, except in Russia, corresponding to a mostly steady decline in the average annual risk of death.

A Selection of Risks: Historically Calculated

In the tables and graphs that follow the text of this chapter, we present a diverse selection of risks variously calculated. It is often desirable to compare risks of the same type if possible, so we present lists where risks are grouped clearly into categories, within which intercomparison is easily justified and probably moderately accurate. But we also specifically introduce disparate risks to stimulate thought. Most of these tables apply to the U.S. We start in Table 7-1a with a set of occupational risks calculated from historical statistics. Many have been declining steadily over the years. The values given are derived from the statistics given in the various sources noted in the tables (and we include where applicable the table number of a particular source, e.g Statistical Abstract of the U.S. 1999 edition). The values given are crude rates rather than the age-adjusted rates. The calculation is especially simple. All that is required is a knowledge of the numbers who died in the past, and the

TABLE 7-1A

Occupational Risks

Deaths per Year of Risky Activity (Disabling Injuries Not Included Except When Stated)

Occupation or Industry	Annual per Capita Risk per 100,000	Annual Trend per 100,000	Source Based On	Ref, #
All Industries	7	-0.2	1955–98	4
Women in Industry	1	+0.1	1992–94	11
Women in industry (homicide)	0.4		1992–94	11
Colorado industry (average)	7		1982–94	10
Colorado industry (homicide)	0.6		1982–94	10
Manufacturing	3.2	–0.2	1955–98	3#705
Retail trade	1.7	–0.2	1955–98	3#705
Service	1.5	–0.3	1955–98	3#705
Government	1.7		1998	3#705
Transport and public utilities	12	–1.2	1955–98	3#705
Construction	14	–2.4	1955–97	3#710
Construction (women)	6		1992–94	11
Mining and quarrying	24	-7.5	1955–98	3#705
Coal mining (accidents)	24	-3	1977–99	5
Coal Mining (China)	500		2000	text
Metal mining and milling	56	–2.2	1959–98	5
Stone Quarries	40	–1	1959–98	5
Stone (underground)	9	1	1978–98	5
Nonmetal mining undergnd	46	–2	1979–98	5
Nonmetal mining surface	18	1	1978–98	5
Agriculture	23	–1.8	1955–98	7,3#716

continued

populations at risk. In Table 7-1a the risk (and rate of decline, where applicable) is as given for the last year in the range shown. In principle the rates of decline should be obtained by regressing the logarithm of the rate against time, and the variability is the year-to-year variability around this regression line. In many cases a simple visual approximation is used.

In the first edition of this book we presented tables such as Table 7-1a in "scientific notation" $1*10^{-5}$ or 1×10^{-5} instead of in "ordinary" notation, 1 in a hundred thousand. For a specialist risk assessor this can be useful, particularly for comparison of wide ranges of risks. However, here we are deliberately expressing the risks as fatalities per year per 100,000 persons at risk, so that

T A B L E   7 - 1 A
Occupational Risks *(continued)*
Deaths per Year of Risky Activity (Disabling Injuries Not Included Except When Stated)

Occupation or Industry	Annual per Capita Risk per 100,000	Annual Trend per 100,000	Source Based On	Ref, #
Tractor fatalities	10	−1	1969–98	7
Police officers killed in line of duty				
Total	32	+0.5	1975–98	3#355
By felons	15	+0.3	1975–97	4, text
Railroad employees	15	−0.4	1975–00	9
Steel workers (accidents only)	28		1969–72	2
Assassination, murder, or battle injury				
President of United States	1,900		1789–2000	text
President of Egypt	1,900		1948–2000	text
President of France	1,400		1848–2000	text
King/Queen of England	430		1066–2000	text
Spouse of King/Queen	210		1066–2000	text
Government office worker	9		1997	text
Airline pilot (accidents only)	10		1997	text
Frequent flying professor (accident only)	3		2000	text
Astronaut Space launch (per launch):				
From direct data (Including Challenger)	4,000		1975–86	text
O-ring failure at 31°F	13,000			text
O-ring failure at 60°F	2,000			text
Fire fighters (buildings)	40	-0.7	1972-99	8
Wildfire fighters				
Total	21		2000	6, 8
Per 12 months work	100		2000	6, 8

Sources: [Ref (1) #19 means table 19 of reference 1]

(1) Murphy (2000); also available on the web at: *www.cdc.gov/nchs/data/nvs48_11.pdf*

(2) Baldewiicz et al. (1974)

(3) Statistical Abstract of the United States 2000 edition (and earlier editions for the trends)

(4) NSC (Annual)

(5) Mine Safety and Health at www.msha.gov/centurystats/centurystats.htm

(6) Mangan (1999) see also *www.fs.fed.us/fire/safety/fatalities/*

(7) Runyan (1990) report on NM agriculture

(8) National Fire Data Center (1999) *www.usfa.fema.gov/nfdc*

(9) Federal Railroad Aministration (Office of Safety) *safetydata.fra.dot.gov/*)

(10)Vassalo et al. (1997) also: stats.bls.gov/opub/cwc/1997/spring/art5abs.htm/)

(11)Knestaut (1996) also at: stats.bls.gov/opub/cwc/1997/summer/brief3.htm/)

TABLE   7 - 1 B

Occupational Risks

Deaths per Year of Risky Activity Involving Uncertain Dose-Response Relationship.
These risks could be zero if there is a threshold. (Disabling injuries not included
except when stated.)

Occupation	Annual Risk per 100,000	Uncertainty Factor	Year	Source
Coal miner with black lung disease	500	⅓ to 3	2000	text
Smoking asbestos worker at 0.1 fiber/ml	18	⅓ to 3	2000	text
Teacher (female age 25–55) in typical school with 0.0002 fibers/ml average asbestos level				
Total (smoker)	0.013		2000	text
Total (non smoker)	0.006		2000	text
Mesothelioma	0.005		2000	text
Lung cancer (smoker)	0.008		2000	text
Lung cancer (non smoker)	0.001		2000	text
Mesothelioma if risk reduced for chrysotile	0.0002		2000	text
Smoking (male) office worker with asbestos at 0.001 fiber/cc	0.1		2000	text
Nuclear power plant worker (exposed at NRC maximum)	20		2000	text
Airline pilot (cosmic ray exposure)	14		2000	text
Hospital X-ray technician (world average)	10		2000	text

the relative magnitude may be more easily seen, and negligible risks may be seen to be negligible. This approach also has the advantage that it is the standard notation used by the National Center for Health Statistics to present various risks.

Table 7-1b is a further set of estimates of occupational risks due to specific on-the-job exposures, all of which involve an uncertain dose response relationship. As noted in Chapter 2, the dose response is generally unknown when the risk is only a few percent above background risk. If there is a threshold in the dose response relationship, most of these risks could be zero. Even with the pessimism (conservatism) of a linear dose response relationship risk estimates for risks tend to be lower than the historically derived total occupational risks for which the relationship between years of "exposure" and death rate is clearly linear. Nonetheless the cancer risks arouse particularly strong emotions as noted in Chapter 4.

The number of persons who are exposed to the risk is obviously important both for deciding the total cost of reducing a risk, and the desirability of

TABLE   7-2A

Risks of Death Due to an Action
(Public Risks Historically Calculated)

Occupation or Industry	Annual per Capita Risk per 100,000	Annual Trend per 100,000	Source Based On	Ref, #
Total crude death rate (U.S.)	870	–79	1980–98	3#1355
Heart disease	271	–3.6	1980–98	1#B, 3#126
Diabetes mellitus	24	+0.4	1980–98	1#B, 3#126
Pneumonia and influenza	35	+0.5	1980–98	1#B, 3#126
Chronic pulmonary disease42	+0.9		1980–98	1#B, 3#126
Cigarette smoking (per smoker)	300			text
All fatal cancers	200	–4	1978–98	1#B, 3#126
Respiratory	59	-0.6	1978–98	3#126
Digestive Organs	47	–1.3	1978–98	3#126
Genital Organs	22	–0.5	1978–98	3#126
Breast	16	–0.7	1978–98	3#126
Cancer from arsenic at 500 ppb in water	140		2000	text
Motor vehicle accident (total)	15	–0.4	1972–98	1#19, 3#1036
Alcohol related (BAC>0.01)	6			9
Pedestrian deaths	2	–0.1	1972–98	1#19, 3#1035
Cyclist per total pop.	0.30	–0.01	1980–98	1#19, 3#1035
Cyclist at night	0.1		1985	6
Collision with animals	0.5		1998	
Using cell phone	0.15		2000	2
Motor vehicle accident (New Mexico)	35		2000	
Rail grade crossing acc. (total)	0.18		1996	8
Not involving automobiles	0.027		1996	8
Rail trespassing accidents	0.15		1999	10
All other accidents	19	0	1990–97	3#126
Home accidents (all ages)	11	0	1978–98	4, 11, text
All toys (under 15)	0.027	-0.001	1985-99	6, 3#12
Garage door (age 2–14)	0.009		1982–89	6, 3#12
Toy chest lids (age 0.5–1.5)	0.06		1973–82	6, 3#12
Electrocution	0.18	–0.02	1980–96	3#135
Illegal drugs (per total population)	5.6	+0.1	1980–97	3#141
Alcohol (direct)	6.3	–0.1	1980–96	3#142
Cirrhosis of the liver (alcohol-related)	4	–0.4	1974–97	text
Objects inhaled and ingested	1.2	+0.001	1968–96	3#135
Misadventures during medical care, etc., complications	1.1	+0.001	1980–98	1, 3#135

continued

TABLE   7 - 2 A
Risks of Death Due to an Action *(continued)*
(Public Risks Historically Calculated)

Occupation or Industry	Annual per Capita Risk per 100,000	Annual Trend per 100,000	Source Based On	Ref, #
Falls: (includes unidentified fractures)				
General population	6	−0.009	1977–98	11, 3#12
Over 70 years old	43		1998	11, 3#12
Drowning (unintentional)	1.6	+0.2	1963–98	1#19
Drowning (UK)	1		1998	7
Fires	1.4	−0.07	1963–77	1
Firearms (total)	11	−0.1	1968–98	1#19
Suicide	6.5		1968–98	1#19
Homicide	4.4		1968–98	1#19
Suicides (total)	11	−0.03	1980–98	1#B, 3#138
Homicide (victims) (total)	6.8	−0.4	1979–98	1#B, 3#126
Black males	56	−4.6	1995–7	3#139
Accidental Poisoning (total)	4		1998	1#19
Gases and vapors	0.24	−0.03	1977–96	3#135
Solids and liquids				
(not drugs or medicines)	0.16	−0.02	1977–96	3#135
Suffocation (total)	4.1		2000	1#19
Unintentional	1.7		2000	1#19
Babies in adult beds	0.24		1990–97	6
Suicide	2.1		2000	1#19
Yearly coast to coast flight (accident risk)	1		2000	text
Being hit by falling aircraft	0.004		1998	text
Being hit by meteorite	0.04		2000	text
Tornadoes	0.015		1950–2000	5, 3#405
Floods	0.045		1950–97	3#405
Lightning	0.016	−0.002	1977–97	3#405
Tropical cyclones and hurricanes	0.009		1952–98	3#405
Drought or heat wave	0.4		1980–00	3#406
Bites and stings by venomous	0.017		1998	11

Sources: [Ref 1#19 means Table 19 of reference 1]

(1) Murphy (2000); also available on the web at: *www.cdc.gov/nchs/data/nvs48_11.pdf*

(2) Harvard Center for Risk Analysis "Risk in Perspective" Summer 2000

(3) Statistical Abstract of the United States 2000 edition (and earlier references with different table numbers)

continued

TABLE   7 - 2 A
Risks of Death Due to an Action *(continued)*
(Public Risks Historically Calculated)

---

(4) NSC (Annual)

(5) Storm reduction Center, NOAA also available on the web at: *www.spc.noaa.gov*

(6) Consumer Product Safety Commission reports: *www.cpsc.gov*

(7) Royal Society for Prevention of Accidents (UK) *www.rospa.co.uk*

(8) Bureau of Transportation Statistics: *www.bts.gov*

(9) Mothers Against Drunk driving: *www.madd.org*

(10) Operation Lifesaver: *www.oli.org*

(11) The risk for bites, stings and falls (and many other risks not listed here) is derived from the website. *www.cdc.gov/nchs/datawh/statab/unpubd/mortabs/gmwki.htm*

This includes all the ICD classifications E880-E888. This is 50% greater than the falls attributed in Table 1054 of the statistical abstracts. But classification E888 is for unidentified falls, and E887 for deaths by fracture not otherwise identified. For examining trends consistency is important. The risk of falls for those over 70 is the number of deaths by falls of those over 70 divided by the population over 70 and is 10 times the average risk.

* Factor of $^1/_{10}$ to 10.

doing so. The separation of occupational risks, where a limited number of people are exposed, in Table 7-1a and 7-1b and the public risks in Tables 7-2a and 7-2b is a partial recognition of this. It is noteworthy that most occupational risks have declined and the rate of decline is greater than it was in 1982. One of the ways that risks averaged over an occupation are being reduced is by searching out sub-groups at especially high risk and attending to them. Such attention is encouraged by various workers' protection laws.

The employer indifference of 1906 was exemplified in Upton Sinclair's novel, *The Jungle:* "In the beginning he had been fresh and strong, and he had gotten a job the first day; but now he was second-hand, a damaged article, so to speak, and they did not want him... they had worn him out, with their speeding-up and their carelessness, and now they had thrown him away!" This probably still applies to developing countries, and to perhaps some small groups, particularly immigrants to the U.S.

Table 7-2a is a list of various commonplace public risks of death, also calculated from historical data. Most of these risks would be considered involuntary. There may be some overlapping between categories in this table (home accidents, for example, includes falls within the home).

Although these risk estimates seem very simple, there is often an ambiguity of the definition of the occupation or grout risk. Since the numerator and

TABLE 7-2B

Risks of (an) Action(s)

(Public Risks Involving an uncertain Dose-Response Relationship. Any of These Risks Could Be Zero if a Threshold Exists)

Occupation	Annual Risk per 100,000	Uncertainty Factor	Source Year	Ref, #
Coal miner with black lung disease	500	⅓ to 3	2000	text
Air pollution (average in U.S.)	25	⅟∞to 5	2000	text
Cancer from drinking:				
Arsenic in water at U.S. EPA level of 50 ppb	140		2000	text
Arsenic in water at Fresno levels	2.8		2000	text
Chloroform in water at EPA limit (100 ppb)	0.07		2000	text
Risk from potassium 40 normally in body	1		2000	text
Living in an ordinary southern California house with indoor air pollution (TEAM study)	0.77		2000	text
One way transatlantic flight (cosmic rays)	0.14		2000	text
One drink with alcohol per day:				
Cancer and other adverse	5			Ch. 2, p. 52
Cardiovascular (reduction)	−200			Ch. 2, p. 52
Living near a superfund site:				
Love Canal	500			text
Stringfellow (house)	0.6			text
Stringfellow (school)	35			text
Midvale (Utah) max estimate	4			text
Midvale (Utah) best estimate	0.01			text
Old EPA regulatory limit (10^{-6}/ lifetime pessimistically calculated)	0.0014		2000	text
Authors' estimate of real risk at *old* EPA regulatory limit	<0.0001		2000	text
Eating ice cream daily	19		1999	1

Source:

(1) Cancer risk from dioxin calculated by Gough, M. and S. Milloy, *http://www.junkscience.org/dec99/benjerry2.htm*

denominator often come from different sources, the definition can be different in the two cases leading to an error. For example the deaths in fighting fires includes helicopter crashes and crashing motor vehicles hurrying to the scene. The number of people fighting wildfires in the U.S. should therefore include not only the people registered but these auxiliary people. On the other hand, few if any people are employed for the full year. The choice of group at risk (discussed in Chapter 1 as the boundary of the problem) can

FIGURE 7-4

Age-Adjusted Death Rates for the 15 Leading Causes of Death: U.S., 1950–1998

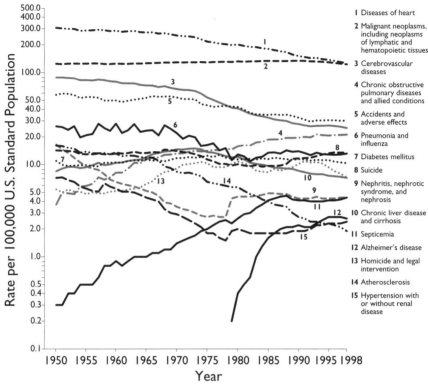

1 Diseases of heart

2 Malignant neoplasms, including neoplasms of lymphatic and hematopoietic tissues

3 Cerebrovascular diseases

4 Chronic obstructive pulmonary diseases and allied conditions

5 Accidents and adverse effects

6 Pneumonia and influenza

7 Diabetes mellitus

8 Suicide

9 Nephritis, nephrotic syndrome, and nephrosis

10 Chronic liver disease and cirrhosis

11 Septicemia

12 Alzheimer's disease

13 Homicide and legal intervention

14 Atherosclerosis

15 Hypertension with or without renal disease

lead to very different values of the risk estimate. This is illustrated in the specific example below of the risk of being killed by bear attack. In comparing risks from one year to the next great care must be taken in using the data to be sure there is consistency. This also applies when one presents, as here, a "raw" risk averaged over the population of all ages, and the age distribution of the population changes. Many risks vary with age. Then the "raw" risk becomes less useful and for purposes of studying the changes with time, an artificial "age adjusted" risk is often constructed valid for a society with a static age distribution (see Appendix III for the methods adopted). In Figure 7-4 we present from Murphy (2000) the age adjusted death rates for various

FIGURE   7 - 5

Annual Fatality in Various Occupations per 100,000 Persons Employed

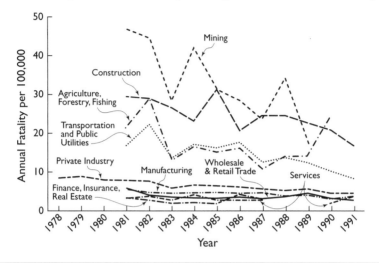

FIGURE   7 - 6

Risk of Cirrhosis of the Liver in U.S. States vs Average Alcohol Consumption

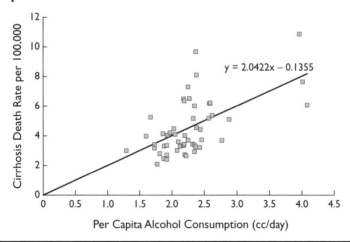

$y = 2.0422x - 0.1355$

TABLE   7-2 C

Lifetime Risk from Action Stated

Action	Lifetime Risk (Parts per 100,000)	Year	Source
Cancer from eating:			
1 tablespoon of peanut butter (if hepatitis B1)	0.0003	2000	text
1 tablespoon of peanut butter (NO hepatitis)	0.00001	2000	text
4 daily tablespoons of peanut butter (if suffering from hepatitis B1)	30	2000	test
4 daily tablespoons of peanut butter (NO hepatitis B1) (cancer risk)	1.3	2000	text
½ lb of charcoal broiled steak a week	3	2000	text
Mesothelioma in female exposed from ages 6–16 to asbestos in school at 0.0002 fibers/cc	0.24	2000	text
Mesothelioma in male school child (5 to 10 times smaller if chrysotile risk is reduced)	0.16	2000	text
Risk of deep space probe (approx.)	0.000001		text
Risk of deep space probe (NASA)	0.00000003		text
EPA regulation range			
Upper end	10	2000	text
Lower end	0.1	2000	text

diseases, showing the trends. This graph also shows breaks in the curves due to changes in definition of the diseases.

Most of the risks have been steadily going down in the 20 years since the first edition of this book. This is illustrated in Figure 7-5 where we plot trends. (OSHA, 1997) for a number of occupations. These trends generally continue those seen in earlier times (shown in the first edition). Figure 7-6 plots cirrhosis of the liver against alcohol consumption in various states showing how that risk is estimated.

Table 7-2b is a further set of everyday risks, expressed on an annual basis, which involve an uncertain- response relationship. They could be zero if there is a threshold.

Table 7-2c shows a set of everyday risks expressed on a lifetime basis. Note that they could be zero if there is a threshold in the relevant dose response relationship.

Table 7-3, in contrast, shows a set of voluntary risks of death—mostly those incurred in sports or in recreational activities. These are shown separately because they are voluntary risks. Most people will voluntarily engage in activities far more risky than activities imposed upon them by other members

TABLE 7 - 3

Recreational Risks

Sport	Average Annual Risk per 100,000	Average Annual Deaths	Estimated Population at Risk	Years of Coverage	Source
All children's toys	0.044	22	60,000	1985	CPSC
Aerial acrobatics (professional)	<~200	0.22	350	1970–78	1
Air show/air racing and acrobatics	500	4.9	1,000	1971–77	1
Flying amateur/home built aircraft	300	25	10,000	1970–77	1
Bicycle racing (registered)	1.4	0.33	10,000	1970–96	1, 5
Boating	5	815	300,000	1972–98	5, 6
Whitewater boating					
(Experienced)	270	27	10,000	1995–99	AWA
(Inexperienced)	70	36	50,000	1995–99	AWA
Waterskiing	47	47	100,000	1995	
Bob sledding	<~70	0	450	1970–78	1
Boxing	40	2	5,000	1995	5
Football (total)	0.6	6	1,000,000	1995	5
Sandlot	0.2	1.7	1,000,000	1970–78	1
Professional and semiprofessional	7	0.11	1,500	1970–78	1
High school	1.2	13	1,000,000	1970–96	1, 5
College	3	1.2	4,000	1970–96	1, 5
Basketball	0.4	4	1,000,000	1995	5
Glider flying	40	7	20,000	1970–77	1
Hang gliding	26	13	50,000	1995	1, 5
Hunting	3	600	2,000,000	1972	2, 3
Ice yachting	5	0.22	5,000	1970–78	1
Balloon flying	90	2.6	3,000	1970–77	1
Mountain recreation:					
Hiking	6.4			1996	5
Casual climbing	57			1996	5
Mountaineering	60	34	60,000	1951–78	1, 4
Dedicated climbing	600			1996	5
Himalayas per ascent	13000		~100	1920–99	text
Bear attack:					
Backpacker	1.3	0.13	10,000	1955–2000	text
Concession worker	10	0.07	500	1955–2000	text
Power boat racing	8	5.2	7,000	1970–78	1
Professional stunting	<~1000	1	200	1975–78	1
Rodeo	<~3	0.33	30,000	1970–78	1
Sail planing	59			1996	

continued

T A B L E   7 - 3
Recreational Risks *(continued)*

Sport	Average Annual Risk per 100,000	Average Annual Deaths	Estimated Population at Risk	Years of Coverage	Source
Scuba diving	42	126	300,000	1970–96	1, 3
Ski racing	2.5	2	80,000	1970–96	1, 3
Sky diving (U.S.)	58	29	50,000	1995–00	
Sky diving (international)	30	74	250,000	1991	
Snow skiing	12	41	300,000	1995	
Snowmobiling	13	60	450,000	1995	5
Spelunking	<~1	44	10,000	1970–78	1
Snowboarding	0.25	5	2,000,000	1991–95	
Sport parachuting	200	41	20,000	1970–78	1
Horseracing (thoroughbred)	100	2.6	2,000	1970–78	1
Swimming	3	2,600	8,000,000	1972–78	2, 3
Tilting soda machines	2.5	5	50000	1985–87	5

Sources:

(1) "Statistical Bulletin" Metropolitan Life Insurance Company (1979) This was the principal source for this table in the first edition but it is no longer being issued. This makes the numbers somewhat less consistent than desirable and much more uncertain than the estimates in the previous two tables.

(2) Bureau of the Census

(3) National Safety Council (annual)

(4) Ferris (1963)

(5) Cosio (1992)

(6) National Boating against Drunk Driving (BADD)

of society. These risks are much harder to quantify. Often the number of deaths can be determined moderately well, but the number of persons engaged in the risky activity is uncertain. Moreover, the risks vary. Usually there is a small "professional" group intensely engaged in the activity with a high risk, and a much larger "amateur" or "non-professional" group, with a smaller one. The average risk is then often dominated by the small group with the high risk.

In general the recreational risks have not been reduced in the last 20 years as as much as occupational risks have. It seems that when a recreation is made safer, individuals begin to engage in hazardous activities that would have been considered too risky before.

Some Risks of "One in a Million"

Time (or Action) to Accumulate a Risk of One in a Million from the Cause Indicated (Historically Calculated)

Motor Vehicle Accident	100 miles
Falls (average over life)	6 days
Falls (average under 70)	15 hours
Drowning	19 days
Fires	13 dqays
Firearms	3 days
Electrocution	200 days
Tornadoes	5½ years
Floods	2 years
Lighting	6 years
Occupational Risks—Working in:	
Manufacturing	100 days
Government	10 days
Transport	3 days
Agriculture	1½ days
Construction	3 days
Coal mine accidents	1½ days
Black lung disease	2 hours
Police officer	1¼ days
Pilot	3 days
Frequent Flying Professor	10 days

Note: the larger risks have a *smaller* number in this table!

Time (or Action) to Reach One in a Million Risk

There are many other ways of presenting these risks, with different ways suited for various purposes. In Figures 7-1 and 7-2 we provided overall background by showing how long in normal life it takes to accumulate a risk of 10^{-6} (one in a million) of dying (depending on age) and given another yardstick to judge a one in a million (10^{-6}) risk, In Tables 7-4a and 7-4b, we list some of the risks that we face, as listed in Tables 7-1a, 7-1b, 7-2a, 7-2b, and 7-3 and put them into a form so that each corresponds to a risk of one in a million—10^{-6}. This table perhaps helps to place different risks in perspective, but some of the interpretations have to be strained a little to get them into this format, so that they are difficult to compare.

TABLE 7-4B

Some Risks of "One in a Million"

Involving Uncertain Dose-Response Relationship

Time (or action) to accumulate a risk of one in a million from the cause indicated. These times could be infinite, or the quantity equal to the threshold dose, if there is a threshold in the dose response relationship. Uncertainties are about a factor of three in addition to the uncertainty of whether or not there is a threshold.

1. Smoking two cigarettes (risk of heart disease included)
2. Drinking thirty diet sodas with saccharin
3. Eating four tablespoons of peanut butter a year if one has hepatitis B1
4. Eating four tablespoons of peanut butter every ten days for a person without hepatitis B1
5. Eating one hundred fifty (½ lb) charcoal broiled steaks (risk of benzopyrene and other aromatic hydrocarbons)
6. Eating one hundred 100 gram servings of shrimp (formaldeyde risk)
7. Eating one hundred 1 gram servings of brown mustard (allylisothiocyanate risk)
8. Eating thirty-five slices of fresh bread (formaldehyde risk)
9. Eating three hundred and fifty slices of stale bread (formaldehyde risk)
10. Eating one-half basil leaf (weighing 1 gram) (estragole risk).
11. Drinking seventy pints of Beer a year (Cancer risk of alcohol)
12. Exposed to Los Angeles or Sacramento water for fifteen years (chloroform risk only— arsenic risk additional)
13. Being exposed to radon in drinking water at typical California central valley levels for six months
14. Drinking water with EPA limit of arsenic (50 ppb) for three days
15. Drinking Fresno water for three weeks (arsenic risk assuming linearity from known risks noted above)
16. One quarter of a typical diagnostic chest X-ray
17. Indoor air pollution risk for living in a typical Dutch house for two weeks (based upon average of four houses—organics only) (Tancrede et al. 1987)
18. Indoor air pollution risk for living in a Southern California house for two weeks, assuming exposures measured in first season of TEAM study; one month for exposures in the second season (Tancrede et al. 1987)
19. Nonsmoker living with average level (1.5 pCi/l) of radon gas in U.S. homes for one week
20. A nonsmoker living in a home with a smoker for two weeks
21. Forty days of living in Denver compared to Philadelphia (radiation)
22. Drinking one-half pint of milk per day for someone without hepatitis B1
23. Drinking one-half pint of milk a month for someone with hepatitis B1

All the above risks of consumption or inhalation are risks relevant to adults consuming this amount. Children consuming half this mount would be at comparable risk.

Loss of Life Expectancy (LOLE)

The risk of death in the Tables 7-1 to 7-3 is not the correct description of a risk for a purist. We all die. The largest single cause of death is birth! The tables are clearly to be interpreted as risks of *premature* death. It would be desirable to calculate how premature (in Years of Life Lost or YOLL by an accident or disease). In a similar way to that described for deriving the expectation of life at birth, we may evaluate the expectation of life at any given age—the expected time to death of a person of that given age and subjected in the future to the age specific risks of 1999. Any changes in the risks to which any person is exposed will change that person's expectation of life, an increase in the risks decreasing their expectation of life, and a decrease in risks increasing it. The magnitude of such changes—the loss of life expectancy—may be computed by using tables of death rates. For our purposes it is straightforward to make a reasonably accurate estimate of the loss of life expectancy due to any given risk. Figure 7-3 shows that most people in the U.S. would survive to their seventies (if they faced current age-specific risks), while few would survive past their early eighties. So we may approximate Figure 7-3 by a curve in which all survive to age 78 (the expectation of life at birth), and then all die. Then, according to this approximation an excess risk, p at age t leads to a loss of life expectancy of just $(78 - t) \times p$ years and if we average over the population (i.e. over all ages) an excess risk p leads to an average loss of life expectancy of $39 \times p$ years, i.e. approximately 20 minutes for a risk of 10^{-6}. If the risk is a continuing one, say p per year, the loss of life expectancy is just

$$\sum_{t=0}^{t=78} (78 - t)\, p \approx 39 \times 78\, p = 3{,}042\, p \tag{7-1}$$

since there is a probability p of a loss of $(78 - t)$ years for each of the ages t from 0 to 78. An excess risk of one in a million (10^{-6}) per year thus corresponds to a loss of life expectancy of $3{,}042 \times 10^{-6}$ year = 1 day. An excess risk of one in a million (10^{-6}) per life corresponds to a loss of life expectancy of 20 minutes, just 78 times smaller.

This works when the risk is roughly constant throughout the lifetime as it is for many accidents. But cancer, a disease primarily of old age, results in an average loss of life (YOLL) of 18 years for each victim. The average loss of life due to air pollution probably varies with the exposure. At one time the air pollution incidents (such as the London fog in December 1952) were believed to "merely" cause death premature by a few days, but that view is now

FIGURE 7-7

Loss of Life Expectancy for Various Risks (from Cohen)

(a)

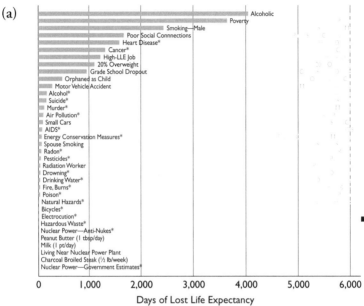

(b)

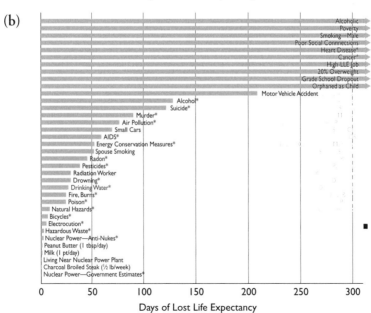

continued

FIGURE 7 - 7

Loss of Life Expectancy for Various Risks (from Cohen) *(continued)*

(c)

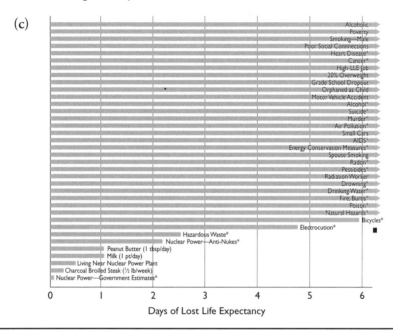

Days of Lost Life Expectancy

unsustainable, and a year or more is considered likely. The concept of risk needs a little care in definition when the deleterious effect is delayed from the cause.

Next, we present in Figures 7-7a, 7-7b, and 7-7c, modified from Cohen (1991), the average reduction in life expectancy from several risks (each figure shows the same information, but with different scales to allow comparisons over a very wide range). As noted in earlier chapters this is often a very useful way of illustrating the risks. The figures also show the smallness of many of the risks with which the public are concerned.

The Human Exposure/Rodent Potency (HERP) list of carcinogenic risks, prepared by Gold, Slone and Ames (2001) is shown in Table 7-5. Recall from Chapter 2 that this is related to RISK in our notation by

$$RISK = HERP \ln 2/100 . \tag{7-2}$$

T A B L E   7 - 5

Ranking Possible Carcinogenic Hazards from Average U.S. Exposures to Rodent Carcinogens (Gold et al. 2001)

[Chemicals that occur naturally in foods are in bold.] *Daily human exposure:* Reasonable daily intakes are used to facilitate comparisons. The calculations assume a daily dose for a lifetime. *Possible hazard:* The human dose of rodent carcinogen is divided by 70 kg to give a mg/kg/day of human exposure, and this dose is given as the percentage of the TD_{50} in the rodent (mg/kg/day) to calculate the Human Exposure/Rodent Potency index (HERP). TD_{50} values used in the HERP calculation are averages calculated by taking the harmonic mean (see Section VIII) of the TD_{50}s of the positive tests in that species from the Carcinogenic Potency Database. Average TD_{50} values, have been calculated separately for rats and mice, and the more potent value is used for calculating possible hazard.

HERP (%)	Possible hazard	Average Daily Exposure	"Potency" TD_{50} (mg/kg/day)[a] Rats	Mice
140	EDB: production workers (high exposure) (before 1977)	Ethylene dibromide, 150 mg	1.52	(7.45)
17	Clofibrate	Clofibrate, 2 g	169	•
14	Phenobarbital, 1 sleeping pill	Phenobarbital, 60 mg	(+)	6.09
6.8	1,3-Butadiene: rubber industry workers (1978–86)	1,3-Butadiene, 66.0 mg	(261)	13.9
6.2	**Comfrey-pepsin tablets, 9 daily (no longer recommended)**	**Comfrey root, 2.7 g**	626	•
6.1	Tetrachloroethylene: dry cleaners with dry-to-dry units (1980–90)	Tetrachloroethylene, 433 mg	101	(126)
4.0	Formaldehyde: production workers (1979)	Formaldehyde, 6.1 mg	2.19	(43.9)
2.4	Acrylonitrile: production workers (1960–1986)	Acrylonitrile, 405 µg	16.9	•
2.2	Trichloroethylene: vapor degreasing (before 1977)	Trichloroethylene, 1.02 g	668	(1,580)
2.1	**Beer, 257 g**	**Ethyl alcohol, 13.1 ml**	9110	(16,300)
1.4	Mobile home air (14 hrs./day)	Formaldehyde, 2.2 mg	2.19	(43.9)
1.3	**Comfrey-pepsin tablets, 9 daily (no longer recommended)**	**Symphytine, 1.8 mg**	1.91	•
0.9	Methylene chloride: workers, industry average (1940s–80s)	Methylene chloride, 471 mg	724	(1,100)

continued

TABLE   7-5

Ranking Possible Carcinogenic Hazards from Average U.S. Exposures to Rodent Carcinogens (Gold et al. 2001) *(continued)*

HERP (%)	Possible hazard	Average Daily Exposure	"Potency" TD_{50} (mg/kg/day)[a] Rats	"Potency" TD_{50} (mg/kg/day)[a] Mice
0.5	Wine, 28.0 g	Ethyl alcohol, 3.36 ml	9110	(16,300)
0.5	Dehydroepiandrosterone (DHEA)	DHEA supplement, 25 mg	68.1	•
0.4	Conventional home air (14 hrs./day)	Formaldehyde, 598 μg	2.19	(43.9)
0.2	Omeprazole	Omeprazole, 20 mg	199	(–)
0.2	Fluvastatin	Fluvastatin, 20 mg	125	•
0.1	Coffee, 13.3 g	Caffeic acid, 23.9 mg	297	(4,900)
0.1	*d-Limonene in food*	*d-Limonene, 15.5 mg*	204	(–)
0.04	Lettuce, 14.9 g	Caffeic acid, 7.90 mg	297	(4,900)
0.03	Safrole in spices	Safrole, 1.2 mg	(441)	51.3
0.03	Orange juice, 138 g	*d-Limonene, 4.28 mg*	204	(–)
0.03	Comfrey herb tea, 1 cup (1.5 g root) (no longer recommended)	Symphytine, 38 μg	1.91	•
0.03	Tomato, 88.7 g TAS (1989); Schmidtlein and	Caffeic acid, 5.46 mg	297	(4,900)
0.03	Pepper, black, 446 mg	*d-Limonene, 3.57 mg*	204	(–)
0.02	Coffee, 13.3 g	Catechol, 1.33 mg	88.8	(244)
0.02	Furfural in food	Furfural, 2.72 mg	(683)	197
0.02	Mushroom (*Agaricus bisporus* 2.55 g)	Mixture of hydrazines, etc. (whole mushroom)	(–)	20,300
0.02	Apple, 32.0 g	Caffeic acid, 3.40 mg	297	(4,900)
0.02	Coffee, 13.3 g	Furfural, 2.09 mg	(683)	197
0.01	BHA: daily U.S. avg (1975)	BHA, 4.6 mg	606	(5,530)
0.01	Beer (before 1979), 257 g	Dimethylnitrosamine, 726 ng	0.0959	(0.189)
0.008	Aflatoxin: daily U.S. avg. (1984–89)	Aflatoxin, 18 ng	0.0032	(+)

continued

TABLE 7-5

Ranking Possible Carcinogenic Hazards from Average U.S. Exposures to Rodent Carcinogens (Gold et al. 2001) *(continued)*

HERP (%)	Possible hazard	Average Daily Exposure	"Potency" TD_{50} (mg/kg/day)[a] Rats	Mice
0.007	Cinnamon, 21.9 mg	Coumarin, 65.0 µg	13.9	(103)
0.006	Coffee, 13.3 g	Hydroquinone, 333 µg	82.8	(225)
0.005	Saccharin: daily U.S. avg. (1977)	Saccharin, 7 mg	2140	(–)
0.005	Carrot, 12.1 g	Aniline, 624 µg	194[b]	(–)
0.004	Potato, 54.9 g	Caffeic acid, 867 µg	297	(4,900)
0.004	Celery, 7.95 g	Caffeic acid, 858 µg	297	(4,900)
0.004	White bread, 67.6 g	Furfural, 500 µg	(683)	197
0.003	*d-Limonene*	Food additive, 475 µg	204	(–)
0.003	Nutmeg, 27.4 mg	*d-Limonene, 466 µg*	204	(–)
0.003	Conventional home air (14 hrs./day)	Benzene, 155 µg	(169)	77.5
0.002	Coffee, 13.3 g	4-Methylcatechol, 433 µg	248	•
0.002	Carrot, 12.1 g	Caffeic acid, 374 µg	297	(4900)
0.002	Ethylene thiourea: daily U.S. avg. (1990)	Ethylene thiourea, 9.51 µg	7.9	(23.5)
0.002	BHA: daily U.S. avg (1987)	BHA, 700 µg	606	(5530)
0.002	DDT: daily U.S. avg. (before 1972 ban)[d]	DDT, 13.8 µg	(84.7)	12.8
0.001	Plum, 2.00 g	Caffeic acid, 276 µg	297	(4900)
0.001	Pear, 3.29 g	Caffeic acid, 240 µg	297	(4900)
0.001	[UDMH: daily U.S. avg (1988)]	[UDMH, 2.82 µg (from Alar)]	(–)	3.96
0.0009	Brown mustard, 68.4 mg	Allyl isothiocyanate, 62.9 µg	96 (–)	
0.0008	DDE: daily U.S. avg. (before 1972 ban)[d]	DDE, 6.91 µg	(–)	12.5
0.0007	TCDD: daily U.S. avg (1994) (0.000156)	TCDD, 12.0 pg	0.0000235	

continued

TABLE 7-5

Ranking Possible Carcinogenic Hazards from Average U.S. Exposures to Rodent Carcinogens (Gold et al. 2001) *(continued)*

HERP (%)	Possible hazard	Average Daily Exposure	"Potency" TD$_{50}$ (mg/kg/day)[a] Rats	Mice
0.0006	Bacon, 11.5 g (+)	Diethylnitrosamine, 11.5 ng		0.0266
0.0006	Mushroom (*Agaricus bisporus* 2.55 g)	Glutamyl-*p*-hydrazino-benzoate, 107 μg	•	277
0.0005	Bacon, 11.5 g	Dimethylnitrosamine, 34.5 ng	0.0959	(0.189)
0.0004	Bacon, 11.5 g	*N-Nitrosopyrrolidine, 196 ng*	(0.799)	0.679
0.0004	EDB: Daily U.S. avg. (before 1984 ban)[d]	EDB, 420 ng	1.52	(7.45)
0.0004	Tap water, 1 liter (1987–92)	Bromodichloromethane, 13 μg	(72.5)	47.7
0.0003	Mango, 1.22 g	*d-Limonene, 48.8 μg*	204	(–)
0.0003	Beer, 257 g	Furfural, 39.9 μg	(683)	197
0.0003	Tap water, 1 liter (1987–92)	Chloroform, 17 μg	(262)	90.3
0.0003	Beer (1994–1995), 257 g	Dimethylnitrosamine, 18 ng	0.0959	(0.189)
0.0003	Carbaryl: daily U.S. avg (1990)	Carbaryl, 2.6 μg	14.1	(–)
0.0002	Celery, 7.95 g	8-Methoxypsoralen, 4.86 μg	32.4	(–)
0.0002	Toxaphene: daily U.S. avg. (1990)[d]	Toxaphene, 595 ng	(–)	5.57
0.00009	Mushroom (*Agaricus bisporus*, 2.55 g)	*p-Hydrazinobenzoate, 28 μg*	•	454[b]
0.00008	PCBs: daily U.S. avg. (1984–86)	PCBs, 98 ng	1.74	(9.58)
0.00008	DDE/DDT: daily U.S. avg. (1990)[d]	DDE, 659 ng	(–)	12.5
0.00007	Parsnip, 54.0 mg	8-Methoxypsoralen, 1.57 μg	32.4	(–)
0.00007	Toast, 67.6 g	Urethane, 811 ng	(41.3)	16.9
0.00006	Hamburger, pan fried, 85 g	PhIP, 176 ng	4.22[b]	(28.6[b])

continued

T A B L E 7 - 5

Ranking Possible Carcinogenic Hazards from Average U.S. Exposures to Rodent Carcinogens (Gold et al. 2001) *(continued)*

HERP (%)	Possible hazard	Average Daily Exposure	"Potency" TD$_{50}$ (mg/kg/day)[a] Rats	Mice
0.00006	Furfural	Food additive, 7.77 µg	(683)	197
0.00005	**Estragole in spices**	**Estragole, 1.99 µg**	•	51.8
0.00005	**Parsley, fresh, 324 mg**	**8-Methoxypsoralen, 1.17 µg**	32.4	(–)
0.00005	Estragole	Food additive, 1.78 µg	•	51.8
0.00003	**Hamburger, pan fried, 85 g**	**MeIQx, 38.1 ng**	1.66	(24.3)
0.00002	Dicofol: daily U.S. avg (1990)	Dicofol, 544 ng	(–)	32.9
0.00001	**Beer, 257 g**	**Urethane, 115 ng**	(41.3)	16.9
0.000006	**Hamburger, pan fried, 85 g**	**IQ, 6.38 ng**	1.65[b]	(19.6)
0.000005	Hexachlorobenzene: daily U.S. avg. (1990)	Hexachlorobenzene, 14 ng	3.86	(65.1)
0.000001	Lindane: daily U.S. avg. (1990)	Lindane, 32 ng	(–)	30.7
0.0000004	PCNB: daily U.S. avg (1990)	PCNB (Quintozene), 19.2 ng	(–)	71.1
0.0000001	Chlorobenzilate: daily U.S. avg. (1989)[d]	Chlorobenzilate, 6.4 ng	(–)	93.9
0.00000008	Captan: daily U.S. avg (1990)	Captan, 115 ng	2080	(2110)
0.00000001	Folpet: daily U.S. avg (1990)	Folpet, 12.8 ng	(–)	1550
<0.00000001	Chlorothalonil: daily U.S. avg. (1990)	Chlorothalonil, <6.4 ng	828[c]	(–)

[a] • = no data in CPDB; a number in parentheses indicates a TD$_{50}$ value not used in the HERP calculation because TD$_{50}$ is less potent than in the other species. (–) = negative in cancer tests; (+) = positive cancer test(s) not suitable for calculating a TD$_{50}$.

[b] TD$_{50}$ harmonic mean was estimated for the base chemical from the hydrochloride salt.

[c] Additional data from the EPA that is not in the CPDB were used to calculate this TD$_{50}$ harmonic mean.

[d] No longer contained in any registered pesticide product (USEPA, 1998).

A Partial List of Catastrophes

Many people are particularly concerned with major catastrophes, and the news media bring these catastrophes to public attention. Table 7-7 (see page 221) lists numbers of deaths involved in some catastrophes. Table 7-7 lists numbers of deaths involved in some catastrophes. This is not a complete list or even a systematic selection, but a list of some accidents that we believe have had a significant influence on public decisions. The accident at Three Mile Island is included for the latter reason because although it killed no one, either promptly or by delayed cancers, it raised a fear of something worse.

A large disaster can often have an effect upon public policy that seems out of line with the numerical value of the risk. Often there is a legislative call for increased regulation as a result—as happened after the coal mining accident of 1969 discussed in Chapters 1 and 2 and shown on Figure 1-4. The most thoughtful risk managers will seize the opportunity to reduce other related risks (black lung disease) not immediately at issue. In this section we list a number of disasters and our estimate of the overall effect. But we have picked cases that seem, in our view to have permeated public consciousness and had a major impact on public decisions. For a clear discussion on how they might be managed we refer to the books by Lagadec (1985). For a listing of accidents in the energy sector see Hirshberg et al. (1998).

Amounts Paid to Avert Deaths

We present a summary (promised earlier in Chapter 4), taken from the early work of Cohen (Table 7-6). In preparing this paper Cohen reviewed each source and modified each entry as he thought appropriate at the end of this chapter to make the methods and numbers consistent between risks. We also show a table (Table 7-8) from a later paper by Tengs et al. of the amounts society has been willing to pay to avert deaths (save lives). The later paper of Tangs et al. merely *quoted* some of the original sources, so that although there are over 600 entries, the reliability and consistency is not as good as in the smaller list of Cohen. Many of the amounts listed are the costs of saving lives by medical treatment. Such costs are incurred after the fact—some risk-has already been realized—so that such costs do not quite correspond with our definition of risk reduction. In other cases, however, the amount is for direct risk reduction. Especially interesting is the increasing use of the risk assessment by the National Highway Safety Administration (NHTSA) in deciding how much to spend on road safety improvements.

T A B L E   7 - 6
Cost per Fatality Averted Implied by Various Societal Activities

Calculated by Cohen in 1975 Dollars and Numbers Doubled by Us for Inflation

Item	Dollars per Fatality Averted
Overseas Activities	
Expanded immunization in Indonesia	200
Food for overseas relief	10,600
Medical Screening and Care	
Cervical cancer	50,000
Breast cancer	160,000
Lung cancer	140,000
Colorectal cancer:	
Fecal blood cancer	20,000
Proctoscopy	60,000
Multiple screening	52,000
Hypertension control	150,000
Mobile intensive care units	60,000
Kidney dialysis	400,000
Traffic Safety	
Highway construction-maintenance practice	40,000
Regulatory and warning signs	68,000
Guardrail improvements	68,000
Skid resistance	84,000
Bridge rails and parapets	92,000
Wrong way entry avoidance	100,000
Rescue helicopters	130,000
Driver education	180,000
Auto safety equipment—1966-70	260,000
Steering column improvement	200,000
Passive torso belt-knee bar	220,000
Impact absorbing roadside devices	216,000

continued

We conclude this list of risks with two graphs (Figures 7-8a and 7-8b) that show a selection of risks presented graphically. The x axis measures the size of the risk, and the y axis the number of people affected (both on linear scales). The lines (rectangular hyperbolae) are lines of a constant product of the number of people affected and the risk. This is the number of people expected to die form the action, or inaction.

On Figure 7-8a, most of the risks shown in the tables are in a small dot so close to the origin that they cannot be separated. Even the major catastrophes that titillate us in the morning newspaper can barely be seen. The major risks are those to the top (large number of people affected) and particularly to the right (high risk) of the graph. The product of the probability of the event or

TABLE 7-6

Cost per Fatality Averted Implied by Various Societal Activities *(continued)*

Calculated by Cohen in 1975 Dollars and Numbers Doubled by us for Inflation

Item	Dollars per Fatality Averted
Breakaway sign, lights posts	232,000
Median barrier improvement	456,000
Passive 3-point harness	500,000
Clear roadside recovery area	568,000
Air bags (driver only)	640,000
Tire inspection	800,000
Miscellaneous Non-radiation	
Sulfur scrubbers in power plants	1,000,000
Smoke alarms in homes	500,000
Higher pay for risky jobs	520,000
Air Force pilot safety	4,000,000
Civilian aircraft (France)	2,400,000
Coke fume standards	9,000,000
Very Hazardous Occupations	
Coal mine safety	44,000,000
Other mine safety	68,000,000
Radiaton Related Activities	
Radium in drinking water	5,000,000
Medical X-ray equipment	7,200
ICRP recommendations	640,000
OMB guidelines	14,000,000
Radwaste practice—general	20,000,000
Radwaste practice—^{131}I	200,000,000
Defense high level waste	400,000,000
Civilian high level waste	
No discounting	36,000,000
Discounting (1%/year)	2,000,000,000
NRC ALARA regulation (with LNT)	6,000,000

risk and the number of people affected (x × y) is the "expectation" of the number of annual deaths. The rectangular hyperbolae displayed are plots of constant numbers of annual deaths.

There is some ambiguity on the number of people at risk since in reality the risk varies across the population. These entries in the tables are therefore very approximate. The risk of nuclear war was estimated in Chapter 2 as 0.02 per year. We estimate that ⅓ of the human race is at risk (number affected 2,000 million), with underdeveloped areas relatively unaffected. Half of these will die in a war, a probability of dying = 0.02 x ½ = 0.01 which is the probability shown on the graph. The product of the probability and the number of people affected is then 2 million for the statistical expectation of

TABLE   7 - 7
Effects of Catastrophes

(Selected List—Large Catastrophes and Influential Ones)

Incident	Place	Year	Deaths < 1 Month	Deaths Delayed
Black Death	World	1347–51	75,000,000	—
Yellow River flood	China	1887	900,000	—
Coal Mine explosion	France	1905	1,050	?
Ship sinking	Canada	1914	1,624	
Ammunition explosion	Halifax NS	1917	1,900	—
Nitrate Fertilizer explosion	Germany	1921	600	—
Night Club Fire	Boston	1942	492	?
Cleveland (natural gas)	USA	1944	136	
Dresden (firebombing)	Germany	1945	200,000	
Hiroshima/Nagasaki	Japan	1945	300,000[a]	500[b]
Tornado (single)	TX and OK	1947	167	—
Nitrate Fertilizer explosion	Texas City	1947	561	—
Chemical (Ludwigshaven)	FRG	1948	245	
Coal tip slide	Aberfan	1966	144	?
(Chemical) Feyzin	France	1966	16	
(Chemical) La Salle	Canada	1966	11	
Chemical (Osaka)	Japan	1970	92	
Chemical (New York)	USA	1973	40	
Chemical (Bohemia)	Czechoslovakia	1973	47	
Chemical (Potchefstroom)	South Africa	1973	18	
Chemical (Flixborough)	GB	1974	28	?
Beek	Holland	1976	14	
Pasacabalo, near Cartagena	Columbia	1977	30	
Seoul	South Korea	1977	58	
Los Alfaques, LPG	Spain	1978	216	
Waverley, Tennessee	USA	1978	12	
Nuclear (Three Mile Island)	Pennsylvania	1978	0	<0.3[b]
Youngstown, Florida	USA	1978	8	
Paris	France	1978	13	
Xilatopec	Mexico	1978	100	
Bantry Bay	Ireland	1979	48	
Warsaw	Poland	1979	41	
Islamabad	Pakistan	1979	26	
Nuclear (Chornobyl)	Ukraine	1986	31	20,000[b]
Chemical (Bhopal)	India	1987	~1,500	~70,000
Igongwe	Tanzania	2000	33	10–50,000
Shuicheng	China	2000	118	

[a] Deaths due to explosion
[b] Estimated cancers due to radiation

FIGURE   7 - 8
Risks of Different Events

(a)

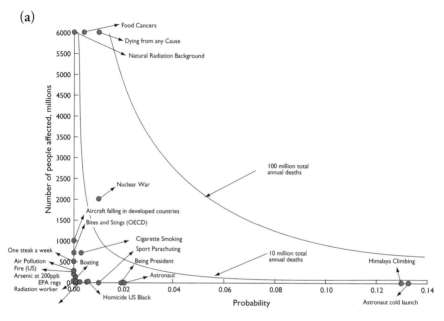

(b)

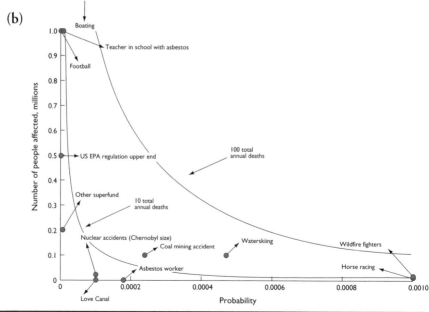

the number of people killed in a nuclear war. Some of the smaller risks may be seen on the chart of figure 7-8b when the scales of the x and y axes are substantially expanded in Figure 7-8b (by factors of 140 for risk, and 6,000 for population affected). Even on this plot it can be seen that few entries in the tables cause even 100 deaths per year.

Some important risks are not put on the table. The number of people affected by global warning is an appreciable fraction of the human race. The number of people affected by HIV virus is about 1% of the human race, even though predominantly in Africa and Asia. But we do not have reliable data on either to place them upon the plot.

Variation and Uncertainties

The reader will note that in addition to the estimates of risks given in Tables 7-1 to 7-5 there are some estimates of the uncertainties. For Tables 7-1a and 7-2a these uncertainties may be derived from variations in the historical data, for we are using models which assume that current trends will continue. In Table 7-5, the cancer risks, the uncertainty estimates are both much larger and also much more difficult to make. Usually they correspond to a factor of about 3 for uncertainties in estimating how potent the various carcinogens are from human data, together with an estimate of the uncertainty in dose of carcinogen. In estimating carcinogenic potency in animals, the uncertainty is less (the experiments are better controlled), but there is then an uncertainty of a factor of about 10 in extrapolating from animals to humans. In addition, in estimating risk from a particular dose, one has to also incorporate uncertainties in the estimation of the dose.

Detailed Discussions of Some Risks

In the sections that follow, and in the appendices we discuss some of these risks where the reference to earlier chapters or to data sources is not obvious. We hope that these discussions will assist and encourage the reader in evaluating risks with which he or she is personally concerned.

Being King or President

The average annual risk of being President of the U.S. is simply calculated by dividing the number of times a President has been assassinated (4) by the number of years there has been a President (211=2000-1789). The average annual risk of being King or Queen of England is similarly calculated back to the year 1066. Although being President of the United States of America is almost the largest occupational risk in the table, it is interesting that every four years people struggle to be elected to this position rather than struggle to avoid it.

Meteorite Impact

The calculation of risk due to meteorite impact is simple, and more accurate than for many other risks, but the magnitude is surprising to many people. About once in a million years a large meteorite is calculated to fall upon the earth and reach the ground. It will cause enough havoc to destroy a quarter to a half of the human race. The estimate was calculated by Chapman and Morrison (1994) using the data and perspective gained in Gehrels (1994). The calculation depends upon a knowledge of the distribution of meteorites, and the measurements of the frequency of impacts. These are now well known. The estimate is historically bounded because an impact larger than required for this result actually occurred approximately 70 million years ago. The risk will remain the same unless and until a decision is made to reduce the probability of impact by early detection (with sensitive telescopes) and intervention (by sending up a rocket and "nudging" the incoming meteorite into a safe trajectory) with appropriate explosives (although this is probably not the best method for "nudging" it is currently the only available option).

Aircraft Falling from the Sky

The risk from an aircraft falling from the sky and killing someone on the ground is non-negligible. It has been calculated by Solomon et al. (1974, 1975) and more recently by Goldstein et al. (1992), and their calculations are updated here. Eleven people are killed by falling aircraft in the U.S. each year. Dividing this by the U.S. population of 281 million gives an average *annual* risk of 4×10^{-8}. Multiplying by the average lifetime of 78 years this becomes a lifetime risk of 3×10^{-6}. This number is an average over the risk for all persons in the United States. It would be possible to estimate the risk for those persons who are those in line with an airport runway or near a "spotting point" (a point used by a pilot to determine his location). For these the risk is likely to be somewhat higher. We note that the risk of an aircraft striking the containment vessel of a nuclear reactor is similar to the risk of killing a person. Striking a containment vessel will not usually lead to any additional fatalities due to radiation releases, but it must be (and usually is in the western world) taken into account in estimations of the risk of nuclear reactor accidents.

Risk of Air Travel

The risk of being killed in an "ordinary" aircraft accident of commercial aircraft comes from Table 1074 of the Statistical Abstract of the U.S. taken from *Civil Aviation Statistics of the World*. The death rate listed there for 1998 was about 0.03 per 100 million passenger miles (3×10^{-10} per passenger mile), although it was 10 times higher in 1972. A one way trip NY to San Francisco is about 3,000 miles. The risk per trip then becomes $3 \times 10^{-10} \times 3 \times 10^{+3} = 1 \times 10^{-6}$ or twice this for a round trip. The risk of a transatlantic trip is about 2×10^{-6}. A "frequent flying professor" might take 15 such round trips a year for an annual risk of 3×10^{-5}. Of course this is averaged over flights of all lengths. To the extent that many accidents occur on take off or landing it is likely that shorter flights have proportionately more accidents per passenger mile. In addition the risk of travel in private aircraft (general aviation) is about 10 times higher.

Automobile Accident

There are a total of about 40,000 fatalities per year from automobile accidents (41,501 in 1998). The total vehicle-miles traveled in the US is about 2.63×10^{12} per year (again in 1998). Thus the vehicle-miles per fatality is about 1×10^8, corresponding to 100 vehicle-miles for a 10^{-6} risk. This number has increased over the years. Car travel is getting safer!

Falling Soda Machines

It has always been popular to "tilt" various machines to make them do what one wants. In the U.S. Army in Germany and Japan there were several examples of servicemen deliberately tilting soda pop machines because this would upset the mechanism and give them a free bottle. Several times the machine fell over. There were 3 deaths in 2 years and two cases where victims were sufficiently badly hurt that early death was inevitable (Cosio 1988). This was clearly not an occupational risk; it was voluntary, and we classify it among recreational risks. Soda machines in US forces facilities are now supposed to be chained down, so this risk may have been reduced for US forces. Soda machines in US forces facilities are now supposed to be chained down, so this risk may have been reduced for US forces.

Failure of Manned Spacecraft

The failure of a manned spacecraft is clearly a new technology for which the discussion in Chapter 2 is appropriate. The risk of failure of a Challenger spacecraft could have been estimated before the launch of January 27, 1986 by examining the 23 earlier launches. It would not be possible statistically to disprove a risk of $^1/_{23}$ by direct evidence. Since the nation desired that the risk be less than this, the safety of the mission had to be assessed by indirect methods but these that were used were not adequate. Some indirect evidence was not used. The accident has been attributed to the catastrophic failure of an O-ring seal during launch. Dalal et al. (1989) calculate the probability of failure of the O-ring seal as a function of temperature from data on the 23 pre-accident launches. They find a probability of 0.13 at 31°F but only 0.02 or less at 60°F. We assume here that a catastrophic O-ring failure will always lead to launch failure. We also assume that a launch failure will always lead to death of the astronauts. This calculation should have been performed or understood by managers in advance of the launch which took place at 31°F. The ensuing catastrophe emphasizes the importance of carrying out analyses of new technologies *before* deployment.

Risk of Bear Attack

This risk, listed in Table 7-3, illustrates two important issues. Those creating risky conditions were not those subject to the risk, and the risk estimate increases with the restriction of the denominator in the calculation (the group actually at risk). The feeding of bears was by one group of people, living in safety in a high altitude hut, for example, and that encouraged the bears to attack others who are campers.

To illustrate the way in which the risk varies with the group considered to be at risk, we consider the risk of death from bear attack in or near Glacier National Park. During the 30-year period from 1970 to 2000 there have been 6 cases. If this is averaged over the 1.6 million yearly park visitors, the risk is seen to be very small (10^{-7} per visitor). But the deaths have all been among back-packers—whose number we can judge from the number of back-country camping permits, 10,000 per year. In this group the risk is thus 200 times greater (2×10^{-5} per year). This is still about the same as driving a car 2,000 miles, and so perhaps comparable to (and maybe two or three times greater than) the risk in driving to and from the Park. It might be possible to identify a specific characteristic of backpackers which places them at risk, and so identify a smaller group at maximum risk. 3 of the 6 cases were among back-packers who were employees of park concessions, a smaller group still—perhaps 500—leading to a still larger risk estimate of 2×10^{-4} in this smaller group, and a correspondingly smaller one in the larger group of non-employee back-packers. To be more precise and find the exact characteristics would require data that are much harder to obtain. But great care must be taken not to reduce the denominator still further and take it as the number of park concession employees actually killed by bears. That would lead to a risk of unity. Unfortunately, such errors are often made in disguised form even by the best of analysts.

In this case greater caution may have recently reduced the risk considerably, although numbers are sufficiently small that there is no statistically discernible trend.

Mountain Climbing

The wide variation in the risk of sports between different practitioners is especially clear in mountain climbing, one of the more dangerous sports. The risk can be minimized but that only leads the adventurous to bigger risks. The risks of climbing the highest mountains has been summarized in Anon (1999). For example, from 1921 to 1998 there have been 1,052 individual ascents of Mt. Everest and 160 deaths above base camp for a risk (per ascent) of 0.15. Expressing the risk per year has little meaning. The risk can be divided into two parts—the risk of dying during ascent, and the risk of dying during descent. Even the risk at descent is high—0.034—from which we find (by subtraction) the risk of ascent at 0.12. For the other 4 most dangerous Himalayan peaks (K2, Annapurna, Makalu, and Kangchenjunga) the risk at descent is even higher—0.107. But the risks among the less adventurous climbers are considerably less, as noted in Table 7-3. These risks are especially interesting because there are clearly voluntary risks. Yet society often endeavors to prevent the adventurous from taking these risks. The question has always been with us: to what degree and with what justification may one risk one's life *and the life of others* when the motive is entirely pleasure? For mountain climbing, the question has been said to date from 1854 when Alfred Wills was the first to climb the Wetterhorn with no scientific, economic, religious or warlike aim.

Risks Involving an (Uncertain) Low-Dose Extrapolation: Using Human Data

Before discussing these risks in more detail and indicating how they are all estimated, we would like to extend one example in a way that may help place them in perspective. Four tablespoons of peanut butter/day are shown as giving a risk of liver cancer of 4×10^{-6} per year, or a lifetime risk of 3×10^{-4}

even for someone with hepatitis B. But four tablespoons of peanut butter corresponds to 400 Kcal, so if one was to eat only peanut butter, it would only require about 26 tablespoons/day, giving a lifetime liver cancer risk of 2 × 10^{-3}, or 0.002. This should be compared with a lifetime probability of any kind of cancer of about 0.25, even in the absence of peanut butter. Such an increase in total cancers would be difficult to observe. It would probably be hard to observe even among liver cancers alone, since the average lifetime risk of liver cancer is about 0.005 in the whole U.S. population, and much higher in those with hepatitis B. It is important to carry out calculations of this sort. We have seen risk assessments where the number of people that are estimated to die exceeds the number of people at risk—a flat impossibility.

The evaluation of the cancer and air and water pollution risks of Tables 7-1b and 7-2b presents the greatest challenge, so we discuss them in more detail. Each case is treated using the model outlined in Chapter 2. For the purposes of these lists a linear relationship ($R = \beta \times d$) is assumed between dose of, or exposure to, a carcinogen, and the response. In the first of these, the potency, β, is derived from human epidemiology and therefore is the slope of the dose response curve at high doses.

Radiation Risks

Radiation cancers have been extensively studied in humans and animals, and are the largest effect of chronic radiation exposure. There are tens of thousands of references, but comparatively few well analyzed situations. A review for physicists is in Wilson (1999). It is usual to take the numbers for cancer induced by radiation from the effects of the exposures to radiation from the atomic bombs in Hiroshima and Nagasaki. The latest analysis of the data is Pierce et al. (1996), with an especial look at effects of low doses by Pierce and Preston (2000). The analysis results must be modified slightly to allow for the fact that in the situations discussed below the radiation exposure takes place over a period of time, whereas the exposure to the direct radiation from the bombs lasted less than a second. This "dose rate reduction factor" can be taken from animal data and is about 2 to 5. Such a value is also consistent with experience from the Russian radiation accidents in the Techa River in 1948 (Burmistrov, Kossenko and Wilson, 2000). We use a linear dose response with a slope of 1 cancer per 3,000 Rems.

There is an appreciable radiation risk for a pilot due to his extensive travel at a cosmic ray level higher than on the ground. Cross-country airplanes travel at an altitude of about 35,000 feet (10 kilometers), at which height there is an appreciable radiation dose due to cosmic radiation, including neutrons. The calculated risk that is applicable to an airline pilot flying the maximum that is allowed can be obtained from direct measurements of radiation dose. Bagshaw (1998) quotes measurements taken by British Airways of a typical 6 microSievert per hour in a Boeing 747-300. This varies by a factor of 2.5 depending upon latitude of the flight. If a pilot flies for 50 hours per month (600 hours per year), his dose becomes 3.6 milliSievert or 360 milliRems per year. This gives a risk of $0.36/3,000 = 1.2 \times 10^{-4}$ or one in 8,000 per year.

The radiation risk for an airline passenger for a passenger flying a single transatlantic flight for 6 hours is 1% of the pilot's risk calculated in the preceding paragraph or 1.2×10^{-6} per year. This is smaller than ($1/_6$ of) the risk of accident and is normally neglected in any discussion of the risks of airplane travel. But it is derived on a comparable basis to the other cancer risks discussed here and helps to put them in perspective.

The radiation risk for a hospital X-ray technician can be calculated if one assumes his or her annual dose. We here assumed it to be 2.5 milliSievert (250 milliRems) per year. This is half the world average dose for hospital technicians (UNSCEAR 1993 Fig. XXIII). We take half the number for two reasons.

1. U.S. practice of radiology is believed to be superior to practice in many countries; and

2. the number has been decreasing with time.

The corresponding risk estimate is 10^{-4} (1 in 10,000) per year.

The risk of a being exposed to a chest X-ray has varied over the last 50 years. In 1948 a chest X-ray was often taken on 35 mm film with few precautions, and the dose could be 1 Rem (0.01 Sv). In 1998 a "typical" chest X-ray at a good hospital gives an equivalent whole body dose of 10 milliRems (Shapiro 1975). Thus the risk of cancer from a chest X-ray (assuming linearity) is $(10^{-2})/3,000 = 3 \times 10^{-6}$.

The risk from radon in drinking water comes from the calculations of the EPA as described in the Federal Register of July 18th 1991 pp 33050 *et. seq.* In particular in the middle column of p 33076, it is stated that the lifetime individual risk is "5×10^{-7} per pCi" of radon in water (a pCi is a picoCurie; a measure of radioactivity corresponding to one millionth of a millionth of that amount of radon in equilibrium with 1 gram of radium). These calculations are based upon the following assumptions:

■ The hazard is radon evaporated from the water and inhaled in the home.

■ A concentration of 1000 pCi/l in water leads to 1 pCi/l in air.

■ The risk from radon to a person exposed in his home may be related to the risk to uranium miners from their exposure to radon gas.

At 300 pCi/l, the calculated risk using EPA's pessimistic assumptions is 1.5 × 10^{-4} per lifetime, or 150 in a million. A survey by Sakaji (1991) in California was designed to estimate the radon concentrations in California wells. That survey found a median concentration of 1,500 pCi/l, five times the proposed EPA standard of 300 pCi/l; and 95% of the well waters exceeded 300 pCi/l.

Black Lung Disease

Black lung disease is assumed to be sufficiently debilitating that it leads to premature (but delayed by perhaps 15 years) death, and is in this sense like cancer. Historical statistics from the Bureau of Mines on compensation for black lung disease are used. There were 2,959 deaths over 7 years among mining machine operators (perhaps 50,000 total). This is almost as large a number as 20 years ago. There is renewed emphasis on improving conditions. The number may be going down as only 230 new cases were reported in 1999.

Cigarette Smoking

The number of cigarettes smoked that corresponds to a one in a million risk is obtained by dividing the total number of cigarettes manufactured in the U.S., with a correction for those sold overseas, obtained from table 1246 of the Statistical Abstract of the U.S. (1999 edition)—about 700 billion per year—by the number of people who the Surgeon General estimates die prematurely in the U.S. from cigarette smoking (about 430,000 people per year) and multiplying by 10^{-6} (NCHS, 2000). The risk is bigger than the risk from lung cancer alone. Cigarette smoking causes as many cancers at sites other than the lung, and causes heart disease at a rate comparable to the rate of all cancers. The risk to a smoker depends upon how many he smokes but a regular one pack-a-day person will smoke 200,000 to 400,000 cigarette in his lifetime leading to an average annual risk of about 3 in 1000.

The risk of living with a smoker comes from the observation that the risk of lung cancer when living with a smoker is 1.3 times the risk of lung cancer for non smokers. That in turn is 1/10 the risk of lung cancer for a smoker. Smokers have an 8% risk of lung cancer, nonsmokers a 0.8% risk. The increase from living with a smoker is then $(8 \times 0.3)/1,000 = 2.4/1,000$.

Cirrhosis of the Liver

The cases of cirrhosis of the liver are assumed to be entirely due to alcohol consumption, at a rate we assume to be proportional to the consumption. This is suggested by a WHO study in 1975 in which cirrhosis rates for 14 countries showed a very high correlation with average annual per capita intake varying from 4 to 25 liters. Figure 7-6 demonstrates a similar correlation between U.S. state alcohol-related cirrhosis rates (CDC 1998) and average alcohol consumption. These are "simple" correlations where each country or state is weighted equally. Such correlations, which are basically "ecological" studies, do not prove that consumers of moderate quantities of alcohol have a proportionate risk of cirrhosis. It may merely be that the number of alcoholics or heavy drinkers is proportional to the total countrywide consumption. We assume that the correlations are causal. In the U.S. the cirrhosis rate in the year 1998 was 4×10^{-5} per year, down from 1.5×10^{-4} (averaged over men and women) in 1974. Moreover, the NCHS reports distinguish between cirrhosis and alcohol-related cirrhosis, with only half the cases being alcohol-related—presumably because of a knowledge of considerable personal consumption. The numbers may therefore be an underestimate of the true alcohol-related deaths.

Asbestos Exposure

Asbestos is fibrous in nature and it is this fibrous quality that seems to make it carcinogenic. The risks from exposure to asbestos are derived from study of those persons who were exposed in their occupation. These include asbestos miners, those who weaved asbestos fibers into cloth, and later installers of asbestos insulation—increased rates of lung cancer mesothelioma have been observed in all such occupations, in addition to asbestosis. In the U.S. the usual reference for a quantitative analysis is a review by Nicholson (1986) for the U.S. EPA. In this he assumed that all asbestos fibers (of the same length and diameter) are equally potent regardless of their chemical nature and persistence in the body. For occupational exposures he derives a potency (which he calls K_m) of 0.01 lung cancers per (fiber/ml) x years. A recent re-analysis (Lash et al., 1997) shows that the potency derived by Nicholson is higher than the average of all the studies, but less than the maximum. For mesothelioma the latency period is longer, and such a simple approximation is less valid. Appendix 5 contains a detailed analysis for smoking and asbestos that shows many of the problems with the data. Nicholson's tables remain only an approximation, but in Tables 7-1b and 7-2b we assume their validity. See also Wilson and Price (2001).

The assumption that all fibers are equal (until proven different) has been questioned, in particular by a recent review by Hodgson and Darnton (2000) of the U.K. Health and Safety executive. Using an alternate assumption that all fibers are different (until proven equal), they find that amphibole fibers are more carcinogenic than chrysotile fibers, and derive a larger potency of 0.048 lung cancers per (fiber/ml) x years for amphiboles and smaller potency of 0.001 lung cancers per (fiber/ml) x years for chrysotile. Their fits to the epidemiological data are consistent with the idea that fibers must be ranked according to their surface chemical activity and their persistence in the body. The last of these is an indication that the effective dose (integrated over time) to the affected organ (the lung) is more important than the exposure (concentration of fibers in the air). A risk assessment for glass wool (Wilson et al. 1999) follows this approach and assumes that glass wool fibers will produce cancers, but with a potency 5 times less than chrysotile because of less persistence in the body and less chemical activity.

Saccharin

Saccharin causes cancer in rats under certain conditions. When saccharin was placed in the diet of rats at 3.5 g/day (2.5 g/day for every kg of body weight, or 2,500 mg/kg-day or about 3,500 mg/day for a rat), 24% develop cancer in their lifetimes. Each diet drink contains about 150 mg of saccharin, so 1 diet drink/day in humans is 150/70 mg/kg-day. For a rat, and assuming a linear dose response relationship, that would give a lifetime risk of cancer of 2×10^{-4}, or an annual average risk of 3×10^{-6}. The number quoted in Table 7-4b assumes that humans are about 3 times more sensitive than rats (the factor currently used by EPA, based on the ¼ power of bodyweight ratios). This might be high. A more important uncertainty, however, is the present belief by many toxicologists, based on extensive further testing of saccharin in rats, that the bladder cancers in rats are caused by bladder stones, which appear only at high doses in rats and may not appear at all in man. Unless there is a compensating type of cancer that appears in man and not in rats, the risk would be zero.

Chloroform in Drinking Water

The risk of carcinogens in drinking water has occupied many volumes. However, we follow (but update) here the calculations in Wilson, Crouch and Zeise (1983). One principal carcinogen in drinking water is chloroform, produced by action of chlorine on organic matter in water purification systems (Morris, 1975). Chlorination is performed, of course, to remove the (far higher) risk of spreading disease through the water supply. In 1977 concentrations of chloroform of 200 ppb (μg/l) were found in drinking water of Miami and New Orleans. More recent and more usual numbers are around 50 ppb (μg/l) and the EPA regulatory limit is 100 ppb (μg/l). A risk estimate can be calculated directly from the potency, β [0.005(mg/kg b.w × day)$^{-1}$], derived from the rat and mice data given in Table 4-3 using the usual EPA-style approach. For anyone ingesting 2 liters per day (which is about the U.S. average if inhalation in showers and the dermal absorption in bathing is expressed as equivalent ingestion) the lifetime risk is:

$$0.005 \text{ (mg/kg b.w} \times \text{day)}^{-1} \times 2{,}000 \text{ gms/day} \times 1{,}000 \text{ mg/gm}$$
$$\times 50 \times 10^{-9}/70 \text{ kg b.w.} = 7 \times 10^{-6}, \tag{7-3}$$

or an annual risk of one in ten million. However, low dose linearity, which is a basis for this risk assessment, has recently been seriously questioned (Butterworth, Kedderis and Connolly 1998), and U.S. EPA concurs in the belief that low-dose linearity does not apply for chloroform (EPA 1998). Chloroform is *not* directly mutagenic, and there are indications that, for chloroform, cell proliferation may be a prerequisite for cancer, and Butterworth et al. suggest that this leads to a non-linear dose response relationship. But if the cell proliferation is similar to that caused by natural (background) processes, linearity could still result as discussed in Chapter 2. Butterworth et al. failed to make a clear discussion of the relationship to background cancers, so the actual dose response is still unclear. We assume linearity here.

Air Pollution

The risk of air pollution in the U.S. risk is taken from the risk coefficient listed in Table 7-5 of the book edited by Wilson and Spengler (1996) combined with the concentrations listed in Table 3-4 or Figure 3-5 of Wilson and Spengler (these listed concentration measurements are mostly in urban areas and higher than the average). Figure 7-5 of that book shows a linear relationship between chronic mortality and average air pollution concentrations, as measured by PM10. The more reliable cohort studies have a coefficient of between 3% and 9% increase in mortality rate per 10 micrograms per cubic meter (10 μg/m^3) of PM10. But the measurement of PM10 is recent, and all indications are that the relevant exposures are those of 20 and more years ago when exposures were twice as great. We therefore divide the coefficient obtained from the correlation by two. We must multiply by an average concentration of 20 microgram per cubic meter (20 μg/m^3)to get a risk between 3% and 9% increment in mortality rate averaged over the population of the U.S. The risk is likely to be as high in most of the major urban areas of the world. However, we repeat the cautionary words in Chapter 2. Although fine particulate matter is currently considered to be a proximate cause of the adverse effects of air pollution, this is far from certain. We therefore state the risk somewhat vaguely as a risk of air pollution (from fossil fuel burning), rather than assign it to a particular proximate cause.

Charcoal-Broiled Foods

Many carcinogens are produced in detectable amounts when steaks are charcoal broiled. Char-broiled chicken and broiled fish are also covered with polyaromatic hydrocarbons (PAH) which are known carcinogens. Some of the carcinogens may come from the charcoal, for it is well known that burning carbonaceous materials produces carcinogens and the first cases of environmental carcinogenesis (cancer of the scrotum), noted by Percival Pott 200 years ago, were associated with the burning of coal. Alternatively they can come from pyrolization of the meat at high temperature. The carcinogens examined-here are confined to the PAH, although there may be other carcinogens present on char-broiled foods. Two measurements are needed for a risk assessment. Firstly the determination of how much PAH are produced and secondly what is the effect of the PAH on animals, and by extension on people.

Lijinsky and Shubik (1964) detected over a dozen polyaromatic hydrocarbons from broiling steaks. Of these benzo(a)pyrene is the best known, and we use only this for this calculation, but compensate at the end by multiplying the estimate by three to account for other PAH. They found that 2 μg (0.002 mg) of benzopyrene was produced in broiling a ½ lb. (230 gms), giving a concentration of 8 μg/kg. In a more complete study, Larsson et al. (1983) found 212 μg/kg when frankfurters were grilled over the flames of a log fire and 7.7 μg/kg over embers. Charcoal broiling frankfurters gave 1 μg/kg and charcoal broiling whole meat gave 2.3 to 6.6 μg/kg. We take here 8 μg/kg benzopyrene and add in the effect of other PAH.

The Chinese hamsters studied by Lijinsky and Shubik ingested 100 μg (0.1 mg) benzo(a)pyrene for each kg of body weight per day for a lifetime. 50% developed tumors. The potency (β) (in Chinese hamsters) is then 7 $[mg/kg\text{-}day]^{-1}$. We used this value in our first edition. More recent data (summarized by Gold et al., 1997) gives a potency in rats of 0.7 $[mg/kg\text{-}day]^{-1}$ which we use here. We multiply the potency by an interspecies factor of 3 to extrapolate to humans. Then our estimate of the risk for a person eating ½ lb. (0.25 kg) of charcoal-broiled steak per week is given by potency × dose:

$$= (0.7 \times 3)\ [mg/kg\ b.w. \times day]^{-1} \times 0.25\ (kg/wk) \times 8\ (\mu g/kg) \div 7\ (days/wk)$$
$$\div 1{,}000\ [\mu g/mg] \div 70\ [kg\ b.w.] kg\ b.w. = 10^{-5}. \tag{7-4}$$
[note as a check that units cancel]

We multiply again by 3 to allow for the effect of the many other poly-aromatic hydrocarbons to get 3×10^{-5}. This cancer risk (although large by EPA regulatory standards) is small, and eating charcoal broiled steaks to excess will give far higher risks of other problems (e.g. heart disease caused by cholesterol or related to obesity).

Natural Carcinogens: Risk of Eating Mushrooms
We first illustrate the risks due to natural carcinogens in foods by discussing the carcinogenicity of mushrooms (outlined in more detail in Appendix 4). Extreme eating of mushrooms has been shown to increase cancer rates in rodents, and according to the standard procedure outlined in Chapter 2 might be assumed to be carcinogenic in people. The lifetime cancer risk from eating then becomes one in five hundred (2×10^{-3}) for an average American or one percent (10^{-2}) for a Russian or Ukrainian who eats more mushrooms, often of his own gathering. This seems large but it is still probably smaller than could be detected in an epidemiological study.

Natural Carcinogens: Human Exposure/Rodent Potency (HERP) List
Ames and collaborators have made similar calculations for a large number of natural carcinogens. We use their most recent compilation Gold, Slone and Ames (2001) and attach their table in its entirety as Table 7-5. We note that what we call the "risk" for the rodent is the HERP calculated by Ames multiplied by (ln 2)/100 or 0.007. Ames suggests a serving of 5 grams of brown mustard a day to get a HERP of 0.07 or a lifetime risk of 0.007×0.07 or 5×10^{-4}. The average might be substantially less, perhaps 1 gram of brown

mustard every 150 days. This would give a lifetime risk of 0.7×10^{-6}. But an interspecies factor of 3 (approximately what we believe can now be justified) brings the human risk to 2×10^{-6}. Ames suggests a 1 gram basil leaf a day gives a HERP of 0.1 and therefore a risk of 7×10^{-4}. With an interspecies factor of 3 this becomes 2×10^{-3}. One basil leaf every 3 years gives therefore a risk of 2×10^{-6}.

Aflatoxin

Aflatoxins, already discussed in Chapter 4 (Table 4-2), are produced by mold and occur extensively in nature. Some are potent carcinogens. We consider the risk for the most potent, aflatoxin B1. From Table 4-4 we find the potency in humans is 150 $[\text{mg/kg.day}]^{-1}$ for someone with hepatitis B1, and 7 $[\text{mg/kg.day}]^{-1}$ for someone without. Assuming an average concentration of aflatoxin B1 in peanut butter of 2 ppb ($^1/_{10}$ of the regulatory limit), 4 tablespoons (64 g) of peanut butter contains 0.13 µg (0.00013 mg) of aflatoxin B1. Then a person eating 4 tablespoons per day has a lifetime risk of liver cancer of 3×10^{-4} (300 in a million) if he has hepatitis B1 and 1.3×10^{-5} if he does not. The average annual risk would be 4×10^{-6} and 2×10^{-7} respectively. The risk per tablespoonful is 2×10^{-9} or 10^{-10} respectively.

A different congener of aflatoxin appears in cow's milk—aflatoxin M, after the cows have eaten corn with mold thereon. Although the carcinogenic potency of this congener has not been measured, we estimate it by noting that it is less toxic than aflatoxin B1 by a factor of 10 and presumably a factor of 10 less carcinogenic. A 1977 survey (FDA 1977) of milk found aflatoxin levels of 0.1 ppb and above in 177 out of 302 samples. An average level might thus be 0.1 ppb, so that 1 pint (~500 g) per day of milk gives a dose of 0.05 µg/day (5×10^{-5} mg/day). This leads to a lifetime risk of 10^{-4} for someone with hepatitis B1 and 2×10^{-6} for someone without.

Aflatoxin need not be present in either peanut butter or milk and the amount can be reduced by careful control. The peanuts should be dried rapidly to avoid mold. Purchasing peanut butter in health food stores is not a panacea. Sometimes such peanut butter comes from nuts deliberately dried in the sun, instead of by machine, and may develop *more* mold. Aflatoxin could be regarded as a food additive, and therefore could have been regulated by FDA under the Delaney Clause (see Chapter 6). But FDA decided not to do so and no one objected. Nonetheless this risk has often been compared with other risks in toxic tort cases in what some lawyers have termed "the peanut butter defense."

Cancers Caused by Arsenic

Cancers in arsenic contaminated areas of Taiwan were analyzed in the paper by Chen et al. (1996) and plotted by Byrd et al. (1996). A more complete risk analysis using a variety of models was done by Morales et al. (2000), but still using the same basic ecological data (average health effect vs. average concentration, in Taiwan. The total rate of all cancers (lung, bladder and kidney being the principal ones) increases by 10% at about 500 ppb in the water. Since about ⅓ of all people develop cancer, this is an excess relative risk of about 30%. Confirming this number in a cohort study, Smith et al. (1998) note that Chileans who drank water with about 500 ppb of arsenic for several years have a 10% addition to the rate. Assuming linearity, (and the curves look more linear than the curves of animal cancer incidence from most carcinogens) the risk is 1% at the U.S. EPA MCL of 50 ppb. However, Morales et al. find a range of possible values for the risk at 50 ppb from above 1% to less 0.1%, and the U.S. EPA took the smaller number. That this risk is international in character is supported by the data of Cussick et al. (1992) who find 5 bladder cancers where 1.6 were expected among British patients who had routinely used (arsenic containing) Fowler's solution. Their average dose was equivalent to drinking water with arsenic at 30 ppb. More up-to-date information on the rapidly developing understanding of arsenical cancers can be found in a website: *http://phys4.harvard.edu/~wilson/arsenic_project_main.html.*

A feature of arsenic that is not widely discussed is that it appears to be carcinogenic in all chemical forms. The lifetime of the carcinogen is therefore infinite: longer than the time for breakdown of most chemical carcinogens, and even longer than long-lived nuclear waste. This leads to a suggestion by one of us (Wilson 2001b) that disposal of arsenic and disposal of nuclear wastes be discussed–similarly.–Even though the U.S. EPA in summer 2000 used the lower risk rather than the higher risk from Morales et al. (2000), a bill (Domenia, 2001) was introduced in the U.S. Senate to "render void" this new EPA regulation and asserting that the proposed 10 ppb standard lacks "a foundation of sound science." The evidence is under review once more both by the National Academy of Sciences and the EPA. Up-to-date information is posted on the above arsenic website.

Carcinogenic Effect of Alcohol

The evidence for carcinogenicity of alcohol is confusing. It is unclear whether alcohol functions as a carcinogen, co-carcinogen, or through an indirect mechanism such as alteration of bacterial flow through the gastro-intestinal tract. Moreover, some or all of any effect may be due to impurities in the beer or wine. But for our purposes, these caveats do not matter. People drink beer or wine, impurities and all, and the intake is large enough that the dose for any alcohol drinker is almost certainly above any threshold. If one uses the animal data from Ames et al. (1986), a consumption of 350 ml/day (a little less than ¾ pint) of beer leads to a HERP of 2.8 (see also Table 7-5) and a risk estimate (due to ethyl alcohol) of 0.02. 1.5 pints a year would then give a risk estimate of 10^{-4}. An interspecies extrapolation factor of 3 would increase the estimate to 3×10^{-4} (which is 100 times the estimate used in the tables). This is another case where the animal data probably *overstate* the risk. There are epidemiological correlations between cancer and alcohol intake for the mouth, pharynx, larynx, esophagus, liver and possibly rectum. For oral cancer there is a very strong synergism between smoking and alcohol. Rothman (1977) estimates the overall risk as follows. In 1968, 14,454 cancers occurred at sites with which alcohol has been associated. This gives a risk of 7×10^{-5} per year for an individual with average alcohol consumption. If the 14,454 cancers were concentrated in the 20% of heavy drinkers (who are usually also smokers) they would have a risk of 3.5×10^{-4} per year. The average beer consumption in the U.S. is ⅔ pint/day, and approximately double the corresponding amount of alcohol is consumed in wine and spirits. A light drinker (1 pint beer per day only) still has a cancer risk of 3.5×10^{-5}/year or 2.8×10^{-3} in a lifetime. Epidemiology listed in Chapter 2 includes more adverse effects and another study (Thun et al. 1997c) shows a risk of 5×10^{-5} per year for 1 drink a day or 3.5×10^{-3} in a lifetime. We must stress here that alcohol has many effects on people in addition to those discussed here. It is implicated in many automobile accidents and alcoholism causes many problems other than cirrhosis and cancer. The numbers here are therefore lower limits on the total risks of imbibing large quantities of alcohol.

But beneficial effects of alcohol have been known for centuries. As also noted in Chapter 2 modest alcohol drinking *reduces* the risk of cardiovascular disease. This effect is large—a reduction of 30% (-2×10^{-3} annual risk or 1.5×10^{-1} lifetime risk). This is not inconsistent. Cardiovascular disease is a different medical outcome to the other risks of alcohol, and the total risk at small doses is the algebraic sum of the different risks; there is clearly a net benefit at doses up to between 1 and 3 drinks a day (Figure 2-9).

Toxic Waste Facilities

The calculations of the risk of living near waste sites assume that the situation at those waste sites gets no worse than when it is first measured, but also that it gets no better. Exposures are estimated from measured concentrations or concentrations calculated from measured releases, then risks are estimated by multiplying by a carcinogenic potency, as discussed in Chapter 2. For Love Canal the risk estimates are taken from a paper by Murray, Harrington and Wilson (1982) who used measured concentrations in a badly contaminated house and added the calculated risks. The lifetime cancer risk for lifetime exposure was estimated at 5 in a thousand (5×10^{-3}). For a lead smelter site in Midvale, Utah the risk estimate is 10^{-7}, based on a calculation presented to a court (Wilson, 1988) correcting an EPA calculation. For the Stringfellow site, the estimates come from (uncontested) calculations presented to a court in a toxic substances lawsuit (Wilson, 1993) using exposure figures presented by the plaintiff's experts. For continuous exposure at the home of the highest exposed plaintiff the risk was 6 in a million in a lifetime and at the elementary school 36 in a million (3.6×10^{-5}) (both caused mainly by measured or postulated hexavalent chromium dust). Similar numbers were estimated by EPA and were (presumably) the reason that an EPA official dismissed the situation as being unimportant, as mentioned in Chapter 4.

Such figures suggest that the Probability of Causation for ailments for anyone actually living near a dump site is likely to be much less than 50%. However, these small numbers did not stop the complaints of nearby residents about the Stringfellow dumpsite being raised as an urgent action matter in the presidential bid of Michael Dukakis. Larger numbers can be obtained by pessimistic assumptions about future exposures and future occupancy. This discussion raises an interesting issue already hinted at in Chapter 6. It is hard to find a reason based solely on public health for removal of a dump site. However, just as many persons tidy their living room when they invite their friends for dinner, so do most people want the dump sites cleaned up—if someone else will pay for it.

Deep Space Probes

There are obvious occupational risks of space launches when a person (astronaut) is involved as noted above. If the spacecraft fails on launch the astronaut will often die—as in the Challenger disaster of 1985. Astronauts are also exposed to much higher levels of cosmic radiation than ordinary pilots so that there is a correspondingly high cancer risk. However, here we concentrate on the risk to the public of unmanned space probes. If such a probe fails upon launch, it will usually fall harmlessly into the ocean, or if it hits the ground, is unlikely to strike people. But the deep space probes, Galileo, Ulysses and now Cassini, come back to near earth on a "swing-by" to gain speed as they swing around the earth. There is a possibility that the orbit is incorrect at this point and that the probe will strike the earth. If the probe does strike the earth the speed is high enough that the probe is likely to break up in the upper atmosphere. In that case the radioactive (plutonium) thermoelectric generators would be evaporated, increasing the radioactive contamination of the upper atmosphere and leading to an eventual hazard to man. The probability of orbit failure and the probability that an individual develops cancer from exposure to plutonium are obviously independent, so this becomes an interesting example of multiplication of small probabilities.

There are several volumes (NASA, 1997) of calculations on the risk from each one of these three space probes, but a simple calculation of the order of magnitude of the risk can illustrate the main features in a simple way. Although for many members of the public the earth swing-by is a frightening prospect, we believe that the risk has been demonstrated to be small independently of the details of the calculation. Even the contingent risk, in the event of an earth impact, is small enough that it would never be directly measurable.

The probability of hitting the earth on an earth swing-by seems to be the most reliable of the components of the overall risk assessment. The basic geometrical point is that the earth is very small compared with the whole of space. NASA adopt the technique of making the initial trajectory pass far from the earth, and then correcting the trajectory in several small steps, by radio command from the ground. The sizes of these steps are limited by hardware on the space probe so that even if radio contact is lost (by meteorite impact for example) the time in which problems can occur is very small. Thus it easy to accept that this probability is less than one in a million—10^{-6}.

If there is an inadvertent impact on the earth during the attempted swing-by, there are two extreme possibilities. One that the plutonium capsules break open in the upper atmosphere and evaporate some or all of the plutonium oxide, and the other that some or all of the capsules fall to earth intact and break open on impact but without sufficient driving force to scatter the material (as in the launch failure case). The impact could be anywhere on earth, but the several capsules would be spread over a wide area. It is then easy to see that the worst effect from the point of view of public health and risk will be the first—upper atmosphere release. Even if *all* the material were released in the upper atmosphere this would not be an observable catastrophe. The amount of plutonium 238 released (less than 500 thousand Curies) would be similar to the amount of the biologically similar plutonium 239 released into the atmosphere by evaporation from the many above ground bomb tests. The distribution of Pu in people would be widespread, varying perhaps by a factor of 3 over the population, as is suggested by the distribution of fallout of strontium 90 (Sr^{90}). The average effect of that on people can be gauged by the fact that there is a body burden of Pu^{239} in all of us (as a consequence of the plutonium put in the atmosphere by atomic bomb tests) of about 20 picoCuries. Not until exposure is 10,000–100,000 as great, as occurred at Mayak (Khohryakov, et al. 1998), where the Russians overexposed their workers in their haste to make an atomic bomb, do we find appreciable increases in cancer. This leads to a contingent risk of less than one in one hundred thousand or 10^{-5} in a person's lifetime.

Combining the two independent calculations leads to an overall risk from the swing-by of the Cassini space probe, approximately equal for every person on earth, given by:

$$R = 10^{-6} \times 10^{-5} = 10^{-11} \tag{7-5}$$

This is a negligible risk by any standard, and the more accurately calculated numbers in the detailed reports give a risk (3×10^{-13}) which is even less. Although this is an extraordinarily low risk, there were 80 websites set up by people who opposed the Cassini space probe as being too dangerous. The risk was discussed as if the risk contingent upon an earth impact was the actual overall risk. It seems that the low overall risk was not understood, and that NASA failed to explain it properly. This is one of many examples of the difficulty that people have in understanding contingent probabilities.

Chornobyl Accident

The accident at Chornobyl was about as bad a nuclear power accident as is reasonable to imagine. Almost all of the radioactive gases, the noble gases, and the iodine were released. Much of the solid cesium was evaporated. Only the high melting point materials remained, and not all of them. Moreover these evaporated materials were spread around the world in fine particles which are easily inhaled. From a local perspective it could have been worse if the wind had blown the radioactive cloud directly over the local town of

Pripyat. Measurements of radioactivity combined with dispersion calculations and a linear dose response relationship for cancer incidence lead to the estimate that 20,000 people might get cancer in the 50 years subsequent to the accident. This calculated number, which could be much smaller if there is a threshold, is nonetheless a small fraction of the natural incidence. About 150 people associated with the plant developed acute radiation sickness, and 31 died, but no one in the general populace got a radiation dose large enough to develop acute radiation sickness. The only large effect (that is believed by radiation experts) has been about 1,500 childhood thyroid cancers, of which only 3 were fatal at the last count. (There are some scientists who believe that about 12,000 thyroid cancers, including cancers in adults, which actually occurred are attributable to Chornobyl. The difference of opinion is because of a lack of reliable knowledge of the *base line* number of thyroid cancers in the absence of radiation.) The fear of Chornobyl may have caused more deaths than the calculated (hypothetical) effects of the radiation. There are, for example, some estimates of 10,000 deliberate abortions. These risks due to fear are not estimated here.

Bhopal

In Bhopal, some tens of tons of methyl isocyanate were accidentally released and drifted over the local populace, causing death and injury (methyl isocyanate especially attacks the respiratory tract). The accident took place in a country where public health is poor in an area of poverty. We assume here that there were 1,500 immediate deaths and about 50,000 persons with varying degrees of disability, although some reports put the death toll as high as 5,000, with up to 200,000 persons affected.

Kuwait Oil Fires

In February 1992 demolition experts from the Iraqi army set fire to over 600 oil wells in Kuwait as they retreated before the armies assembled by the United Nations. The number of oil wells on fire was 100 times the maximum known before in any one year. In an unprecedented technological feat all of these fires were extinguished within 6 months. Meanwhile, 3% of the world's annual consumption of oil had been burned in one small region and burned in a dirty manner. Predictions were made that there would be massive respiratory problems among the population, particularly in Kuwait. Although increases in hospital admissions for respiratory problems were observed after the fire, this increase could not be distinguished from an increase due to a resumption of ordinary medical care after the end of the Iraqi occupation. There were several factors that seem to have contributed to reduce the impact on Kuwait. Firstly, the prevailing wind (during these 6 months) was from the NW, and blew the plume from the fires SE over the countries of Saudi Arabia and Bahrein (where one of us observed that the sun was obscured at midday 6 weeks later). In addition, the pollution was lofted above a temperature inversion layer, and was only deposited slowly. Only on a few days did the wind blow towards the city, at which times the air pollution was probably comparable to the London fog of December 1952. The paucity of direct measurements on the ground of particle density, size, and acidity, and the widespread nature of the pollution, means that the effect can only be calculated very approximately. We have estimated that if all particles were equal in their adverse effect, 50,000 respiratory fatalities might have occurred throughout the region over a 10-year period. This number is small compared with the large fluctuation in medical outcomes due to the confusion following the Iraqi invasion and withdrawal. But since the particles were mostly alkaline, and not acidic (as measured in Dharhan), the number might well be 5 times lower.

TABLE   7-8

Five Hundred Life-Saving Interventions and Their Cost-effectiveness from Tengs et al. (1995)

Life-saving intervention[a]	Cost/life-year[b]
Fatal Injury Reduction	
Airplane safety	
Automatic fire extinguishers in airplane lavatory trash receptacles	$16,000
Fiberglass fire-blocking airplane seat cushions	$17,000
Smoke detectors in airplane lavatories	$30,000
Emergency signs, floor lighting etc. (vs. upper lighting only) in airplanes	$54,000
Automobile design improvements	
Install windshields with adhesive bonding (vs. rubber gaskets) in cars	$0
Dual master cylinder braking system in cars	$13,000
Automobile dummy acceleration (vs. side door strength) tests	$63,000
Collapsible (vs. traditional) steering columns in cars	$67,000
Side structure improvements in cars to reduce door intrusion upon crash	$110,000
Front disk (vs. drum) brakes in cars	$240,000
Dual master cylinder braking system in cars	$450,000
Automobile occupant restraint systems	
Driver automatic (vs. manual) belts in cars	$0
Mandatory seat belt use law	$69
Mandatory seat belt use and child restraint law	$98
Driver and passenger automatic shoulder belt/knee pads (vs. manual belts) in cars	$1,300
Driver and passenger automatic shoulder/manual lap (vs. manual lap) belts in cars	$5,400
Airbag/manual lap belts (vs. manual lap belts only) in cars	$6,700
Airbag/lap belts (vs. lap/shoulder belts)	$17,000
Driver and passenger automatic (vs. manual) belts in cars	$32,000
Driver airbag/manual lap belt (vs. manual lap/shoulder belt) in cars	$42,000
Driver and passenger airbags/manual lap belts (vs. airbag for driver only and belts)	$61,000
Driver and passenger airbags/manual lap belts (vs. manual lap belts only) in cars	$62,000
Child restraint systems in cars	$73,000
Rear outboard lap/shoulder belts in all (vs. 96%) cars	$74,000
Airbags (vs. manual lap belts) in cars	$120,000
Rear outboard and center (vs. outboard only) lap/shoulder belts in all cars	$360,000

continued

TABLE 7-8

Five Hundred Life-Saving Interventions and Their Cost-effectiveness from Tengs et al. (1995) *(continued)*

Life-saving intervention[a]	Cost/life-year[b]
Construction safety	
Full (vs. partial) compliance with 1971 safety standard for concrete construction	$0
1988 (vs. 1971) safety standard for concrete construction	$0
1989 (vs. no) safety standard for underground construction	$30,000
1989 (vs. 1972) safety standard for underground construction	$30,000
1989 safety standard for underground gassy construction	$30,000
Revised safety standard for underground non-gassy construction	$46,000
Install canopies on underground equipment in coal mines	$170,000
Safety standard to prevent cave-ins during excavations at construction sites	$190,000
Full compliance with 1989 (vs. partial with 1971) safety standard for trenches	$350,000
Full (vs. partial) compliance with 1971 safety standard for trenches	$400,000
Fire, heat, and smoke detectors	
Federal law requiring smoke detectors in homes	$0
Fire detectors in homes	$0
Federal law requiring smoke detectors in homes	$920
Smoke and heat detectors in homes	$8,100
Smoke and heat detectors in bedroom area and basement stairwell	$150,000
Smoke detectors in homes	$210,000
Fire prevention and protection, other	
Child-resistant cigarette lighters	$42,000
Flammability standards	
Flammability standard for children's sleepwear size 0–6X	$0
Flammability standard for upholstered furniture	$300
Flammability standard for children's sleepwear size 7–14	$45,000
Flammability standard for upholstered furniture	$68,000
Flammability standard for children's sleepwear size 7–14	$160,000
Flammability standard for children's clothing size 0–6X	$220,000
Flammability standard for children's clothing size 7–14	$15,000,000
Helmet promotion	
Mandatory motorcycle helmet laws	$0
Federal mandatory motorcycle helmet laws (vs. state-determined policies)	$2,000
Mandatory motorcycle helmet laws	$2,000
Promote voluntary helmet use while riding All-Terrain Vehicles	$44,000

continued

T A B L E   7 - 8

Five Hundred Life-Saving Interventions and Their Cost-effectiveness from Tengs et al. (1995) *(continued)*

Life-saving intervention[a]	Cost/life-year[b]
Highway improvement	
Grooved pavement on highways	$29,000
Decrease utility pole density to 20 (vs 40) poles per mile on rural roads	$31,000
Channelized turning lanes at highway intersections	$39,000
Flashing lights at rail-highway crossings	$42,000
Flashing lights and gates at rail-highway crossings	$45,000
Widen existing bridges on highways	$82,000
Widen shoulders on rural two-lane roads to 5 (vs. 2) feet	$120,000
Breakaway (vs. existing) utility poles on rural highways	$150,000
Widen lanes on rural roads to 11 (vs. 9) feet	$150,000
Relocate utility poles to 15 (vs. 8) feet from edge of highway	$420,000
Light truck design improvements	
Ceilings of 0–6,000 lb light trucks withstand forces of 1.5 x vehicle's weight	$13,000
Ceilings of 0–10,000 lb light trucks withstand forces of 1.5 x vehicle's weight	$14,000
Ceilings of 0–8,500 lb light trucks withstand forces of 1.5 x vehicle's weight	$78,000
Ceilings of 0–10,000 lb light trucks withstand 5000 lb of force	$170,000
Side door strength standard in light trucks to minimize front seat intrusion	$190,000
Ceilings of 0-6000 lb light trucks withstand 5000 lb of force	$1,100,000
Side door strength standard in light trucks to minimize back seat intrusion	$10,000,000
Light truck occupant restraint systems	
Driver and passenger nonmotorized automatic (vs. manual) belts in light trucks	$14,000
Push-button release and emergency locking refractors on truck and bus seat belts	$14,000
Driver and passenger motorized automatic (vs. manual) belts in light trucks	$50,000
Driver airbag (vs. manual lap/shoulder belt) in light trucks	$56,000
Driver and passenger airbags (vs. manual lap/shoulder belts) in light trucks	$67,000
Natural disaster preparedness	
Soils testing and improved site-grading in landslide-prone areas	$0
Ban residential growth in tsunami-prone areas	$0
Strengthen unreinforced masonry San Francisco bldgs to LA standards	$21,000
Strengthen unreinforced masonry San Francisco bldgs to beyond LA standards	$1,000,000
Triple the wind resistance capabilities of new buildings	$2,600,000
Construct sea walls to protect against 100-year storm surge heights	$5,500,000
Strengthen buildings in earthquake-prone areas	$18,000,000

continued

T A B L E   7 - 8

Five Hundred Life-Saving Interventions and Their Cost-effectiveness from Tengs et al. (1995) *(continued)*

Life-saving intervention[a]	Cost/life-year[b]
School bus safety	
Seat back height of 24" (vs. 20") in school buses	$150,000
Crossing control arms for school buses	$410,000
Signal arms on school buses	$430,000
External loud speakers on school buses	$590,000
Mechanical sensors for school buses	$1,200,000
Electronic sensors for school buses	$1,500,000
Seat belts for passengers in school buses	$2,800,000
Staff school buses with adult monitors	$4,900,000
Speed limit	
National (vs. state and local) 55 mph speed limit on highways and interstates	$6,600
Full (vs. 50%) enforcement of national 55 mph speed limit	$16,000
National (vs. state and local) 55 mph speed limit on highways and interstates	$30,000
National (vs. state and local) 55 mph speed limit on highways	$59,000
National (vs. state and local) 55 mph speed limit	$89,000
National (vs. state and local) 55 mph speed limit on rural interstates	$510,000
Traffic safety education	
Driver improvement schools (vs. suspending/revoking license) for bad drivers	$0
Media campaign to increase voluntary use of seat belts	$310
Public pedestrian safety information campaign	$500
Improve traffic safety information for children grades K-12	$710
Motorcycle rider education program	$5,700
Improve motorcycle testing and licensing system	$8,700
Improve basic driver training	$20,000
Alcohol safety programs for drunk drivers	$21,000
Multimedia retraining courses for injury-prone drivers	$23,000
Improve educational curriculum for beginning drivers	$84,000
First aid training for drivers	$180,000
Improve pedestrian education programs for school bus passengers grades K–6	$280,000
Warning letters sent to problem drivers	$720,000
Vehicle inspection	
Random motor vehicle inspection	$1,500
Compulsory annual motor vehicle inspection	$20,000
Periodic motor vehicle inspection	$21,000
Periodic motor vehicle inspection	$57,000

continued

TABLE   7 - 8

Five Hundred Life-Saving Interventions and Their Cost-effectiveness from Tengs et al. (1995) *(continued)*

Life-saving intervention[a]	Cost/life-year[b]
Periodic inspection of motor vehicle sample focusing on critical components	$390,000
Periodic motor vehicle inspection	$1,300,000
Injury reduction interventions, miscellaneous	
Terminate sale of three-wheeled All-Terrain Vehicles	$0
Require front and rear lights to be on when motorcycle is in motion	$1,100
Selective traffic enforcement programs at high-risk times and locations	$5,200
Insulate omnidirectional CB antennae to avert electrocution	$8,500
Oxygen depletion sensor systems for gas space heaters	$13,000
Require employers to ensure employees' motor vehicle safety	$25,000
"American" oxygen depletion sensor system for gas space heaters	$51,000
Workplace practice standard for electric power generation operation	$59,000
Pedestrian and bicycle visibility enhancement programs	$73,000
Lock out or tag out of machinery in repair	$99,000
"French" oxygen depletion sensor system for gas space heaters	$130,000
Redesign chain saws to reduce rotational kickback injuries	$230,000
Ground fault circuit interrupters	$1,100,000
Ejection system for the Air Force B-58 bomber	$1,200,000
Equipment, work practices, and training standard for hazardous waste cleanup	$2,000,000

Toxin Control

Arsenic control	
Arsenic emission standard (vs. capture and control) at high-emit copper smelters	$36,000
Arsenic emission control at high-emitting copper smelters	$74,000
Arsenic emission standard (vs. capture and control) at glass plants	$2,300,000
Arsenic emission control at low-ernitting ASARCO/El Paso copper smelter	$2,600,000
Arsenic emission control at glass plants	$2,900,000
Arsenic emission standard (vs. capture and control) at low-emit copper smelters	$3,900,000
Arsenic emission control at secondary lead plants	$7,600,000
Arsenic emission control at low-emitting copper smelters	$16,000,000
Arsenic emission control at low-ernitting copper smelters	$29,000,000
Arsenic emission control at primary copper smelters	$30,000,000
Arsenic emission control at glass manufacturing plants	$51,000,000
Arsenic emission control at low-emitting Copper Range/White Pine copper smelter	$890,000,00

continued

TABLE 7-8

Five Hundred Life-Saving Interventions and Their Cost-effectiveness from Tengs et al. (1995) *(continued)*

Life-saving intervention[a]	Cost/life-year[b]
Asbestos control	
Ban asbestos in brake blocks	$29,000
Asbestos exposure standard of 1.0 (vs. 2.0) fibers/cc in asbestos cement industry	$55,000
Ban asbestos in pipeline wrap	$65,000
Ban asbestos in specialty paper	$80,000
Ban products containing asbestos (vs. 0.2 fibers/cc standard)	$220,000
Phase in ban of products containing asbestos (vs. 0.2 fibers/cc standard)	$240,000
Asbestos exposure standard of 1.0 (vs. 2.0) fibers/cc in textile industry	$400,000
Asbestos exposure standard of 0.2 (vs. 2.0) fibers/cc in ship repair industry	$410,000
Ban asbestos in roofing felt	$550,000
Ban asbestos in friction materials	$580,000
Ban asbestos in non-roofing coatings	$790,000
Ban asbestos in millboard	$920,000
Asbestos exposure standard of 0.2 (vs. 0.5) fibers/cc in friction products industry	$1,200,000
Asbestos exposure standard of 0.2 (vs. 0.5) fibers/cc in cement industry	$1,900,000
Ban asbestos in beater-add gaskets	$2,000,000
Ban asbestos in clutch facings	$2,700,000
Ban asbestos in roof coatings	$5,200,000
Ban asbestos in sheet gaskets	$5,700,000
Ban asbestos in packing	$5,700,000
Ban products containing asbestos (vs. 0.5 fibers/cc) in textile industry	$6,800,000
Ban asbestos in reinforced plastics	$8,200,000
Ban asbestos in high grade electrical paper	$15,000,000
Asbestos exposure standard of 0.2 (vs. 2.0) fibers/cc in construction industry	$29,000,000
Ban asbestos in thread, yarn, etc.	$34,000,000
Asbestos exposure standard of 1.0 (vs. 2.0) fibers/cc in friction products industry	$41,000,000
Ban asbestos in sealant tape	$49,000,000
Ban asbestos in automatic transmission components	$66,000,000
Ban asbestos in acetylene cylinders	$350,000,000
Ban asbestos in missile liner	$420,000,000
Ban asbestos in diaphragms	$1,400,0000,000
Benzene control	
Benzene exposure standard of I (vs. 10) ppm in rubber and tire industry	$76,000
Control of new benzene fugitive emissions	$230,000

continued

TABLE   7-8

Five Hundred Life-Saving Interventions and Their Cost-effectiveness from Tengs et al. (1995) *(continued)*

Life-saving intervention[a]	Cost/life-year[b]
Control of existing benzene fugative emissions	$240,000
Benzene exposure standard of I (vs. 10) ppm	$240,000
Benzene emission control at pharmaceutical manufacturing plants	$460,000
Benzene emission control at coke by-product recovery plants	$1,400,000
Benzene exposure standard of I (vs. 10) ppm in coke and coal chemicals industry	$3,000,000
Benzene emission control during transfer operations	$4,100,000
Control of benzene storage vessels	$14,000,000
Benzene emission control at ethylbenzene/styrene process vents	$14,000,000
Benzene emission control during waste operations	$19,000,000
Benzene emission control at rnaleic anhydride plants	$20,000,000
Benzene emission control at service stations storage vessels	$91,000,000
Control of benzene equipment leaks	$98,000,000
Benzene emission control at chemical manufacturing process vents	$180,000,000
Benzene emission control at bulk gasoline plants	$230,000,000
Benzene emission control at chemical manufacturing process vents	$530.000.000
Benzene emission control at rubber tire manufacturing plants	$20,000,000,000
Chlorination	
Chlorination of drinking water	$3,100
Chlorination, filtration and sedimentation of drinking water	$4,200
Coal and coke oven emissions control	
Coal-fired power plants emission control through high stacks etc.	$0
Coal-fired power plants emission control through coal beneficiation etc.	$37,000
Coke oven emission standard for iron- or steel-producing plants	$130,000
Acrylonitrile emission control via best available technology	$9,000,000
Formaldehyde control	
Ban urea-formaldehyde foam insulation in homes	$11,000
Ban urea-formaldehyde foam insulation in homes	$220,000
Formaldehyde exposure standard of I (vs. 3) ppm in wood industry	$6,700,000
Lead control	
Reduced lead content of gasoline from 1.1 to 0.1 grams per leaded gallon	$0
1,3 Butadiene control	
1,3 Butadiene exposure standard of 10 (vs. 1000) ppm PEL in polymer plants	$340,000
1,3 Butadiene exposure standard of 2 (vs. 1000) ppm PEL in polymer plants	$770,000

continued

TABLE   7 - 8

Five Hundred Life-Saving Interventions and Their Cost-effectiveness from Tengs et al. (1995) *(continued)*

Life-saving intervention[a]	Cost/life-year[b]
Pesticide control	
Ban chlorobenzilate pesticide on noncitrus	$0
Ban amitraz pesticide on apples	$0
Ban amitraz pesticide on pears	$350,000
Ban chlorobenzilate pesticide on citrus	$1,200,000
Pollution control at paper mills	
Chloroform emission standard at 17 low cost pulp mills	$0
Chloroform private well emission standard at 7 papergrade sulfite mills	$25,000
Chloroform private well emission standard at 7 pulp mills	$620,000
Chloroform reduction by replacing hypochlorite with chlorine dioxide at I mill	$990,000
Dioxin emission standard of 5 lbs/air dried ton at pulp mills	$4,500,000
Dioxin emission standard of 3 (vs. 5) lbs/air dried ton at pulp mills	$7,500,000
Chloroform emission standard of 0.001 (vs. 0.01) risk level at pulp mills	$7,700,000
Chloroform reduction by replace hypochlorite with chlorine dioxide at 70 mills	$8,700,000
Chloroform reduction at 70 (vs. 33 worst) pulp and paper mills	$15,000,000
Chloroform reduction at 33 worst pulp and paper mills	$57,000,000
Chloroform private well emission standard at 48 pulp mills	$99,000,000,000
Radiation control	
Automatic collimators on X-ray equipment to reduce radiation exposure	$23,000
Radionuclide emission control at underground uranium mines	$79,000
Radionuclide emission control at Department of Energy facilities	$730,000
Radionuclide control via best available technology in uranium mines	$850,000
Radiation standard "as low as reasonably achievable" for nuclear power plants	$1,100,000
Radiation levels of 0.3 (vs. 1.0) WL at uranium mines	$1,600,000
Radiation standard "as low as reasonably achievable" for nuclear power plants	$2,500,000
Radionuclide emission control at surface uranium mines	$3,900,000
Radionuclide emission control at elemental phosphorous plants	$9,200,000
Radionuclide emission control at operating uranium mill tailings	$11,000,000
Radionuclide control via best available technology in phosphorous mines	$16,000,000
Radionuclide emission control at phosphogypsum stacks	$29,000,000
Radionuclide emission control during disposal of uranium mill tailings piles	$40,000,000

continued

TABLE   7-8

Five Hundred Life-Saving Interventions and Their Cost-effectiveness from Tengs et al. (1995) *(continued)*

Life-saving intervention[a]	Cost/life-year[b]
Radiation emission standard for nuclear power plants	$100,000,000
Radiation emission standard for nuclear power plants	$180,000,000
Thin, flexible, protective leaded gloves for radiologists	$190,000,000
Radionuclide emission control at coal-fired industrial boilers	$260,000,000
Radionuclide emission control at coal-fired utility boilers	$2,400,000,000
Radionuclide emission control at NRC-licensed and non-DOE facilities	$2,600,000,000
Radionuclide emission control at uranium fuel cycle facilities	$34,000,000,000
Radon control	
Radon remediation in homes with levels ≥ 21.6 pCi/L	$6,100
Radon remediation in homes with levels ≥ 8.11 pCi/L	$35,000
Radon limit after disposal of uranium mill tailings of 20 (vs. 60) pCi/m^2	$49,000
Radon remediation in homes with levels ≥ 4 pCi/L	$140,000
Radon limit after disposal of uranium mill tailings of 2 (vs. 6) pCi/m^2	$260,000
Radon emission control at Department of Energy facilities	$5,100,000
S02 control	
S02 controls by installation of capacity to desulphurize residual fuel oil	$0
Trichloroethylene control	
Trichloroethylene standard of 2.7 (vs. 1) microgram/L in drinking water	$34,000,000
Vinyl chloride control	
Vinyl chloride emission control at EDCVNC and PVC plants	$1,600,000
Vinyl chloride emission standard	$1,700,000
VOC control	
South Coast of California ozone control program	$610,000
Toxin control, miscellaneous	
Process safety standard for management of hazardous chemicals	$77,000
Medicine	
Alpha antitrypsin replacement therapy	
Alpha antitrypsin replacement (vs. med) therapy for smoking men age 70	$31,000
Alpha antitrypsin replacement (vs. med) therapy for smoking women age 40	$36,000
Alpha antitrypsin replacement (vs. med) therapy for nonsmoking women age 30	$56,000
Alpha antitrypsin replacement (vs. med) therapy for nonsmoking men age 60	$80,000

continued

TABLE 7-8

Five Hundred Life-Saving Interventions and Their Cost-effectiveness from Tengs et al. (1995) *(continued)*

Life-saving intervention[a]	Cost/life-year[b]
Beta-blocker treatment following myocardial infarction	
Beta blockers for myocardial infarction survivors with no angina or hypertension	$360
Beta-blockers for myocardial infarction survivors	$850
Beta-blockers for high-risk myocardial infarction survivors	$3,000
Beta-blockers for low-risk myocardial infarction survivors	$17,000
Breast cancer screening	
Mammography for women age 50	$810
Mammography every 3 years for women age 50–65	$2,700
Annual mammography and breast exam for women age 35–49	$10,000
Annual physical breast cancer exam for women age 35–49	$12,000
Annual mammography and breast exam (vs. just exam) for women age 40–64	$17,000
Annual mammography and breast exam for women age 40–49	$62,000
Annual mammography and breast exam (vs. just exam) for women age 40–49	$95,000
Annual mammography for women age 55–64	$110,000
Annual mammography (vs. current screening practices) for women age 40–49	$190,000
Breast cancer treatment	
Postsurgical chemotherapy for premenopausal women with breast cancer	$18,000
Postsurgical chemotherapy for women with breast cancer age 60	$22,000
Bone marrow transplant and high (vs. standard) chemotherapy for breast cancer	$130,000
Cervical cancer screening	
Cervical cancer screening every 3 years for women age 65+	$0
Cervical cancer screening every 9 (vs. 10) years for women age 30–39	$410
One time mass screening for cervical cancer for women age 38	$1,200
Cervical cancer screening every 5 years for women age 65+	$1,900
One time cervical cancer screening for women age 65+	$2,100
Cervical cancer screening every 2 (vs. 3) years for women age 30-39	$2,300
Cervical cancer screening every 3 years for women age 65+	$2,800
Annual (vs. every 2 years) cervical cancer screening for women age 30–39	$4,100
One time cervical cancer screening for never-screened poor women age 65	$5,000
Annual cervical cancer screening for women beginning at age 60	$11,000
Cervical cancer screening every 4 years (vs. never) for women age 20	$12,000

continued

TABLE   7 - 8

Five Hundred Life-Saving Interventions and Their Cost-effectiveness from Tengs et al. (1995) *(continued)*

Life-saving intervention[a]	Cost/life-year[b]
One time mass screening for cervical cancer	$13,000
Cervical cancer screening every 5 years for women age 35+ with 3+ kids	$32,000
Cervical cancer screening every 3 years for regularly-screened women age 65+	$41,000
Annual (vs. every 3 years) cervical cancer screening for women age 65+	$49,000
Annual cervical cancer screening for women beginning at age 21	$50,000
Annual cervical cancer screening for women beginning at age 20	$82,000
Cervical cancer screening every 3 (vs. 4) years for women age 20	$220,000
Annual cervical cancer screening for women beginning at age 20	$220,000
Cervical cancer screening every 2 (vs. 3) years for women age 20	$310,000
Annual (vs. every 2 years) cervical cancer screening for women age 20	$1,500,000
Childhood immunization	
Immunization for all infants and pre-school children (vs. scattered efforts)	$0
Pertussis, diphtheria, and tetanus (vs. just diphtheria and tetanus) immunization	$0
Measles, mumps, and rubella immunization for children	$0
Polio immunization for children age 0–4	$0
Rubella vaccination for children age 2	$0
National measles eradication program for children	$0
Cholesterol screening	
Cholesterol screening for boys age 10 and their first-degree relatives	$4,600
Cholesterol screening for boys age 10	$6,500
Cholesterol treatment	
Lovastatin for men age 35–54 with heart disease and > 250 mg/dL	$0
Low-cholesterol diet for men age 60 and 180 mg/dL	$12,000
Low-cholesterol diet for men age 30	$19,000
Lovastatin for men age 55-64 with heart disease and < 250 mg/dL	$20,000
Oat bran cholesterol reduction for men age 48 and > 265 mg/dL	$24,000
Lovastatin/low cholesterol diet (vs. diet) for men age 60 and 300 mg/dL	$26,000
Cholestyramine/low cholesterol diet (vs. diet) for men age 60 and 300 mg/dL	$31,000
Lovastatin for men age 45–54 with no heart disease and > 300 mg/dL	$34,000
Cholestyramine/low cholesterol diet (vs. diet) for age 35–39 and 290 mg/dL	$100,000
Cholestyramine/low cholesterol diet (vs. diet) for men age 50–54 and 290 mg/dL	$150,000
Cholestyramine for men age 48 and > 265 mg/dL	$160,000
Cholestyramine/low cholesterol diet (vs. cholestyrarnine) age 35–39 290 mg/dL	$200,000

continued

TABLE 7-8

Five Hundred Life-Saving Interventions and Their Cost-effectiveness from Tengs et al. (1995) *(continued)*

Life-saving intervention[a]	Cost/life-year[b]
Cholestyramine for men with cholesterol levels above the 95th percentile	$230,000
Low-cholesterol diet for men age 20 and 180 rng/dL	$360,000
Lovastatin 40 (vs. 20) mg for women age 35–44 with heart disease < 250 mg/dL	$360,000
Cholestyramine/low cholesterol diet (vs. diet) for men age 65–69 and 290 mg/dL	$920,000
Lovastatin for women age 35–44 with no heart disease and > 300 mg/dL	$1,200,000
Cholestyramine/low cholesterol diet (vs. diet) for men age 20 and 240 mg/dL	$1,300,000
Cholestyramine/low cholesterol diet (vs. diet) for men age 20 and 240 mg/dL	$1,800,000
Clinical trials	
Women's Health Trial to evaluate low-fat diet in reducing breast cancer	$18,000
Clinical trial to evaluate alpha antitrypsin replacement therapy	$53,000
Colorectal screening	
Annual stool guaiae colon cancer screening for people age 55+	$0
One stool guaiac colon cancer screening for people age 40+	$660
One hemoccult screening for colorectal cancer for asymptomatic people age 55	$1,300
Colorectal cancer screening for people age 40+	$4,500
Colonoscopy for colorectal cancer screening for people age 40+	$90,000
Six (vs. five) stool guaiaes colon cancer screening for people age 40+	$26,000,000
Coronary artery bypass graft surgery (CABG)	
Left main coronary artery bypass graft surgery (vs. medical management)	$2,300
Left main coronary artery bypass graft surgery (vs. medical management)	$5,600
3-vessel coronary artery bypass graft surgery (vs. medical management)	$12,000
3-vessel coronary artery bypass graft surgery (vs. PTCA) for severe angina	$23,000
2-vessel coronary artery bypass graft surgery (vs. medical management)	$28,000
2-vessel coronary artery bypass graft surgery (vs. medical management)	$75,000
3-vessel coronary artery bypass graft surgery (vs. PTCA) for mild angina	$100,000
2-vessel coronary artery bypass graft surgery (vs. PTCA) for severe angina	$430,000
Drug and alcohol treatment	
Occupational assistance programs for working problem-drinkers	$0
Detoxification for heroin addicts	$0
Methadone maintenance for heroin addicts	$0
Narcotic antagonists for heroin addicts	$0

continued

TABLE   7 - 8

Five Hundred Life-Saving Interventions and Their Cost-effectiveness from Tengs et al. (1995) *(continued)*

Life-saving intervention[a]	Cost/life-year[b]
Emergency vehicle response	
Defibrillators in emergency vehicles for resuscitation after cardiac arrest	$39
Defibrillators in emergency vehicles staffed with paramedics (vs. EMTS)	$390
Defibrillators in ambulances for resuscitation after cardiac arrest	$460
Emergency vehicle response for cardiac arrest	$820
Advanced life support paramedical equipped vehicle	$5,400
Advanced resuscitative care (vs. basic emergency services) for cardiac arrest	$27,000
Combined emergency medical services for coordinated rapid response	$120,000
Gastrointestinal screening and treatment	
Sclerotherapy (vs. medical therapy) for esophageal bleeding in alcoholics	$0
Truss (vs. elective inguinal herniorrhaphy) for inguinal hernia in elderly patients	$0
Expectant management of silent gallstones in men age 30	$0
Home (vs. hospital) parenteral nutrition for patients with acute loss of bowels	$0
Home parenteral nutrition for patients with acute loss of bowels	$0
Pre-operative total parenteral nutrition in gastrointestinal cancer patients	$0
Ulcer therapy (vs. surgery) for duodenal ulcers	$6,600
Medical or surgical treatment for advanced esophageal cancer	$12,000
Surgery for liver cirrhosis patients with acute variceal bleeding	$17,000
Ulcer (vs. symptomatic) therapy for episodic upper abdomen discomfort	$41,000
Misoprostol to prevent drug-induced gastrointestinal bleed in at-risk patients	$47,000
Medical management for liver cirrhosis patients with acute variceal bleeding	$61,000
Misoprostol to prevent drug-induced gastrointestinal bleed	$210,000
Upper gastrointestinal X-ray and endoscopy (vs. ulcer therapy) for gastric cancer	$300,000
Upper gastrointestinal X-ray and endoscopy (vs. antacids) for gastric cancer	$420,000
Heart disease screening and treatment, miscellaneous	
Exercise stress test for asymptomatic men age 60	$40
Pacemaker implant (vs. medical management) for atrioventricular heart block	$1,600
Reconstruct mitral valve for symptomatic mitral valve disease	$6,700
Exercise stress test for age 60 with mild pain and no left ventricular dysfunction	$13,000
Implantable cardioverter-defibrillator (vs. medical therapy) for cardiac arrest	$23,000
Coronary angiography (vs. medical therapy) in men age 45–64 with angina	$28,000
Regular leisure time physical activity, such as jogging, in men age 35	$38,000
Replace (vs. reconstruct) mitral valve for symptomatic mitral valve disease	$150,000

continued

T A B L E   7 - 8

Five Hundred Life-Saving Interventions and Their Cost-effectiveness from Tengs et al. (1995) *(continued)*

Life-saving intervention[a]	Cost/life-year[b]
Heart transplantation	
Heart transplantation for patients age 55 or younger and favorable prognosis	$3,600
Heart transplantation for patients age 50 with terminal heart disease	$100,000
HIV/AIDS screening and prevention	
Voluntary (vs. limited) screening for HIV in female drug users and sex partners	$0
Screen blood donors for HIV	$14,000
Screen donated blood for HIV with an additional FDA-licensed test	$880,000
Universal (vs. category-specific) precautions to prevent HIV transmission	$890,000
HIV/AIDS treatment	
Zidovudine for asymptomatic HIV+ people	$0
Oral dapsone for prophylaxis of PCP in HIV+ people	$16,000
Aerosolized pentamidine for prophylaxis of PCP in HIV+ people	$20,000
AZT for people with AIDS	$26,000
Prophylactic AZT following needle stick injury in health care workers	$41,000
Zidovudine for asymptomatic HIV+ people	$45,000
Hormone replacement therapy	
Estrogen for menopausal women age 50	$0
Estrogen-progestin for symptomatic menopausal women age 50	$15,000
Estrogen for symptomatic menopausal women age 50	$26,000
Estrogen-progestin for 15 years in asymptomatic menopausal women age 50	$30,000
Estrogen-progestin for 5 years in asymptomatic menopausal women age 50	$32,000
Estrogen for post-menopausal women age 55–70	$36,000
Estrogen for menopausal women age 50	$42,000
Estrogen for asymptomatic post-menopausal women age 50–65	$77,000
Estrogen for symptomatic post-menopausal women age 50–65	$81,000
Estrogen for asymptomatic menopausal women age 50	$89,000
Hormone replacement for asyrnptomatic perimenopausal white women age 50	$120,000
Estrogen-progestin for post-menopausal women age 60	$130,000
Estrogen for asymptomatic post-menopausal women age 55–70	$250,000
Hypertension drugs	
Antihypertensive drugs for men age 25+ and 125 mmHg	$3,800
Antihypertensive drugs for men age 25+ and 85 mmHg	$4,700
Beta-blockers for hypertensive patients age 35–64 no heart disease and ≥ 95 mmHg	$14,000

continued

T A B L E   7 - 8

Five Hundred Life-Saving Interventions and Their Cost-effectiveness from Tengs et al. (1995) *(continued)*

Life-saving intervention[a]	Cost/life-year[b]
Antihypertensive drugs for patients age 40 and ≥ 105 mmHg	$16,000
Antihypertensive drugs for patients age 40 and 95–104 mmHg	$32,000
Captopril for people age 35–64 with no heart disease and ≥ 95 mmHg	$93,000
Hypertension screening	
Hypertension screening for Black men age 55–64 and ≥ 90 mmHg	$5,000
Hypertension screening for men age 45–54	$5,200
Hypertension screening for White men age 45–54 and ≥ 90 mmHg	$6,500
Hypertension screening for Black women age 45–54 and ≥ 90 mmHg	$8,400
Hypertension screening for asymptomatic men age 60	$11,000
Hypertension screening for asymptomatic women age 60	$17,000
Hypertension screening for asymptomatic men age 40	$23,000
Hypertension screening every 5 years for men age 55–64	$31,000
Hypertension screening for asymptomatic women age 40	$36,000
Hypertension screening for White women age 18–24 and ≥ 90 mmHg	$37,000
Hypertension screening for asymptomatic men age 20	$48,000
Hypertension screening for asyrnptomatic women age 20	$87,000
Hysterectomy to prevent uterine cancer	
Hysterectomy without oopherectomy for asymptomatic women age 35	$0
Hysterectomy with oopherectomy for asymptomatic women age 40	51,000
Hysterectomy for asymptomatic women age 35	230,000
Influenza vaccination	
Influenza vaccination for all citizens	$140
Influenza vaccination for high risk people	$570
Influenza vaccination for people age 5 +	$1,300
Intensive care	
Coronary care unit for patients under age 65 with cardiac arrest	$390
Intensive care for young patients with barbiturate overdose	$490
Intensive care and mechanical ventilation for acute respiratory distress syndrome	$3,100
Intensive care for young patients with polyradiculitis	$3,600
Intensive care and mechanical ventilation for acute respiratory failure	$4,700
Intensive care for unstable patients with unpredictable clinical course	$21,000
Intensive care for patients with heart disease and respiratory failure	$21,000
Intensive care for patients with multiple trauma	$26,000

continued

T A B L E   7 - 8

Five Hundred Life-Saving Interventions and Their Cost-effectiveness from Tengs et al. (1995) *(continued)*

Life-saving intervention[a]	Cost/life-year[b]
Coronary care unit for emergency patients with acute chest pain	$250,000
Intensive care for very ill patients undergoing major vascular surgery	$300,000
Intensive care for very ill patients with operative complications	$390,000
Intensive care for seriously ill patients with multiple trauma	$460,000
Intensive care for very ill patients undergoing neurosurgery for head trauma	$490,000
Intensive care for men with advanced cirrhosis, kidney and liver failure	$530,000
Intensive care for very ill patients with emergency abdominal catastrophes	$660,000
Intensive care for very ill patients undergoing neoplastic disease operations	$820,000
Intensive care for very ill patients undergoing major vascular operations	$850,000
Intensive care for very ill patients with gastrointestinal bleeding, cirrhosis etc.	$950,000
Leukemia treatment and infection control	
Bone marrow transplant (vs. chemotherapy) for acute nonlyrmphocytic leukemia	$12,000
Bone marrow transplant for acute nonlymphocytic leukemia in adults	$20,000
Chemotherapy for acute nonlymphocytic leukemia in adults	$27,000
Therapeutic leukocyte transfusion to prevent infection during chemotherapy	$36,000
Prophylactic (vs. therapeutic) leukocyte transfusion to prevent infection	$210,000
Intravenous immune globulin to prevent infections in leukemia patients	$7,100,000
Neonatal intensive care	
Neonatal intensive care for infants weighing 1000–1499 grams	$5,700
Neonatal intensive care for infants weighing 751–1000 grams	$5,800
Neonatal intensive care for infants weighing 500–999 grams	$18,000
Neonatal intensive care for low birth weight infants	$270,000
Newborn screening	
PKU genetic disorder screening in newborns	$0
Congenital hypothyroidism screening in newborns	$0
Sickle cell screening for Black newborns	$240
Sickle cell screening for non-Black high risk newborns	$110,000
Sickle cell screening for newborns	$65,000,000
Sickle cell screening for non-Black low risk newborns	$34,000,000,000
Organized health services	
Special supplemental food program for women, infants, and children	$3,400
Comprehensive (vs. fragmented) health care services	$5,700
Comprehensive (vs. fragmented) health care services for mothers and children	$11,000

continued

TABLE   7 - 8

Five Hundred Life-Saving Interventions and Their Cost-effectiveness from Tengs et al. (1995) *(continued)*

Life-saving intervention[a]	Cost/life-year[b]
Organized family planning services for teenagers	$16,000
No cost sharing (vs. cost sharing) for health care services	$74,000
Community health care services for women and infants	$100,000
Osteoporosis screening	
Bone mass screening and treat if < 0.9 g/(cm)^2 for perimenopausal women age 50	$13,000
Bone mass screening and treat if < 1.0 g/(cm)^2 for perimenopausal women age 50	$18,000
Bone mass screening and treat if < 1. 1 g/(cm)^2 for perimenopausal women age 50	$41,000
Percutaneous transluminal coronary angioplasty (PTCA)	
PTCA (vs. medical management) for men age 55 with severe angina	$5,300
PTCA (vs. medical management) for men age 55 with severe angina	$7,400
PTCA (vs. medical management) for men age 55 with mild angina	$24,000
PTCA (vs. medical management) for men age 55 with mild angina	$110,000
Pneumonia vaccination	
Pneumonia vaccination for people age 65+	$1,800
Pneumonia vaccination for people age 65+	$2,000
Pneumonia vaccination for people age 65+	$2,200
Pneumonia vaccination for people age 65+	$2,200
Pneumonia vaccination for high risk immunodeficient people age 65+	$6,500
Pneumonia vaccination for people age 45–64	$10,000
Pneumonia vaccination for high risk people age 25–44	$14,000
Pneumonia vaccination for high-risk immunodeficient people age 45–64	$28,000
Pneumonia vaccination for low risk people age 25–44	$66,000
Pneumonia vaccination for children age 2–4	$160,000
Pneumonia vaccination for children age 2–4	$170,000
Pneumonia vaccination for children age 2–4	$170,000
Prenatal care	
Term guard uterine activity monitor (vs. self-palpation) to detect contractions	$0
Financial incentive of $100 to seek prenatal care for low risk women	$0
Universal (vs. existing) prenatal care for women with < 12 years of education	$0
Universal (vs. existing) prenatal care for women with >12 years of education	$0
Universal (vs. existing) prenatal care for women with 12 years of education	$0
Prenatal screening for hepatitis B in high risk women	$0

continued

TABLE 7-8

Five Hundred Life-Saving Interventions and Their Cost-effectiveness from Tengs et al. (1995) *(continued)*

Life-saving intervention[a]	Cost/life-year[b]
Brady method screening for group B streptococci colonization during labor	$0
Prenatal care for pregnant women	$0
Antepartum Anti-D treatment for Rh-negative primiparae pregnancies	$1,100
Prenatal care for pregnant women	$2,100
Antepartum Anti-D treatment for Rh-negative multiparae pregnancies	$2,900
Isada method screening for group B streptococci colonization during labor	$5,000
Renal dialysis	
Home dialysis for chronic end-stage renal disease	$20,000
Home dialysis for end-stage renal disease	$22,000
Home dialysis for end-stage renal disease	$23,000
Home dialysis for people age 45 with chronic renal disease	$24,000
Home dialysis for people age 64 or younger with chronic renal disease	$25,000
Hospital dialysis for end-stage renal disease	$31,000
Home dialysis for people age 55–60 with acute renal failure	$32,000
Dialysis for people age 35 with end-stage renal disease	$38,000
Hospital dialysis for people age 55–64 with chronic renal failure	$42,000
Home dialysis for end-stage renal disease	$46,000
Hospital dialysis for people age 55–60 with acute renal failure	$47,000
Dialysis for end-stage renal disease	$51,000
Center dialysis for end-stage renal disease	$55,000
Center dialysis for end-stage renal disease	$63,000
Center dialysis for end-stage renal disease	$64,000
Center dialysis for people age 45 with chronic renal disease	$67,000
Center dialysis for end-stage renal disease	$68,000
Center dialysis for end-stage renal disease	$71,000
Hospital dialysis for end-stage renal disease	$74,000
Home dialysis (vs. transplantation) for end-stage renal disease	$79,000
Renal dialysis and transplantation	
Home dialysis then transplant for end-stage renal disease	$40,000
Hospital dialysis then transplant for end-stage renal disease	$46,000
Renal transplantation and infection control	
Cytomegalovirus immune globulin to prevent infection after renal transplant	$3,500
Cytomegalovirus immune globulin to prevent infection after renal transplant	$14,000
Kidney transplant for end-stage renal disease	$17,000

continued

TABLE   7 - 8

Five Hundred Life-Saving Interventions and Their Cost-effectiveness from Tengs et al. (1995) *(continued)*

Life-saving intervention[a]	Cost/life-year[b]
Kidney transplant and dialysis for people age 15–34 with chronic renal failure	$17,000
Kidney transplant for people age 45 with chronic renal disease	$19,000
Kidney transplant from live-related donor for end-stage renal disease	$19,000
Kidney transplant from cadaver with cyclosporine (vs. azathioprine)	$27,000
Kidney transplant from cadaver with cyclosporine	$29,000
Kidney transplant from cadaver with azathioprine	$29,000
Cytomegalovirus immune globulin to prevent infection after renal transplant	$200,000
Smoking cessation advice	
Smoking cessation advice for pregnant women who smoke	$0
Smoking cessation among patients hospitalized with myocardial infarction	$0
Smoking cessation advice for men age 50–54	$990
Smoking cessation advice for men age 45–49	$1,100
Smoking cessation advice for men age 35–39	$1,400
Smoking cessation advice for women age 50–54	$1,700
Smoking cessation advice for women age 45–49	$1,900
Smoking cessation advice for women age 35–39	$2,900
Nicotine gum (vs. no gum) and smoking cessation advice for men age 45–49	$5,800
Nicotine gum (vs. no gum) and smoking cessation advice for men age 35–69	$7,500
Nicotine gum (vs. no gum) and smoking cessation advice for men age 65–69	$9,100
Nicotine gum (vs. no gum) and smoking cessation advice for women age 50–54	$9,700
Smoking cessation advice for people who smoke more than one pack per day	$9,800
Nicotine gum (vs. no gum) and smoking cessation advice for women age 35–69	$11,000
Nicotine gum (vs. no gum) and smoking cessation advice for women age 65–69	$13,000
Tuberculosis treatment	
Isoniazid chemotherapy for high risk White male tuberculin reactors age 20	$0
Isoniazid chemotherapy for low risk White male tuberculin reactors age 55	$17,000
Venous thrornboembolism prevention	
Heparin (vs. anticoagulants) to prevent venous thromboembolism	$0
Compression stockings to prevent venous thromboembolism	$0
Compression stockings to prevent venous thromboembolism	$0
Heparin to prevent venous thromboembolism	$0
Heparin and dihydroergotamine to prevent venous thromboembolism	$0
Intermittent pneumatic compression to prevent venous thromboembolism	$0
Heparin and stockings to prevent venous thromboembolism	$0

continued

TABLE   7 - 8

Five Hundred Life-Saving Interventions and Their Cost-effectiveness from Tengs et al. (1995) *(continued)*

Life-saving intervention[a]	Cost/life-year[b]
Warfarin sodium to prevent venous thromboembolism	$0
Intermittent pneumatic compression and stockings to prevent thromboembolism	$400
Dextran (vs. anticoagulants) to prevent venous thromboernbolism	$640
Heparin to prevent venous thromboembolism	$960
Heparin and stockings to prevent venous thromboembolism	$1,000
Heparin and dihydroergotamine to prevent venous thromboembolism	$1,700
Intermittent pneumatic compression to prevent venous thromboembolism	$2,400
Heparin, I day, for women with prosthetic heart valves undergoing surgery	$5,100
Heparin/dihydroergotamine (vs. stockings) to prevent venous thromboembolism	$42,000
Heparin, 3 days, for women with prosthetic heart valves undergoing surgery	$4,300,000
Medicine miscellaneous	
Broad-spectrum chemotherapy for cancer of unknown primary origin	$0
Cefoxitin/gentamicin (vs. ceftizoxime) for intra-abdominal infection	$880
Mezlocillin/gentamicin (vs. ceftizoxime) for hospital acquired pneumonia	$1,400
Computed tomography in patients with severe headache	$4,800
Continuous (vs. nocturnal) oxygen for hypoxemic obstructive lung disease	$7,000
Preoperative chest X-ray to detect abnormalities in children	$360,000

Source: Tengs et al. 1995

[a]   Due to space limitations, life-saving interventions are described only briefly. When the original author compared the intervention to a baseline of "the status quo" or "do nothing" the baseline intervention is omitted here. Other baseline interventions appear as "(vs. _____)." Cost-effectiveness estimates are based on the particular life-saving intervention, base case intervention, target population, data, and methods as detailed by the original author(s). It is suggested the reader review the original document to gain a full appreciation of the origination of the estimates.

[b]   All costs are in 1993 U.S. dollars and were updated with the general consumer price index. To emphasize the approximate nature of estimates, they are rounded to two significant figures. When the cost is negative, it is entered here as $0.

8

Bibliography

BOOKS

In risk assessment the most important books are those that contain data. We therefore start this chapter with a selection of data sources. Primary among them are:

Census (annual). "Statistical Abstract of the United States: National Data Book and Guide to Sources." U.S. Bureau of the Census, U.S. Department of Commerce, U.S. Government Printing Office.

DOT (2001) "Bureau of Transportation Statistics, BTS01-01" U.S. Department of Transportation, National Transportation Statistics 2000, BTS01-01, U.S. Government Printing Office, Washington, D.C.; also at http://www.bts.gov/btsprod/nts/

NSC (annual). "Accident Facts." National Safety Council, Chicago, IL.

USBM (annual). "Minerals Yearbook." U.S. Bureau of Mines, Washington D.C.

USDA (annual). "Agricultural Statistics." U.S. Department of Agriculture, Washington, D.C.

NCHS (annual). "Vital Statistics of the United States." National Center for Health Statistics, U.S. Department of Health, Education and Welfare, Washington, D.C.

NIH (1976). "Cancer Rates and Risks." U.S. Department of Health, Education and Welfare. DHEW publication No. 76–691.Washington, D.C.

NIH (1985). "Report of the National Institutes of Health ad hoc Working Group to develop Radioepidemiological Tables." National Institutes of Health publication 85-2748 U.S. Department of Health and Human Services, Washington, D.C.

NIH (2001) update to NIH 1985, in preparation.

NVSR (annual). Statistical information is compiled into a national data base through the Vital Statistics Cooperative Program of the National Center for Health Statistics (NCHS) and Centers for Disease Control and Prevention. National Vital Statistics Reports, National Center for Health Statistics, Hyattsville, MD.

IARC (regular) "IARC Monographs on the Evaluation of Carcinogenic Risk of Chemicals to Humans," Volumes 1–76 plus supplements 1–7 International Agency for Research on Cancer, Lyon, France: also at http://www.iarc.fr

UNSCEAR (1993). United Nations Scientific Committee on the Effects of Atomic Radiation. Sources, Effects and Risks of Ionizing Radiation, UNSCEAR 1993 Report, United Nations.

Gangolli, S. and M. Richardson, Eds. "Dose: dictionary of Substances and their effects" 7 volumes plus index; Royal Society of Chemistry, Cambridge, UK.

Gold, L.S., and Zeiger, E. (Eds.), (1997), "Handbook of Carcinogenic Potency and Genotoxicity Databases." CRC Press.

Gold, L.S., et al. (1984). "Carcinogenic Potency Data Base of the Standardized Results of Animal Bioassays." *Environmental Health Perspectives* 58:9–319.

———(1986) "chronological supplement…" *Environmental Health Perspectives* 67:161–200

———(1987) "second supplement…" *Environmental Health Perspectives* 74:237–329

———(1990) "third supplement…" *Environmental Health Perspectives* 84:11–15:

———(1993) "fifth plot…" *Environmental Health Perspectives* 100:65–135

———(1995) "sixth plot…" *Environmental Health Perspectives* 103:1–122

———(1999) "supplement …" *Environmental Health Perspectives* 107S4:527–600.

Hirschberg, S., Spiekerman, G. and Dones, R. (1998). "Severe Accidents in the Energy Sector," PSI 98-16 ISSN 1019-0643 Paul Scherrer Institute, CH-5232 Villigen, Switzerland.

Metropolitan Life Insurance Company, many years before 1985. "Statistical Bulletins."

Murray, C.J.L. and A.D. Lopez (1996). "The Global Burden of Disease: a Comprehensive Assessment of Mortality and Disability from Diseases, Injuries and Risk Factors in 1990 and projected to 2020" Harvard University Press Cambridge, MA.

NRPB 1995. "Risk of radiation-induced cancer at low doses and low dose rates for radiation protection purposes." Documents of the NRPB, volume 6, No.1. National Radiological Protection Board, Chilton, Didcot, Oxon OX11 0RQ, United Kingdom.

A number of books have been written about risk analysis and cost benefit analysis:

ACS (1984). "Assessment and Management of Chemical Risks," edited by American Chemical Society, Washington, D.C.

Arrow, K.J. (1974). "Essays in the Theory of Risk Bearing," North Holland, Amsterdam, Netherlands.

Baker, R.F., R.M. Michels, and E. Preston. (1975). "Public Policy Development: Linking the Technical and Political Processes." John Wiley, New York.

Baumol, W.J. and W.E. Oates. (1975). "The Theory of Environmental Policy: Externalities, Public Outlays and Quality of Life." Prentice-Hall, Englewood Cliffs, New Jersey.

Bernstein, P.L. (1996). "Against the Gods: The Remarkable Story of Risk. "John Wiley & Sons, Inc. New York/Chichester/Brisbane/Toronto/Singapore.

Bunker, J.P., B.A. Barnes; and F. Mosteller (Eds.) (1977). "Costs, Risks and Benefits of Surgery." Oxford University Press, Oxford and New York.

Burton, I., R. Kates, and G. White. (1975). "The Environment as Hazard." MIT Press, Cambridge, Massachusetts.

Byrd, D.M. and C.R. Cothern (2000). "Introduction to Risk Analysis." *Government Institutes*, Rockville, MD.

CA: A cancer journal for Physicians 6 times a year. American Cancer Society. This is a very readable small journal. One issue each year gives cancer statistics for the previous year.

Calabrese, E.J. (1983). "Principles of Animal Extrapolation." Wiley, New York.

Calabresi, G. (1970). "The Cost of Accidents: A Legal and Economic Analysis." Yale University Press, New Haven, Connecticut.

Caldwell, L.K., Ed. "Science, Technology and Public Policy: A Selected and Annotated Bibliography." (3 vols.) Bloomington, Indiana: Program in Public Policy for Science and Technology, Department of Government, Indiana University, 1968–1972.

CalEPA (1997).

Calow, P., Ed. (1998). "Handbook of Environmental Risk Assessment and Management." Government Institutes, Rockville MD.

Clark, E.M. and A.J. Van Horn (1976) "Risk Benefit Analysis and Public Policy: a Bibliography." Energy and Environment Policy Center Report, Harvard University, Cambridge, MA.

Clayson, D.B., D. Krewski and I. Munro (eds.) (1985). "Toxicological Risk Assessment." CRC Press. Boca Raton, FL.

Clayson, D.B., (2000) "Toxicological Carcinogenesis." CRC Press, FL.

Cohrssen, J.J. and Covello V.T. (1989). "Risk Analysis: a Guide to Principles and Methods for Analyzing Health and Environmental Risks." *U.S. Council of Environmental Quality* NTIS, U.S. Department of Commerce.

Dacy, D., and H. Kunreuther. (1969). "The Economics of Natural Disasters." The Free Press, New York.

Dasgupta, A.K., and D.W. Pearce. (1972). "Cost-Benefit Analysis." Harper & Row, New York.

Davies, J.C., V.T. Covello and F.W. Allen, Eds., "Risk Communication." The Conservative Foundation, Washington, D.C.

East-West Environment and Policy Institute (1987) "Workshop on Risk Assessment of Hazardous Chemical Systems in Developing Countries." Honolulu, Hawaii, July 6–24. East-West Environment and Policy Institute, Occasional Paper No. 5.

Ebbin, S., and R. Kaspar (1974). "Citizen Groups and the Nuclear Power Controversy: Uses of Scientific and Technological Information." MIT Press, Cambridge, MA.

EPA (1979) "National Interim primary drinking water regulation for trihalomethanes in drinking water." *Federal Register* 44; 68642 11/13.

EPA (1980) *Federal Register* 45FR79318.

EPA (1985) *Federal Register* 50FR46880, 11/13/85.

EPA (1987) *Federal Register* 52FR35690.

EPA (1989a) *Federal Register* 54FR38044 (Sept. 14, 1989). In this the agency has defined acceptable risk targets under the Clean Water Act, the Comprehensive Environmental Response, Compensation and Liability Act ("Superfund"), the Resource Conservation and Recovery Act, the Federal Insecticide, Fungicide & Rodenticide Act, and the Safe Drinking Water Act 5.

EPA (1989b) "National Emission Standards for Hazardous Air Pollutants; benzene Rule and Proposed Rule." 40CFR Part 61 September 14.

EPA (1990). "Drinking water toxics under Safe Drinking Water Act" *Federal Register* 55(143):30409.

EPA (1991). "Section 409 Food Additive Regulations: order responding to Objectives to EPA Response requesting Revocation of Food Additive Regulations." *Federal Register* 56:7750.

EPA (1992a). Draft Report: A cross-species scaling factor for carcinogen risk assessment based on equivalence of mg/kg33/43/day; Notice." *Federal Register* 57:24141–24173.

EPA (1992b). "Seven Cardinal Rules of Risk Communication." EPA 230-K-92-01 U.S. Environmental Protection Agency, Washington, D.C.

EPA (1994). "RCRA Hazardous Waste Listings." *Federal Register* 59(24) December 22.

EPA (1995). "Risk Assessment Methodologies for Toxic Air Pollutants." *Government Institutes*, Rockville, MD.

EPA (1996a). "Proposed Guidelines for Carcinogen Risk Assessment: notice." *Federal Register* 61:17960–18011 (note that in summer 2000 no final guidelines have appeared).

EPA (1996b). "Corrective Action for Releases from Solid Waste Management Units at Hazardous Waste Management Facilities: Proposed Rule." 40CFR Chapter 1.

EPA (1996c). "For your information: the Food Quality Protection Act of 1996." U.S. Environmental Protection Agency, Washington, D.C.

EPA (1996d). "Major issues in the Food Quality Protection Act of 1996." U.S. Environmental Protection Agency, Washington, D.C.

EPA (1997). "Exposure Factors Handbook." EPA/600/P-95/002Fa-c (EPA has a continuing program at *http://www.epa.gov/ncea/jmprog.htm*). U.S. Environmental Protection Agency, Office of Research and Development. Washington, D.C.

EPA (1998a). "National primary drinking water regulations: disinfectants and disinfection byproducts: notice of data availability." *Federal Register* 63:15674–15692.

EPA (1998b). *Federal Register* FR 69390.

EPA (1998c)"Hazardous Waste Combustors; Revised Standards; Final Rule – Part 1: RCRA Comparable Fuel Exclusion; Permit Modifications for Hazardous Waste Combustion Units; Notification of Intent to Comply; Waste Minimization and Pollution Prevention Criteria for Compliance Extensions. June 19.

EPA (1999a). "Risk Assessment Guidance for Conducting Probabilistic Risk Assessment" RAGS3A U.S. Environmental Protection Agency, Office of Research and Development. Washington, D.C.

EPA (1999b). "Hazardous Waste Identification Rule (HWIR): Identification and Listing of Hazardous Wastes; Proposed Rule." *Federal Register* 64:63381-63461, November 19, 1999. See also; *http://www.epa.gov/OSWRCRA/hazwaste/id/hwirwste/* that links to the supporting analysis and modeling system.

EPA (2000a). "National Primary Drinking Water Regulations; Arsenic and Clarifications to Compliance and New Source Contaminants Monitoring; Proposed Rule." *Federal Register*: June 22, 65(121) 38887–38983.

EPA (2000b) "Arsenic in Drinking water: Economic Analysis." EPA 815 R-00-026

Federal Focus, Inc. (1996a). "Principles for Evaluating Epidemiologic Data in Regulatory Risk Assessment—Developed by an Expert Panel." At a Conference in London, England, October 1995, Federal Focus, Inc., Washington, D.C.

Federal Focus, Inc. (1996b). "Epidemiologic Data in Regulatory Risk Assessment—Recommendations for Implementing the "London Panel" and for Risk Assessment Guidance." Federal Focus, Inc., Washington, D.C.

Finkel, A.M. (1990). "Confronting Uncertainty in Risk Management, A Guide for Decision-Makers." *Center for Risk Management, Resources for the Future,* Washington, D.C.

Flynn, J., P. Slovic and H. Kunreuther, Eds. (2001). "Risk, Media and Stigma: Understanding Challenges to Modern Science and Technology." Earthscan, London, U.K.

Fraumeni, J. F., Ed. (1975). "Persons at High Risk of Cancer: An Approach to Cancer Etiology and Control." Academic Press, New York.

Fumento, M. (1993). "Science Under Siege: Balancing Technology and the Environment." William Morrow, New York.

Gehrels, T., Ed. (1994). "Hazards Due to Comets and Asteroids." University of Arizona Press, Tucson, AZ.

Glickman, T.S. and M. Gough, Eds. (1990). "Readings in Risk." Resources for the Future, Washington, D.C.

Gold, M.R., J.E. Siegel, L.B. Russell, and M.C. Weinstein (1996). "Cost-Effectiveness in Health and Medicine." Oxford University Press, Oxford.

Graham, J.D., Green L.C. and Roberts M.J. (1988). "In search of safety: chemicals and cancer risk." Harvard University Press, Cambridge, MA.

Graham, J.D. Ed. (1991). "Harnessing Science for Environmental Regulation." Westport, CT: Praeger.

Graham, J.D. and J.B. Wiener, Eds. (1995). "Risk versus risk: tradeoffs in protecting health and the environment." Harvard University Press, Cambridge, MA.

Graham, J.D., Ed. (1997). "The role of epidemiology in regulatory risk assessment." Elsevier, Amsterdam and New York.

Graubard, S., Ed. 1994 (Fall). *"*Health & Wealth.*" Journal of the American Academy of Arts and Sciences*, Cambridge, MA.

Green, A.E., and A. J. Bourne. (1972). "Reliability Technology." John Wiley, London.

Green, A.E., Ed. (1982). *"*High Risk Safety Technology." John Wiley, NY.

Greenway, A.R. (1998). "Risk Management Planning Handbook." *Government Institutes*, Rockville MD

Hahn, R.W., Ed. (1996). "Risks, costs, and lives saved: getting better results from regulation." Oxford University Press, New York: AEI Press, Washington, D.C.

Hamilton, J.T. and W.K. Viscusi (1999). "Calculating risks? The spatial and political dimensions of hazardous waste policy." MIT Press Cambridge, MA.

Hart, R.W. (Chairman) (1985). "Report of the Color Additive Scientific Review Panel." NCTR/Food and Drug Administration.

Hartwell, J. (1997). "The Greening of Industry: A Risk Management Approach." Cambridge: Harvard University Press.

Hirschberg, S., G. Spiekerman, and R. Dones (1998). "Comprehensive Assessment of Energy Systems: Severe Accidents in the Energy Sector." First edition (PSI 98-116), Paul Scherrer Institute, Switzerland.

Hollaender, A., Ed. (1971). "Chemical Mutagens." Plenum Press, New York.

Holland, C.D., R.L. Sielken, Jr. (1993). "Quantitative Cancer Modeling and Risk Assessment." PTR Prentice Hall, Englewood Cliffs, NJ.

IAEA (1996). "Electricity, Health and the Environment: Comparative Assessment in Support of Decision Making." Proceedings of an International Symposium held in Vienna. International Atomic Energy Agency, Austria, 16–19 October 1995.

IAEA (1999). "Health and Environmental Impacts of Electricity generation Systems: Procedures for Comparative Assessment." Technical report Series No. 394. International Atomic Energy Agency, Austria.

IARC (1999). "Quantitative Estimation and Prediction of Cancer Risks." Ed. S. Moolgavkar, D. Kreuskai, L. Zeise, E. Cardis, and H. Moller. International Agency for Research on Cancer, Scientific Publications, 131, Oxford University Press.

IPCC (2000). "Methodological and Technological Issues in Technology Transfer." Metz B., O. Davidson, J-W. Martens, S. van Rooijen and L. Van Wie Mcgrory (Eds.) Special Report of the Intergovernmental Panel on Climate Change, Cambridge University Press, UK.

IPCC (1997). "The Regional Impacts of Climate Change: An Assessment of Vulnerability." Watson, R.T., M.C. Zinyowere and R.H. Moss (Eds.) Special Report of the Intergovernmental Panel on Climate Change, Working Group II, Cambridge University Press, UK.

IPCC (2000a). "Emissions Scenarios." Nakicenovic and R. Swart (Eds.) Special Report of the Intergovernmental Panel on Climate Change, Cambridge University Press, UK.

IPCC (2000b). "Land Use, Land-Use Change, and Forestry." Watson R.T., I.R. Noble, B. Bolin, N.H. Ravindranath, D.J. Verardo and D. J. Dokken (Eds.) Special Report of the Intergovernmental Panel on Climate Change, Cambridge University Press, UK.

IPCC (2000c) "Methodological and Technological Issues in Technology Transfer." Metz, B., E. Davidson, J-W. Martens, S. Van Rooijen and L. Van Wie McGrory (Eds.) Special Report of the Intergovernmental Panel on Climate Change, Cambridge University Press, UK.

IPCC (2001)"IPCC Third Assessment Report: Climate Change." Intergovernmental Panel of Climate Change, Geneva, Switz (in press). (Contains the following: Technical Summary and 13 chapters.)

Jarret, H., Ed. (1966). "Environmental Quality in a Growing Economy." The Johns Hopkins University Press, Baltimore, MD.

Kammen, D.M. and D.M. Hassendahl (1999), "Should we risk it?: Exploring Environmental Health and Technological Problem Solving." Princeton University Press, Princeton, NJ.

Keeney, R.L. and H. Raiffa (1976). "Decision Analysis with Multiple Conflicting Objectives." John Wiley, New York.

Lagadec, P., "Major Technological Risk—An Assessment of Industrial Disasters," Pergamon Press, Paris.

Lagadec, P. (1981). "La Civilisation du Risque: Catastrophes Technologiques et Responsabilité Sociale." *Éditions du Seuil,* Paris, France.

Landy, M., Roberts M. & Thomas S.(1990). "The Environmental Protection Agency: Asking the Wrong Questions." Oxford University Press, New York.

Lave, L.B. and E.P. Seskin, with M.J. Chappie. (1977). "Air Pollution and Human Health." The John Hopkins University Press, Baltimore.

Lawless, E. (1976). "Technology and Social Shock." New Brunswick, New Jersey: Rutgers University Press.

Lifton, R.J. (1967). "Death in Life—Survivors of Hiroshima." New York: Vantage Books.

Lifton, R.J. and E. Olson. (1974). "Living and Dying." Praeger, New York.

Loomis, T. A. (1968). "Essentials of Toxicology." Philadelphia.

Lowrance, W. (1976). "Of Acceptable Risk: Science and the Determination of Safety." William Kaufman, Los Altos, CA.

McKnight, A.D., P.K. Marstrand, and J.C. Sinclair, Eds. (1974). "Environmental Pollution Control: Technical, Economic and Legal Aspects." Allen & Unwin, London.

Medford, D. (1973). "Environmental Harassment or Technology Assessment." Elsevier, New York.

Mettler, F.A. and Upton A.C., Eds. (1995). "Medical Effects of Ionizing Radiation," 2nd edition. W.B. Saunders, Philadelphia, PA.

Molak, V., Ed. (1997). "Fundamentals of Risk Analysis and Risk Management." Lewis pubs, Boca Raton, FL.

Moolgavkar, S.H., Ed. (1990). "Scientific Issues in Quantitative Risk Assessment." Birkhauser, Boston, MA.

Morgan, M.G. and M. Henrion (1990). "Uncertainty: A guide to Dealing with Uncertainty in Quantitative Risk and Policy Analysis." Cambridge University Press, UK.

NAS (1982). "Risk and Decision Making: Perspectives and Research." National Academy Press, Washington, D.C.

NAS (1983). "Risk Assessment in the Federal Government: Managing the Process." National Academy Press, Washington, D.C.

NAS (1989). "Improving Risk Communication." National Academy Press, Washington, D.C.

NAS (1994). "Science and Judgment in Risk Assessment." National Academy Press, Washington, D.C.

OECD (1977) "Programme on Long Range Transport of Air Pollution: Measurements and Findings." Organization for Economic Cooperation and Development, Paris.

Paustenbach, D.J. (1989). "The Risk Assessment of Environmental and Human Health Hazards." Wiley-Interscience Publishers, New York.

Paustenbach, D.J. (Editor) (2001). "Human and Ecological Risk Assessment: Theory and Practice." Publication anticipated.

Preston, S.H., N. Keyfitz and R. Shoen (1972). "Causes of Death—Life Tables for National Populations." Seminar Press,New York.

Raiffa, H. (1968). "Decision analysis: introductory lectures on choices under uncertainty." Random House, New York.

Renn, O. (1998). "The Role of Risk Perception for Risk Management." *Reliability, Engineering and System Safety* 59(1) 49–62.

Rodricks, J.V., and R.G. Tardiff (1979). "Colloquium on Risks." NUS Corporation, Rockville, MD.

Rogers, P.P., K.F. Jalal, B.N. Lohani, G.M. Owens, C-C. Yu, C.M. Dufournaud and J. Bi (1997). "Measuring Environmental Quality in Asia." Division of Engineering Sciences, Harvard University and Asian Development Bank.

Rowe, W. D. (1977). "An Anatomy of Risk." Wiley-Interscience, New York.

Royal Society Study Group. (1983). *Risk Assessment.* Royal Society, London, UK.

Schüz, M., Ed. (1990). "Risiko und Wagnis—Die Herausforderung der Industriellen Welt." edited by M. Verlag Günther Neske, Pfullingen, Germany.

Schwing, R.C. and W.A. Albers, Jr., Eds. (1980). "Societal Risk Assessment—How Safe is Safe Enough?" Plenum Press, New York.

Shneidman, E.S. (1974). "Deaths of Man." Penguin Books. Baltimore, MD.

Shrader-Frechette, K.S. (1985). "Risk Analysis and the Scientific Method." D. Riedel Publishing Company, Dordrecht.

Slovic, P. (2000). "The Perception of Risk." Earthscan, London, UK.

SFEN (La Société Française d'Energie Nucléaire) (1980). "Colloque sur les risques sanitaires des différentes énergies." (Colloquium on the Risks of Different Energy Sources.) Gedim, Saint-Etienne, France.

Society of Risk Analysis (Japan) (2000). "Handbook of Risk Research." Ed. T. Morioka, Y. Sakai, S. Ikeda, H. Hirose and I. Uchiyama, TBS Brittania, Tokyo, Japan.

Tversky, A., Slovic P., Kahnemann D. (1982). "Judgment Under Uncertainty: Heuristics and Biases." Cambridge University Press, New York

Tversky, A., and Kahnemann D. (1986). "Judgment and Decision Making: An Interdisciplinary Reader." Ed. Arkes and Hammond. Cambridge University Press, New York

U.S. Surgeon General: "Smoking and Health: a Report of the Surgeon General." PHS79-50066 or any edition, Public Health Service, Washington, D.C.

Urquhart, J., and K. Heilmann (1994). "Risk Watch—The Odds of Life." Facts on File Publications, NY.

Viscusi, W.K. (1992). "Fatal Tradeoffs: Public and Private Responsibilities for Risk." Oxford University Press.

Waller, R.A. and V.T. Covello, Eds. (1984). "Low Probability High-Consequence Risk Analysis—Issues, Methods, and Case Studies." Plenum Press, NY.

Wildawsky, A. (1995). "But Is It True? A Citizen's Guide to Environmental Health and Safety Issues." Harvard University Press, Cambridge, MA.

Wilson, J.D. (1998). *Default and Inference Options: Use in Recurrent and Ordinary Risk Decisions.* Discussion Paper 98-17, Resources for the Future.

Wilson, J.R. (1963). "Margin of Safety." Doubleday, Garden City, New York.

Wilson, R., and Jones W.J. (1974). "Energy, Ecology and the Environment," Academic Press, New York.

Wilson, R., and Crouch E.A.C. (1982). "Risk-Benefit Analysis." *Ballinger Publishing Company*: Cambridge, MA (the first edition of this book).

Wynne, B. (1996). In "Risk, Environment and Modernity." ed S. Lash, B. Szersynski and B. Wynne. Sage, London, UK.

Zervos, C., Ed. (1991). "Risk Analysis: Prospects and Opportunities." Plenum Press, New York.

Ziman, J.M. (1968). "Public Knowledge: An Essay Concerning the Social Dimension of Science" Cambridge University Press, Cambridge, UK.

The first book in this group is a major, classic which alerted the country to the risks of uncontrolled pesticide use. This book was particularly influential because although it has a polemical style it acknowledged the major benefits pesticides had brought. Some later books on environmental and public health issues are less balanced:

Ackerman, B.A., S. Rose-Ackerman, J.W. Sawyer, Jr. and D.W. Henderson (1974). "The Uncertain Search for Environmental Quality." The Free Press, New York.

Ashford, N. A. (1975). "Crisis in the Workplace: Occupational Disease and Injury." MIT Press, Cambridge, MA.

Carson R. (1962). "Silent Spring." Fawcett Pubs. New York.

Commoner Barry (1971). "The Closing Circle: Nature, Man and Technology." Knopf, New York.

Epstein, S.S. (1978). "The Politics of Cancer." Sierra Club Books, San Francisco.

Turner, J. (1970). "The Chemical Feast: Report on the Food and Drug Administration." Grossman, New York.

These critical books have led to books in which the authors criticize what they believe are exaggerations in the earlier work:

Angell, M. (1997). "Science on trial: the clash of medical evidence and the law in the breast implant case." W. W. Norton, London and New York.

Baxter, W. F. (1974). "People or Penguins: The Case for Optimal Pollution." Columbia University Press, New York.

Efron, E. (1984). "The Apocalyptics." Simon and Schuster, New York.

Foster, K.R., D.E. Bernstein and P.W. Huber, Eds. (1993). "Phantom Risk—Scientific Inference and the Law." MIT Press, Cambridge, MA.

Huber, P.W. (1988). "Liability: the Legal Revolution and Its Consequences." Basic Books.

Irwin, A., and B. Wynne, Eds. (1996). "Misunderstanding Science? The Public Reconstruction of Science and Technology." Cambridge University Press, Cambridge, UK.

Milloy, S. "Science without Sense." Junk Science Store, NY.

Milloy, S., and M. Gough. "Silencing Science." Junk Science Store, NY .

Morris, J., and R. Bate. (1994) "Fearing Food: Risk, Health and the Sustainer." Butterworth-Heineman.

Lewis, H.W. (1990). "Technological Risk." Norton, New York.

Whelan, E.M., and F.J. Stare (1976). "Panic in the Pantry: Food Facts, Fads and Fallacies." Atheneum, New York.

There are some important books, which primarily address regulatory procedures:

Beck, U. (1992). "Risk Society: Toward a New Modernity." (Translated by Mark A. Ritter.) Sage, London, UK.

Breyer, S.G. (1993). "Breaking the Vicious Circle: Toward Effective Risk Regulation." Harvard University Press, Cambridge, MA.

The above book is particularly important because its author is now a justice of the Supreme Court.

Clarke, L. (1989). "Acceptable Risk? Making Decisions in a Toxic Environment." University of California Press, Berkeley CA.

Douglas, M., and A. Wildawsky (1982). *Risk and Culture.* University of California Press, Berkeley, CA.

Hutt, P.B. and R.A. Merrill (1991). "Food and Drug Law: Cases and Materials," 2nd ed. Foundation Press, Westbury, New York.

The above book on risk assessment for chemicals was commissioned by the Food and Drug Administration but was used in its early days by the Environmental Protection Agency.

Jasanoff, S. (1986). "Risk Management and Political Culture." Russell Stage Foundation, New York. This book on risk assessment for chemicals was commissioned by the Food and Drug Administration but was used in its early days by the Environmental Protection Agency.

Jasanoff, S. (1990). "The Fifth Branch: Science Advisers as Policymakers." Harvard University Press, Cambridge, MA.

Kates,R., C.Hohenemser and J.X. Kasperson, Ed. (1988). "Perilous Progress: Managing the Hazards of Technology." Westview Press, Boulder, CO. Westview Press, Boulder, CO.

Krimsky, S., and Plough A. (1988). "Environmental Hazards: Communicating Risks as a Social Process." Auburn House, Dover, MA.

Lave, L.B. (1981). "The Strategy of Social Regulation-Decision Frameworks of Policy— Studies in the Regulation of Economic Activity." The Brookings Institution, Washington, D.C.

NAS (1996). "Understanding Risk: Informing Decisions in a Democratic Society." National Academy Press. National Academy of Sciences/National Research Council, Washington, D.C.

Omenn, G.S. (1997). (Chairman, The Presidential/Congressional Commission on Risk Assessment and Risk Management) "Framework for Environmental Health Risk Management" Final Report, Volume 1 "Risk Assessment and Risk Management in Regulatory Decision-Making," Final Report, Volume 2.

Perrow, C. (1984). "Normal Accidents." Basic Books, New York.

Pidgeon, N., C. Hood, D. Jones, B. Turner (1992). "Risk—Analysis, Perception, and Management" The Royal Society, London, 89–134.

The Royal Society (1983). *Risk Assessment—A Study Group Report.* The Royal Society, London, UK.

Shrader-Frechette, K.S. (1980). *Nuclear Power and Public Policy: The Social and Ethical Problems of Fission Technology.* D. Reidel Publishing Co., Dordrecht, Holland.

Shrader-Frechette, K.S. (1991). *Risk and Rationality. Philosophical Foundations for Populist Reforms.* University of California Press, Berkeley and Los Angeles, CA.

Shrader-Frechette, K.S. (1993). *Burying Uncertainty.* University of California Press, Berkeley and Los Angeles, CA.

Slovic, P., S. Lichtenstein, B. Fischhoff (1985). In *Perilous Progress: Managing the Hazards of Technology,* Ed. R.W. Kates, C. Hohenemser and J.X. Kasperson. Westview Press, Boulder, CO.

Stallones, R.A., et al. (1983) "Risk Assessment in the Federal Government: Managing the Process." "The RED BOOK." National Academy Press, Washington, D.C.

Swedish National Institute of Radiation Protection *Proceedings of Management of Risk from Genotoxic Substances in the Environment* (1989). The Swedish National Institute of Radiation Protection, Swedish National Chemicals Inspectorate, and National Swedish Environmental Protection Board, Stockholm, Sweden.

Journals

The scientific literature on risk analysis is exploding. We first list the specialist risk (but interdisciplinary) journals.

> *Risk Analysis: An International Journal*
> *Journal of Risk Research*
> *Human and Ecological Risk Assessment*
> *Risk: Health, Safety, and the Environment*
> *Journal of Risk and Uncertainty*
> *Risk and Decision Policy*

A number of the leading disciplinary journals have articles with important data and articles:

> *Nature*
> *Science*
> *Lancet*
> *Scientific American*
> *Radiation Research*

Journal of the National Cancer Institute (JNCI)
American Journal of Epidemiology
British Journal of Cancer
New England Journal of Medicine (NEJM)
Cancer
Cancer Research
Environmental Health Perspectives
Journal of Toxicology and Environmental Health
Environment
Environment International
Biometrics
Annals of Occupational Hygiene
Journal of Occupational Medicine
Food and Cosmetic Toxicology
Technology

Websites

Most of the institutions involved in understanding and assessing risks have websites. There are several websites where it is possible to access and download data and programs directly. One may either go to the website of the institution, government or other agency which is suspected of having data available, and then browse, or go directly to a site known to have data available. The reader must be alert to the fact that websites change faster than printed pages decay.

In the U.S. government we note that there is an excellent list of sites of U.S. Government Agencies, which have statistical information:

http://www.fedstats.gov/noframe.html

And the site for the Center for Disease Control:

http://www.cdc.gov/

And in particular the data warehouse of the National Center for Health Statistics:

http://www.cdc.gov/nchs/datawh.htm

The fine details of mortality for 1998:

http://www.cdc.gov/nchs/data/gmwki_98.pdf

And final mortality summary for 1998:

http://www.cdc.gov/nchs/data/nvs48_11.pdf

The Bureau of labor statistics has data on employment in various occupations:

http://stats.bls.gov/cpsaatab.htm#charemp

The National Toxicology Program, administered by the National Institute of Environmental Health Sciences, has an excellent site on toxicity and carcinogenicity of chemicals:

http://ntp-server.niehs.nih.gov/

In particular there is an excellent chemical safety data base at:

http://ntp-server.niehs.nih.gov/Main_Pages/Chem-HS.html

The Carcingenic Potency Data Base at Berkeley has a useful website:

http://potency.berkeley.edu/cpdb.html

The International Agency for Research on Cancer, at Lyon has an excellent set of monographs on evaluation of the carcinogenic risks to man at:

http://193.51.164.11/monoeval/crthgr01.html

The Mining Safety and Health Administration of the U.S Department of Labor have statistics for the last century:

http://www.msha.gov/centurystats/centurystats.htm

The U.S. bureau of the census has a useful FERRET program to search census data:

http://ferrett.bls.census.gov:80/cgi-bin/ferrett

The dictionary "Dose" referred to above is available at:

http://www.rsc.org

The United States Environmental Protection Agency has a data base called IRIS: Integrated Risk Information System:

http://www.epa.gov/iris/

The Agency for Toxic Substance and Disease Registry has a website with questions and answers:

http://toxnet.nlm.nih.gov/

The National Library of Medicine:

http://www.atsdr.cdc.gov/toxfaq.html

The National Institutes of Health have two websites for searching the medical literature:

(1) PUBMED:
> *http://www.ncbi.nlm.nih.gov/entrez/query.fcgi*

the PUBMED query brings forth:
> *http://www.ncbi.nlm.nih.gov/entrez/query.fcgi?db=PubMed*

(2) "Internet Grateful Med," which replaces a PC based program:
> *http://igm.nlm.nih.gov*

Pubscience is also a useful site
> *http://pubsci.osti.gov/srchfrm.html*

The National Oceanographic and Atmospheric Administration (NOAA) have a useful storm prediction center:
> *http://www.spc.noaa.gov*

The U.S. Forest Service tells us about fires and other forest hazards:
> *http://fs.fed.us*

The European Organization for Cooperation and Development has a useful website with hazard and risk information:
> *http://www.oecd.org/EHS*

Aircraft accidents are listed in the National Transportation Safety Board website:
> *http://www.ntsb.gov/aviation/Paxfatal.htm*

and, in particular, Chemical Accident Risk Assessment Thesaurus:
> *http://www.oecd.org/EHT/CARAT/v3.0/html/default.htm*

Russian demographic statistics are useful:
> *http://www.demoscope.ru/*

and, in particular:
> *http://www.demoscope.ru/d_f_a/de99005.html*

Many private U.S. organizations have useful websites:
Louisiana State University has a site for medical emergencies with much material:
> *http://toxicology.lsumc.edu/*

There is a U.S. Chemical Safety Hazard and Investigation Board with its website, but statistics are few and far between:
> *http://www.chemsafety.gov*

The Metropolitan Life Insurance Co. has a website with an index of its articles (and member form):

http://www.metlife.com/Sb

Other Insurance data are available:

http://www.insure.com/

The National Safety Council statistical information:

http://www.nsc.org/lrs/statstop.htmhttp://www.nsc.org/lrs/statinfo

Various small organizations have data for their sport:

http://www.awa.com

An environmental group has an excellent list of chemicals:

http://www.scorecard.org/chemical-profiles/

The atlas of cancer mortality is useful to someone trying to determine environmental causes:

http://www.nci.nih.gov/atlas/mortality.html

The Society for Risk Analysis (United States) has a website:

http://www.sra.org

The Center for Risk Analysis at Harvard University is a useful source of information:

http://www.hsph.harvard.edu/Organizations/hcra/hcra.html

The following sites collect various media reports of risks that some people consider to be "junk science."

http://www.cfis.com
http://www.junkscience.org
http://www.cei.org

Internationally the Paul Scherrer Institute in Zurich has a large data base on accidents and other interesting environmental issues:

http://www.psi.ch/gabe

In the United Kingdom of Great Britain and Northern Ireland, the Royal Society for Prevention of Accidents has data:

http://www.rospa.co.uk

The Intergovernmental Program on Climate Change (IPCC) has three websites for the three working groups:

http://www.meto.gov.uk/sec5/CR_div/ipcc/wg1/

http://www.usgcrp.gov/ipcc/

http://www.rivm.nl/env/int/ipcc/

Specific References

Papers referred to in any of the preceding chapters are gathered here in alphabetical order. Also included are references to a few key papers not otherwise mentioned.

Acheson, E.D., M.J. Gardner, P.D. Winter, and C. Bennett (1984). "Cancer in a factory using amosite asbestos." *Int. J. Epidemiol.* 13:3–10.

Allen, B.C., K.S. Crump and A.M. Shipp (1988) "Correlation Between Carcinogenic Potency in Animals and in Humans." *Risk Analysis* 8:531-544.

American Physical Society News, No. 7; See also *Physics Today* July 1995 at page 49.

Ames, B.N. (1975) "Identifying Environmental Chemicals causing Mutations and Cancer." *Science* 204:587–589.

Ames, B.N., R. Magaw, and L.S. Gold (1987). "Ranking Possible Carcinogenic Hazards." *Science* 236:271–275.

Ames, B.N. and L.S. Gold (1990). "Chemical Carcinogenesis: Too Many Rodent Carcinogens." *Proc. Nat. Acad. Sciences,* 87:7772–7776.

Ames, B.N., L.S. Gold and W.C. Willett (1995). "The Causes and Prevention of Cancer." *Proc. Nat. Acad. Sciences,* 92:5258–5265..

Andelman, J.B. (1985). "Human exposures to volatile halogenated organic chemicals in indoor and outdoor air." *Env. Health. Perspect.* 62:313–318.

Andelman, J. B., N.J. Giardino, N. J., J. Marshall, J., N.A. Esmen, J.E. Borrazzo, C.I Davidson, C. Wilkes, C. R., and M.J. Small, M. J. (1989). "Exposure to Volatile Chemicals from Indoor Uses of Water." In "Total Exposure Assessment Methodology," AWMA VIP-16, pages 300-311, Las Vegas, Nevada, U.S. EPA/Air & Waste Management Association.

Anderson, C. (1991). "Cholera Epidemic Traced to Risk Miscalculation." *Nature,* 354:255.

Anderson, E.L. and the Carcinogen Assessment Group of the U.S. Environmental Protection Agency (1983). *Risk Analysis* 3:277–295.

Anon.(1999) Article about mountain climbing statistics *High* 198:48

Armitage, P. and R. Doll (1954). "The Age Distribution of Cancer and a Multistage Theory of Carcinogenesis." *Brit J. Cancer* 8:1–12.

Armitage, P. and R. Doll (1957). "A Two Stage Theory of Carcinogenesis in relation to the Age Distribution of Cancer." *Brit J. Cancer* 11:161–169.

Armstrong, B., C. Tremblay and G. Theriault (1988). "Compensating Bladder Cancer Victims Employed in Aluminum Reduction Plants." *Journal of Occupational Medicine* 30:771-775.

Arrow, K.J., and A.C. Fisher (1974). "Environmental Preservation, Uncertainty and Irreversibility." *Quarterly Journal of Economics* 88:312–319.

Ashby, J. and R.W. Tennant (1991). "Definitive Relationships among Chemical Structure, Carcinogenicity and Mutagenicity for 391 Chemicals Tested by the U.S. NTP." *Mutation Research* 257:229–306.

Bagshaw (1998). Abstract at meeting of National Council of Radiological Protection and Measurements (NRCPM) on April 1st at Crystal City, VA.

Baldewicz, W., G. Haddock, Y. Lee, Prajoto, R. Whitley, and V. Denny (1974). "Historical Perspectives on Risk for Large Scale Technological Systems," UCLA-ENG-7485.

Baram, M.S. (1976). "Regulation of Environmental Carcinogens: Why Cost-Benefit Analysis May be Harmful to Your Health." *Technology Review* 78(8):40–43.

Baris, Y.I., A.A. Sahin, M. Ozesmi, I. Kerse, E. Ozen, B. Kolacan, M. Altinors, and A. Goktepeli (1978). "An outbreak of pleural mesothelioma and chronic fibrosing pleurisy in the village of Karain/Urgup in Anatolia," *Thorax* 33:181–192.

Baris, I., L. Simonato, M. Artvinli, F. Pooley, R. Saracci, J. Skidmore, and C. Wagner, (1987). "Epidemiological and environmental evidence of the health effects of exposure to erionite fibres: a four-year study in the Cappadocian region of Turkey." *Int. Journ. Cancer* 39:10–17.

Belton, V. (1994). "Multiple Criteria Decision Analysis—Practically the Only Way to Choose," Working Paper 90/10 in Operational Research Tutorial Papers: 1990, edited by Hendry, L. C. and Eglese, R. W., Operational Research Society, Birmingham, England.

Berry, G., M.L. Newhouse, and M. Turok (1972). "Combined effect of asbestos exposure and smoking on mortality from lung cancer in factory workers." *The Lancet*, Sept. 2, 1972, 476–479.

Berry, G., M.L. Newhouse, and P. Antonis (1985). "Combined effect of asbestos and smoking on mortality from lung cancer and mesothelioma in factory workers." *Br. J. Indust. Med.* 42:12–18.

Blot, W.J., L.E. Morris, R. Stroube, I. Tagnon, and J.F. Fraumeni, Jr. (1980). "Lung and laryngeal cancers in relation to shipyard employment in Coastal Virginia." *JNCI* 65:571–575.

Blot, W.J., J.M. Harrintgon, A. Toledo, R. Hoover, C.W. Heath and J.F. Fraumeni (1978). "Lung cancer after employment in shipyards during World War II." *N. Engl. J. Med.* 299:620–624.

Bogen, K.T. (1995). "Methods to Approximate Joint Uncertainty and Variability in Risk," *Risk Analysis,* 15:411–419.

Bogen, K.T., G.A. Keating, S. Meissner, and J.S. Vogel (1998). "Initial uptake kinetics in human skin exposed to dilute aqueous trichloroethylene in vitro." *J. Exp. Anal. Environ. Epidemiol.* 8:253-271.

Bond, V.P (1981) "The Cancer Risk Attributable to Radiation Exposure; Some Practical Problems." *Health Physics* 4:108–111

Bouville, A., K. Eckerman, W. Griffith, O. Hoffman, R. Leggett and J. Stubbs. (1994). "Evaluating the reliability of biokinetic and dosimetric models and parameters used to assess individual doses for risk assessment purposes." *Radiation Protection Dosimetry,* 53:211–215.

Boyd, G.J. (2001). "Risk Management Program for the Disposal of Chemical Agents and Munitions." Talk at the *special symposium on Quantitative Risk Assessment,* Irvine, CA; May 31st-June 2nd.

Bozzo, S.R., K.M. Novak, F. Galdos, S.J. Finch, and L.D. Hamilton (1979). "Mortality, Migration, Income and Air Pollution: A Comparative Study." *Soc. Sci. and Med. Geog.,* 13D(2), 95-109.

Braun, D.C., and T.D. Truan (1958). "An epidemiological study of lung cancer in asbestos miners." *Amer. Med. Assoc. Arch. Indust. Health,* 17:634–653.

Bruk, G.J., V.N. Shutov, I.G Travnikova, M.I Balonov, M.V Kaduka, and L.N. Basalaeva (1999). "The role of Forest products in the Formation of Internal Exposure Doses to the Population of Russia after the Chernobyl Accident" in: Contaminated forests; Recent Developments in Risk Identification and Future Perspectives Ed: I. Linkov and W. Schell Nato Science series (2) vol. 58 Kluwer Academic Publishers. Dordrecht, Boston and London.

Bunge, R.L., and R.L.Cleek (1995a). "A new method for estimating dermal absorption from chemical exposure. 2. Effect of molecular weight and octanol-water partitioning." *Pharmaceutical Research*, 12:88-95.

Bunge, R.L., R.L. Cleek, and B.E. Vecchia (1995b). "A new method for estimating dermal absorption from chemical exposure. 3. Methods for prediction and data analysis." *Pharmaceutical Research*, 12:972-982.

Burmistrov, D., M. Kossenko and R. Wilson (2000). "The Techa River Accident and its Effects." *Technology,* in press.

Burns, D.M., T.G. Shanks, W. Choi, M.J. Thun, C.W. Heath, and L. Garfinkel (1997). The American Cancer Society Cancer Prevention Study I: "12-year follow-up of 1 million men and women." In: *Changes in Cigarette-related disease risks and their implication for prevention and control.* Smoking and Tobacco Control Monograph No. 8, NIH Publication 97-4213, February 1997.

Butler, W. and J. Barnes (1968). "Carcinogenic Action of Ground Nutmeal containing Aflatoxins in Rats." *Food and Cosmetic Toxicology* 6:135.

Butler, W., Greenblatt and W. Lijinsky (1969). "Carcinogenesis in Rats by Aflatoxins B1,G1 and B2." *Cancer Research* 29:220.

Butterworth, B.E., G.L. Kedderis, and R.B. Connolly (1998). "CIIT activities." 18:41–10.

Byrd, D.M., M. Luann Roegner, James C. Griffiths, Steven H. Lamm, Karen S. Grumski, Richard Wilson, Shenghan Lai (1996). "Carcinogenic Risks of Inorganic Arsenic in Perspective." *Int. Arch. Occup. Environ. Health* 68, 484–494.

Cairns, J. (1975). "The Cancer Problem." *Scientific American* 233(5):64–78.

Cairns, J. (1999). "Absence of Certainty is Not Synonymous with Absence of Risk." *Environmental Health Perspectives* 107(2): 56-57.

Cairns, J., and K.L. Dickson (1995). "Individual Rights vs. the Rights of Future Generations: Ecological Resource Distribution over Large Temporal time Scales." In *An Aging Population, an Aging Planet, and a Sustainable Future*, Ed. Ingman S.R., X. Pei C.D. Ekstrom, H.J. Friedsam and K.R. Bartlett, Texas Institute of Research and Education on Aging, Denton TX.

Calabrese, E., and L.A. Baldwin (2000). "The Effect of Gamma Rays on Longevity." *Biogerontology*, 1:309-319.

Califano, J. (1978). "Draft summary: estimates of the fraction of cancer incidence in the United States attributable to occupational factors," with 8 contributors but no authors. Presented to AFL-CIO, September 11.

Camus, M. (2001) "An Asbestos Ban must be based upon a Comparative Risk Assessment." *CMAJ* 164(4)491-4

CDC (1990). "The health benefits of smoking cessation: a report of the Surgeon General." DHHS Publication No. (CDC) 90-8416.

Chapman, C.R. and D. Morrison (1994). "Impacts on the Earth by Asteroids and Comets: Assessing the Hazard." *Nature* 367:33–40.

Chase, G.R., P. Kotin, K. Crump, and R.S. Mitchell (1985). "Evaluation for compensation of asbestos-exposed individuals." *J. Occup. Medicine* 27:189–198.

Chen, C.J., Y.C. Chuang, S.L. You, and H.Y. Lin (1986). "A Retrospective Study on Malignant Neoplasms of Bladder, Lung and Liver in Blackfoot Disease Endemic Area in Taiwan." *Br J Cancer*, 53:399–405.

Cheng, W-N., and J. Kong (1992). "A retrospective mortality cohort study of chrysotile asbestos products workers in Tianjin 1972–1987." *Environ. Research* 59:271–278.

Cleek, R.L., and A.L. Bunge (1993). "A new method for estimating dermal absorption from chemical exposure. 1. General approach." *Pharmaceutical Research* 10:497-506.

Cohen, B.L. (1980). "Society's evaluation of Life Saving in Radiation Protection and Other Contexts." *Health Physics* 38:33.

Cohen, B.L. (1989). "Journalism's Failure on Nuclear Power Information." *Journal of Hazardous Materials*, 21:255.

Cohen, B.L. (1991). "Catalog of Risks Extended and Updated." *Health Physics* 61(3): 317–334.

Cohen, B.L. (1995). "Tests of the Linear No-Threshold Theory of Radiation Carcinogenesis for Inhaled Radon Decay Products." *Health Physics* 68:157–174.

Cohen, B.L. (1997). "Problems in the Radon vs. Lung Cancer Test of the Linear No-Threshold Theory and the Procedure for Resolving Them." *Health Physics* 72:623–628.

Condran, G.A. and R.A. Cheney (1982). "Mortality Trends in Philadelphia: Age- and Cause-Specific Death Rates 1870–1930." *Demography* 19:(1) 97–123.

Condran, G.A., and E. Crimmins-Gardner. (1978). "Public Health Measures and Mortality in U.S. Cities in the Late Nineteenth Century." *Human Ecology* 6:27–54.

Congress (1983). "The Orphan Drug Act." Public Law 97-414.

Congress (1984). "Veterans Dioxin and Radiation Exposure Compensation Standards Act." Public Law 98-542.

Congress (1988). "Radiation-Exposed Veterans Compensation Act." Public Law 100-321.

Congress (1990). "Radiation Exposure Compensation Act." Public Law 101-425.

Congress (2000). "National Defense Authorization Act." Public Law 106-698.

Corrosion Proof Fitting et al. (1991). "Corrosion Proof Fitting et al., Petitioners vs. The Environmental Protection Agency and William K. Reilly, Administrator." United States Court of Appeals, Fifth Circuit. Respondent No 89-4596, October 18, 1991, p. 564.

Cox, L.A. (1987) "Statistical Issues in the Estimation of Assigned Shares for Carcinogenesis Liability." *Risk Analysis* 7:71–80.

Cox, L.A. (1996). "More accurate dose-response estimation using Monte Carlo uncertainty analysis." *Human and Ecological Risk Assessment* 2:150–174.

Cropper, M.L. and Portney (1992). "Discounting Human Lives." *Resources* No. 108.

Crawford, M. and R. Wilson. "Low-Dose Linearity: The Rule or the Exception?" *Human and Ecological Risk Assessment* 2:305–330 (1996).

Cross, R.B. (1992). "The risk of reliance on perceived risk." *Risk: Issues in Health and Safety* 3:59–70.

Crouch, E.A.C. and R. Wilson (1981). "The Regulation of Carcinogens." *Risk Analysis* 1:47.

Crouch, E.A.C. and R. Wilson (1987). "Risk Assessment and Comparisons: An Introduction." *Science* 236: 267.

Crouch, E.A.C., and R. Wilson (1979). "Interspecies Comparison of Carcinogenic Potency." *J. Tox. Env. Hlth.* 5: 1095–1118.

Crouch, E.A.C. and R. Wilson (1981). "The Regulation of Carcinogens." *Risk Analysis* 1:47.

Crouch, E.A.C. (1996). "Uncertainty Distributions for Cancer Potency Factors— Laboratory Animal Carcinogenicity and Interspecies Extrapolation." *Hum. Ecol. Risk Assess.* 2:103–129.

Crowther, J. (1924). "Some Considerations Relative to the Action of X-rays on Tissue Cells." *Proc. Roy. Soc. Lond.(B) Biolog Sci.* 96:207–211.

Crump, K.S., Hoel, D.G., Langley, C.H., and Peto, R. (1976). "Fundamental Carcinogenic Processes and their Implications for Low Dose Risk Assessment." *Cancer Research* 36:2973.

Cuzick, J., P. Sasieni, and S. Evans. (1992). "Ingested Arsenic, Keratoses, and Bladder Cancer." *Amer J Epidemiol* 136(4):417–42.

Daubert (1995); Daubert v. Merrell Dow Pharmaceuticals, Inc., 509 U.S. 579, 113 S.Ct. 2786, 125 L. ed. 2d 469 (1993). On remand 43 F.3d 1311 (9th Cir. 1995), cert. denied ___ U.S. ___, 116 S.Ct. 132 L.ed.2d 126 (1995). Also at: http://supct.law.cornell.edu/supct/html/92-102.ZS.html

Dayal, S.R., E.B. Fowlkes, and B. Hoadley (1989) "Risk Analysis of the Space Shuttle:Pre-Challenger Prediction of Failure." *Journ. Amer. Stat. Assoc.* 84(408) 945-957.

De Klerk, J.H., A.W. Misk, B.K. Armstrong, and M.S.T. Hobbs (1991). "Smoking, exposure to crocidolite, and the incidence of lung cancer and asbestosis." *Br. J. Ind. Med.* 48:412–417.

Doll, R. (1971). "Cancer and Ageing: the Epidemiological Evidence." in Oncology, vol. V. Chicago: Year Book Medical Publishers, pp. 1–28.

Doll, R., and R. Peto (1976). "Mortality in relation to smoking: 20 years' observations on male British doctors." *Br. Med. J.* 2:1525–1536.

Doll, R., and R. Peto (1978). "Cigarette smoking and bronchial carcinoma: Dose and time relationships among regular and lifelong non-smokers." *J. Epidemiol. Comm. Health* 32:303–313.

Doll, R. (1979). "The Pattern of Disease in the Post Infection Era: National Trends." *Proc Royal Society of London* B205:47.

Doll, R., and R. Peto (1981). "The Causes of Cancer: Quantitative Estimates of Avoidable Causes of Cancer in The United Sates Today." *J. Nat. Cancer Inst.* 66: 1191-1308.

Doll, R., R Peto, E. Hall, K. Wheatley and R Gray (1994). "Mortality in relation to consumption of alcohol: 13 years' observation on Male British Doctors." *Br. Med. J.* 309:911–918.

Doll, R. (1998). "The Benefit of Alcohol in Moderation." *Drug and Alcohol Review* 17:353–363.

Domenici, P. (2001). Senate bill S 223.

Dutkiewicz, T. and H. Tyras (1967). "A Study of the Skin Absorption of Ethyl Benzene in Man." *Brit. Med. J.* 24:330-332.

Dutkiewicz, T. and H. Tyras (1968). "Skin Absorption of Toluene, Styrene and Xylene by Man." *Brit. J. Ind. Med.* 25:243-246.

Ebbin, S., and R. Kaspar (1974). "Citizens Groups and the Nuclear Power Controversy: Use of scientific and Technological Information." MIT Press, Cambridge, MA.

Eisenbud, M. (1978). "Environmental Causes of Cancer." *Environment* 20(8):1–16.

Elmes, P.C., and M.J.C. Simpson (1971). "Insulation workers in Belfast: 3. Mortality 1940–66." *Br. J. Indust. Med.* 28:226–236.

Elmes, P.C., and M.J.C. Simpson (1977). "Insulation workers in Belfast: A further study of mortality due to asbestos exposure (1940–75)." *Br. J. Indust. Med.* 34:174–180.

English, D.R., et al. (1995). "Quantification of Drug Caused Morbidity and Mortality in Australia." Commonwealth Department of Human Services and Health, Canberra, Australia.

Enterline, P.E. (1982), "Sorting out Multiple Causal factors in Individual Cases." In *Epidemiological Methods for Occupational and Environmental Studies Ed. Chiazze and Lundin,* Ann Arbor Science Publications, Ann Arbor MI.

Enterline, P.E. (1983). Multiple causal factors in individual cases. *In: Methods and issues in occupational and environmental epidemiology.* 177–182. Ann Arbor Science Publications, Ann Arbor MI.

Erren, T.C., M. Jacobsen, and C. Piekarski (1999). Synergy between asbestos and smoking on lung cancer risks. *Epidemiology* 10:405–411.

EPA, All EPA references are under BOOKS (above)

Ershow, A.G., and K.P. Cantor (1989). "Total tap water intake in the United States: population Based estimate of quantities and Sources." Life Sciences Research office, Federation of American Societies for Experimental Biology, Bethesda MD.

European Commission (1999). "ExternE: Externalities of Energy." ISBN 92-827-5210-0. Vols.1–9 and New Results. Published by European Commission, Directorate-General XII, Science Research and Development. L-2920 Luxembourg.

Evans, J., J. Graham, G. Gray & R. Sielken (1994a). "A Distributional Approach Expert Judgment in Distributional Analysis of Carcinogenic Potency." *Regulatory Toxicology and Pharmacology* 14; 1:25–34.

Evans, J., G. Gray, R. Sielken, A. Smith & J. Graham (1994b). "Use of Probabilistic Expert Judgment in Distributional Analysis of Carcinogenic Potency." *Regulatory Toxicology and Pharmacology* 20:15–36.

Ferris, B.G. (1963). "Mountain Climbing Accidents in the United States" *New England Journal of Medicine* 268:430–431.

Feshbach, M., and A. Friendly (1992). "Ecocide in the USSR." Basic Books, New York.

Fischhoff, B. (1984). "Defining Risk." *Policy Sciences* 17:123–139.

Fischhoff, B. (1996). "Public values in risk research." Annals of the American Academy of *Political and Social Science* 545:75–84.

Fischoff, B., C. Hohenemser, R.E. Kasperson and R.W. Kates (1978). "Handling Hazards." *Environment* 20(7) 16–37.

Fischhoff, B., P. Slovic, S. Lichtenstein, S. Read, B. Combs (1977). "How Safe Is Safe Enough?: A Psychometric Study of Attitudes Towards Technological Risks and Benefits." Decision Research, Eugene, OR.

Fischhoff, B. (1995). "Risk Perception and Communication Unplugged: Twenty Years of Progress." *Risk Analysis* 15:137–145.

Food and Drug Administration (FDA). (1977). "Saccharin and its salts: Proposed rule and hearing." *Federal Register* 42FR19996: April 153th.

Food and Chemical News. (1977). November 7, p 22; November 28 p 38.

Fritzsche, A.F. (1989). "The Health Risks of Energy Production." *Risk Analysis* 9:565–577.

Gardner, M.J., M.P. Snee, A.J. Hall, C.A. Powell, S. Downes and J.D. Terell (1990a). "Methods and Basic Data of Case-Control Study of Leukemia and Lymphoma among Young People near Sellafield nuclear plant in West Cumbria." *British Medical Journal* 300:429.

Gardner, M.J., M.P. Snee, A.J. Hall, C.A. Powell, S. Downes and J.D. Terell (1990b). "Results of Case-Control Study of Leukemia and Lymphoma among Young People near Sellafield nuclear plant in West Cumbria." *British Medical Journal* 300:423.

Gawande, A. (1999). "The Cancer Cluster Myth." *New Yorker* February 1999 pp 34–37.

Gehrels, T., Ed. (1994). "Hazards Due to Comets and Asteroids." University of Arizona Press, Tucson, AZ.

General Electric Co. (1997) v. Joiner, ___ U.S. ___, 118 S.Ct. 512,. 139 L. ed. 2d 508. See also: *http://supct.law.cornell.edu/supct/html/96-188.ZO.html*

Giardino, N.J., and J.B. Andelman (1996). "Characterization of the emissions of trichloroethylene, chloroform, and 1,2-dibromo-3-chloropropane in a full-size, experimental shower." *J. Expos. Anal. Environ. Epidem.* 6:413–423.

Gold, L.S., T.H. Slone and B.N. Ames (2001). "Pesticide Residues in Food and Cancer Risk: A Critical Analysis." In: Handbook of Pesticide Toxicology, 2nd Edition (R. Krieger, Ed.) Academic Press.

Gold et al. (1992). "Rodent Carcinogens: setting Priorities." *Science* 258:261–265 Tables 2 and 3.

Goldstein, B.D., M. Denak, M. Northridgen and D. Wartemberg (1992). "Risk to Groundlings of Death due to Airplane Accidents: a Risk Communication Tool." *Risk Analysis* 12(3):339-351.

Goodman, G., and R. Wilson (1992). "Comparison of the Dependence of the TD50 on Maximum Tolerated Dose for Mutagens and Non-mutagens." *Risk Analysis* 12:525–533.

Goodman, G., and R. Wilson. (1991). "Predicting the Carcinogenicity of Chemicals in Humans from Rodent Bioassay Data." *Environ. Health Perspect.* 94: 195–218.

Gottlieb, M.S. and R.B. Stedman (1979). Lung cancer in shipbuilding and related industries in Louisiana. *Southern Medical Journal* 72:1099–1101.

Graham, J.D. et al. (1992). "Poorer is riskier." *Risk Analysis* 12:333–337.

Graham, J.D. (1995). "Historical Perspective on Risk Assessment in the Federal Government." *Toxicology* 102:29–52.

Graham, J.D. et al. (1998). "Evaluating the Cost-Effectiveness of Clinical and Public Health Measures." *Annual Review of Public Health* 19:125–52.

Gray, G.M., P. Li, I. Shlyakhter, R. Wilson (1995). "An Empirical Examination of Factors Influencing Prediction of Carcinogenic Hazard Across Species." *Regulatory Toxicology and Pharmacology* 22: 283–291.

Green, L.C, S.R. Armstrong, E.A.C. Crouch, T.L. Lash, S.J. Luis., K.K. Perkins (1993). "Revised Protocol for a Multi-Pathway Risk Assessment for the WTI Facility in East Liverpool, Ohio. Cambridge Environmental Inc., Cambridge, MA.

Greenland, S. and J.M. Robins (1988) "Conceptual Problems in the Definition and Interpretation of Attributable Fractions." *Amer. J. Epidemiol.* 128:1185–1197.

Grimson, R.C. (1987). "Apportionment of risk among environmental exposures: application to asbestos exposure and cigarette smoking." *J. Occup. Medicine* 29: 253–255.

Gudiksen, P.H., T.F. Harvey, and R. Lange (1989). "Chernobyl Source Term, Atmospheric Dispersion, and Dose Estimation." *Health Physics* 57:697-706.

Guess, H., K. Crump and R. Peto (1977). "Uncertainty Estimates for Low Dose Rate Extrapolation of Animal Carcinogenicity Data." *Cancer Research* 37:3475–3483.

Hafemeister, D. (1996). "Biological Effects of Low-Frequency Electromagnetic Fields." Resource Letter BEL FES-11, *Am. J. Physics* 64: 974.

Hamilton, L.D., S.R. Bozzo, S.J. Finch, K.M. Novak, S.C. Morris, J. Nagy, M.D. Rowe (1980). "Comparative Risks from Different Energy Systems: Evolution of the Methods of Studies." SFEN, Colloquium on the Risks of Different Energy Sources, 516-572.

Hammitt, J.K. (1995). "Can More Information Increase Uncertainty?" *Chance,* Summer, 8:3.

Hammitt, J.K. (2000). "Evaluating Risk Communication: In Search of a Gold Standard." IN: Cottam, Harvey, Pape and Tait (Eds.). *Foresight and Precaution.* Rotterdam: 15–19.

Hammond, E.C. (1966). "Smoking in relation to the death rates of one million men and women. In: Epidemiological study of cancer and other chronic diseases." Editor W. Haenszel. Nat. Cancer Inst. Monograph. 19:127–204. U.S. Government Printing Office.

Hammond, E.C., I.J. Selikoff, and H. Seidman (1979). "Asbestos exposure, cigarette smoking and death rates." *Ann. NY Acad. Sci.* 330:473–490.

Harber, P., and D. Shusterman (1996). "Medical Causation Analysis Heuristics." *Journal of Occupational and Environmental Medicine* 38(6):577–586.

Hardin, G. (1968). "The Tragedy of the Commons." *Science* 162:1243–1248.

Hart, R.W, S.C. Freni, D.W. Gaylor, J.R. Gillette, L.K. Lowry, J.M. Ward, E.K. Weisburger, P. Lepore, and A. Turturro (1985). "Final report of the Color Additive Scientific Review Panel." *Risk Analysis* 6(2):117-54.

Hattis D. and Burmaster D.E. (1994). "Assessment of Variability and Uncertainty Distributions for Practical Risk Analyses." *Risk Analysis* 14:713–730.

Health & Safety Executive (1978). "Canvey: investigation of potential hazards from operation in the Canvey Island/Thurrock Area." Her Majesty's Stationary Office (London, UK).

Heaseman, M.A., I.W Kemp, J.D. Urquart, and P. Black (1986). "Childhood Leukemia in Northern Scotland." *Lancet* 266:385.

Higginson, J., and C.S. Muir (1976). "The Role of Epidemiology in Elucidating the Environmental Importance of Environmental Factors in Human Cancer." *Cancer Detection and Prevention* 1:79–105.

Hill, A.B. (1965). "The Environment and Diseases: Association and Causation." Proc. Royal Soc. Med., Sec. Occup. Med. 58:295.

Hilt, B., S. Langård, A. Andersen, and J. Rosenberg (1985). "Asbestos exposure, smoking habits, and cancer incidence among production and maintenance workers in an electrochemical plant." *Am. J. Ind. Med.* 8:565–577.

Hodgson, J.T, and A. Darnton (2000). "The Quantitative Risks of Mesothelioma and Lung Cancer in Relation to Asbestos Exposure." *Ann. Occup. Hygiene* 44:565–601.

Hoffman, F.O. and Hammonds J.S. (1994). "Propagation of Uncertainty in Risk Assessments: The Need to Distinguish Between Uncertainty Due to Lack of Knowledge and Uncertainty Due to Variability." *Risk Analysis* 14:707–712.

Hoyert, D.L., K.D. Kochanek and S.L. and Murphy (2000) "Final Data for 1997." National Vital Statistics Reports, 48(11), National Center for Health Statistics, Hyattsville, MD. *http://www.cdc.gov/nchs/data/nvs48_11.pdf.*

Hughes, J.M., and H. Weill (1991). "Asbestosis as a precursor of asbestos related lung cancer: results of a prospective mortality study." *Br. J. Ind. Med.* 48:229–233.

Hull, C.J., E. Doyle, J.M. Peters, D.H. Garabrant, L. Bernstein, and S. Preston-Martin (1989). "Case-control study of lung cancer in Los Angeles County welders." *Am. J. Ind. Med.* 16:103–112.

IARC (1997). "Evaluations of Carcinogenic Risks to Humans, Polychlorinated Dibenzo-dioxins and Polychlorinated Dibenzofurans." Volume 69, International Agency for Research on Cancer, IRAC press, Lyon, France. Also available on the web at: *http://193.51.164.11/monoeval/crthgr01.html.*

IARC (2001). "Evaluations of Carcinogenic Risk to Humans. Group 1: Carcinogenic to humans." International Agency for Research on Cancer, IARC press, Lyon. Also available on the web at: *http://193.51.164.11/monoeval/crthgr01.html.*

ICRP (1990). Recommendations of the International Commission on Radiological Protection, Report 60, Annals of the ICRP, Pergamon Press, UK.

IDSP (1990). "Industrial Disease Standards Panel, Second report to the Workers' Compensation Board on certain issues arising from the Report of the Royal Commission on Asbestos." Report No. 7, ISSN 0840-7274, April, 1990. ISBN 0-7729-7105-6.

Industrial Union (1980). "Industrial Union Department, AFL-CIO v. American Petroleum Institute." 448 U.S. 607 (1980) ("Benzene").

IPCC (1995). "Climate Change 1995." *Intergovernmental Panel on Climate Change.* Cambridge University Press, Cambridge, UK.

Jasanoff, S. (1993). "Bridging the two cultures of risk analysis." *Risk Analysis* 13(2):123–130.

Joiner (1997). General Electric Co. v. Joiner. ___ U.S., 118 S.Ct. 512,. 139 L.ed.2d 508. See also: *http://supct.law.cornell.edu/supct/html/96-188.ZS.html*

Kalelkar, A. (1988). "Investigation of Large Magnitude Incidents: Bhopal as a Case Study." Arthur D. Little, Cambridge, MA. *http://www.bhopal.com/casestudy.html*.

Kalia, Y.N., F. Pirot, and R.H. Guy (1996). "Homogeneous transport in a heterogeneous membrane: water diffusion across human stratum corneum in vivo." *Biophysical Journal* 71:2692-2700.

Kammen, D.M., A.I. Shlyakhter, and R. Wilson (1994). "What is the Risk of the Impossible." *Technology: Journal of the Franklin Institute* 331A:97–116.

Kasperson, R., Renn O., Slovic P., Brown H., Emel J., Goble R., Kasperson J., Ratick S. (1988). "The social amplification of risk: a conceptual framework." *Risk Analysis* 8:177–187.

Keeney, R.L., R.B. Kukcani and R. Nair (1978) "Assessing the Risk of an LNG terminal." *Technolgoy Review* 81:64.

Kimbrough, R.D., H Falk, P Stehr, and G Fries. (1984). *J. Toxic. Envir. Hlth* 14:47.

Kinlen, L. (1988). "Evidence for an Infective Cause of Childhood Leukemia: comparison of a Scottish New Town with Nuclear Reprocessing sites in Britain." *Lancet* 10;2(8624):1323-1327.

Khokhryakov, V.F., A.M. Kellerer, M. Kreisheimer and S.A. Romanov (1998). "Lung Cancer in Nuclear Workers of MAYAK." *Radiat. Environ. Biophys.* 37:11-17.

Kjuus, H., R. Skjaerven, S. Langård, J.T. Lien, and T. Aamodt (1986). A case-referent study of lung cancer, occupational exposures and smoking, II Role of asbestos exposure. *Scand. J. Work Environ. Health* 12:203–209.

Kletz, T. (1977). "Evaluate risk in plant design." *Hydrocarbon Processing* 56:297.

Kletz, T. (2000). "By accident—a life preventive theme in industry." PFV Publications, London, UK.

Knestaut, A (1996)"Fewer Women than men die of Work-Related Injuries." *Compensation and Working Conditions* 1(1),1 also at: *stats.bls.gov/opub/cwc/1996/Summer/brief3.htm*

Kociba, R.J., D.G. Keyes, J.E. Beyer, R.M. Carreon, C.E. Wade, D.A. DiHenberger, R.P. Kalnins, L.E. Franson, C.N. Park, S.D. Barnard, R.A. Hummel and C.G. Humiston (1978). "Results of a two-year chronic toxicity and oncongenicity study of 2,3,7,8-tetrachlorobenzo-p-dioxin in rats." *Toxicology of Applied Pharmacology* 46:279–303.

Krewitt, W., Hurley F., Trukenmuller A., Friedrich R. (1998). "Health Risks of Energy Systems." *Risk Analysis* 18(4):377–384.

Kumho (1999). Kumho Tire Company, Ltd., et al. v. Patrick Carmichael, et al. Supreme Court of the United States No. 97-1709 argued December 7, 1998–decided March 23, 1999. Also at: *http://supct.law.cornell.edu/supct/html/97-1709.ZS.html*

Lackner, K.S., R. Wilson and H.-J. Ziock (2001). "Free Market Approaches to Controlling Carbon Dioxide Emissions to the Atmosphere." in Global Warming and Energy Policy, Ed/ B. Kursunuglu. Plenum, FL.

LaDou, J., P.Landrigan, J.C. Bailar, V. Foa, and A. Frank (2001). "A call for an International Ban on Asbestos." *CMAJ* 164(4):491-4.

Lagakos, S.W. and F. Mosteller (1986) "Assigned Shares in Compensation for Radiation-Related Cancer." *Risk Analysis* 6:345–380.

Lamm, S.H., A.S. Walters, R. Wilson, D.M. Byrd and H. Gruenwald (1989). "Consistencies and Inconsistencies Underlying the Quantitative Assessment of Leukemia Risk from Benzene Exposure." *Environ. Health Persp.* 82:289–297.

Lange, R., M.H. Dickerson and P.H. Gudiksen (1988). "Dose Estimates from the Chernobyl Accident." *Nuclear Technology* 82:311-322.

Larsson, B.K, G.P Sahlberg, A.T. Eriksson and L.F Busk (1983). "Polycyclic Aromatic Carbons in Grilled Food." *J. Agric. Food Chem.* 31:867–873.

Lash, T.L., E.A.C. Crouch, and L.C. Green (1997). "A meta-analysis of the relation between cumulative exposure to asbestos and relative risk of lung cancer." *Occup. Env. Med.* 54:254–263.

Lawless, E.W. (1975). "Technology and Social Shock—100 Cases of Public Concern Over Technology." Midwest Research Institute for NSF/RANN, Kansas City, MO.

Leon, D.A., L. Chenet, V.M. Shkolnikov, S. Zakharov, J. Shapiro, G. Rakhmanova, S. Vassin M. and McKee (1997). *Lancet* 350:383–388.

Lichtenstein et al. (1978). "Judged Frequency of Lethal Events." *Journ. Exper. Psychology*, 4:551-578.

Liddell, F.D.K., D.C. Thomas, G.W. Gibbs, and J.C. McDonald (1984). "Fibre exposure and mortality from pneumoconiosis, respiratory and abdominal malignancies in chrysotile production in Quebec, 1926–75." *Singapore Annals Academy of Medicine* 13, No. 2(suppl.):340–344.

Lijinsky, W. and P. Shubik (1964). "Benzo(a)pyrene and other polynuclear hydrocarbons in charcoal broiled meat." *Science* 145:33.

Little, J.C. (1992). "Comment on Human exposure to volatile organic compounds in household tap water: the indoor inhalation pathway." *Environ. Sci. Technol.* 26:836–837; Response by McKone, 26:837–838.

Littlefield, N.A., J.H. Farmer and D.W Gaylor (1979). "Effects of Dose and Time in a long-term low-dose carcinogenic study." *Jour. Envir. Path.Toxicol.* 3:17–34.

Loh, Y.S., A.I. Shlyakhter and R. Wilson (1997). "Electromagnetic Fields and the Risk of Leukemia and Brain Cancer: A Review of Epidemiological Literature." *Journal of the Franklin Institute*, 334A:3–21.

Mangan, R.L, (1999) "Wildland Fire Fatalities in the U.S.: 1990–98." Report 9951-2808-MTDC, March, U.S. Forest Service (*www.fs.fed.us/fire/safety/fatalities/*).

Marmot, M., and E. Brunner (1991). "Alcohol and Cardiovascular Disease: the Shape of the U shaped Curve." *Brit. Med. J.* 303:565–568.

Martischnig, K.M., D.J. Newell, W.C. Barnsley, W.K. Cowan, E.L. Feinmann, and E. Oliver (1977). "Unsuspected exposure to asbestos and bronchogenic carcinoma." *Brit. Med. J.* 1:746–479.

Maslia, M.L., M.A. Mustafa, R.C. Williams, S. Williams-Fleetwood, L.C. Hayes, and L.C. Wilder (1996). "Use of computational models to reconstruct and predict trichloroethylene exposure." *Toxicol. Indust. Health* 12:139–152.

Matsumoto, K., M. Ito, S. Yagyu, H. Ogino, and I. Hirono (1991). "Carcinogenicity examination of Agaricus bisporus, edible mushroom, in rats." *Cancer Lett.* (1-2):87–90.

Mazur, A. (1975). "Opposition to Technological Innovation." *Minerva* 13:58.

McDonald, J.C., F.D.K. Liddell, G.W. Gibbs, E.E. Eyssen and A.D. McDonald (1980). "Dust exposure and mortality in chrysotile mining, 1910–75." *Br. J. Indust. Med.* 37:11–24.

McDonald, J.C., F.D.K. Liddell, A. Dufresne and A.D. McDonald (1993). "The 1891–1920 birth cohort of Quebec chrysotile miners and millers: mortality 1967–88." *Br. J. Ind. Med.* 50:1073–1081.

McKone, T.E and K.T. Bogen (1991). "Predicting the Uncertainties in Risk Assessment." *Envir. Sci. Technol.* 25:26–74.

McKone, T.E. and P.B. Ryan (1989). "Human Exposures to Chemicals through Food Chains: An Uncertainty Analysis." *Environ. Sci. Technol.* 23:1154–1163.

McKone, T.E. (1994). "Uncertainty and Variability in Human Exposures to Soil Contaminants through Home-Grown Food: A Monte Carlo Assessment." *Risk Analysis* 14: 449–464.

McKone, T.E. (1987). "Human exposure to volatile organic compounds in household tap water: the indoor inhalation pathway." *Environmental Science and Technology* 27:1194–1202.

McMurry et al. (1981). Report from Tennesee Valley Authority.

Mertz, P., Slovic and J. Purchase (1998). "Judgments of chemical risks: comparisons among senior managers, toxicologists and the public." *Risk Analysis* 18:391–404.

Moore, R.D., and T.A. Pearson (1986). "Moderate Alcohol Drinking and Coronary Heart Disease." *Medicine* 65:242–267.

Morales, K.H., L. Ryan, T-L Kuo, M-M. Wu, and C-J Chen (2000). "Risk of Internal Cancers from Arsenic in Drinking Water." *Envir. Health Perspectives* 108(7):655–661.

Morgan, G., S.C. Morris, M. Henrion, D.A.L. Amaral and W.R. Rish (1984). "Technical uncertainty in policy analysis: a sulfur air pollution example." *Risk Analysis* 4(3): 201–216.

Morgan, M.G. and Keith D.W. (1995). "Subjective Judgments by Climate Experts." *Environmental Science & Technology* 29:468–476.

Morris, J.M. and Hammitt J.K. "Life Expectancy as an Alternate Risk Communication Format." In: Cottam, Harvey, Pape, and Tait (Eds.). *Foresight and Precaution.* Rotterdam: 29–33.

Murphy, S.L. (2000). "Deaths 1998." National Vital Statistics Report 48(11), Center for Disease Control, Atlanta; and on the web at: *http://www.cdc.gov/nchs/data/nvs48_11.pdf.*

Murray, J.P, J.J. Harrington, and R. Wilson (1982). "Chemical and Nuclear Waste Disposal: Problems and Solutions." *Cato Journal* 2(2):565–606.

National Center for Health Statistics, Hyattsville, MD, USA. 2. *http://www.cdc.gov/nchs/data/nvs48_11.pdf.*

NAS (1987). "Regulating pesticides in foods: the Delaney Paradox." National Academy of Sciences/National Research Council, Washington, D.C.

NAS (1996) "Possible Health Effects of Exposure to Residential Electric and Magnetic Fields." National Research Council of the National Academy of Sciences, Washington, D.C.

NAS (1999). Health Effects of Exposure to Radon I. Committee on Health Risks of Exposure to Radon (BEIR VI), Board on Radiation Effects Research, Commission on Life Sciences, National Research Council. National Academy Press, Washington, D.C. (*http://www.nap.edu/html/beir6/*)

NCRP (1993). "Limitation of Exposure to Ionizing Radiation." NCRP report No.116. National Council on Radiation Protection and Measurements. Bethesda, MD.

Nelkin, D. (1971). "Scientists in an Environmental Controversy," *Science Studies* 1:245.

Nelkin, D. (1974). "The Role of Experts in a Nuclear Siting Controversy." *Bulletin of the Atomic Scientists* 30(9):29–36.

Neutra, R.R. (1990). "Counterpoint from a Cluster Buster" *Amer. J. Epidem.* 132(1):1–8.

NIH (1997). Changes in Cigarette-related disease risks and their implication for prevention and control. Smoking and Tobacco Control Monograph No. 8, NIH Publication 97-4213, February 1997.

Nicholson, W.J. (1983). "Quantitative risk assessment for asbestos-related cancers." Prepared for the Occupational Safety and Health Administration, Office of Carcinogen Standards, Cincinnati: OSHA, (Contract No. J-9-F-2-0074).

Nicholson, W.J., G. Perkel, and I.J. Selikoff (1982). "Occupational exposure to asbestos: population at risk and projected mortality—1980–2030." *Am. J. Ind. Med.* 3:259–311.

Nicholson, W.J. (1986). "Airborne Asbestos Health Assessment Update." Report for the United States Environmental Protection Agency EPA/600/8.84/003F.

NRC (1986). "Safety Goals for Operation of Nuclear Power Plants." Federal Register 51FR28044, Aug. 4.

NRC (1990). "Severe Accident Risks: An Assessment for Five U.S. Nuclear Power Plants." NUREG-1150 (3 volumes). U.S. Nuclear Regulatory Commission, Washington, D.C.

OTA (1985). "Preventing Illness and Injury in the Workplace." OTA-H-256m Office of Technology Assessment, U.S Congress, Washington, D.C.

Otway, H.J. and Cohen (1975). "Revealed Preferences: Comment on the Starr Benefit-Risk Relationships." (Research Memorandum RM 75-5) Laxenburg, Austria: International Institute of Applied Systems Analysis.

Pamuk, E., D. Makuc, K. Heck, C. Reuben, and K. Loeckner (2000). "Socioeconomic Status and Health Chartbook: Health United States, 1998." Center for Health Statistics, Hyattsville, MD. Also on the web at *http://www.cdc.gov/nchs/data/hus00.pdf.*

Parodi, S., M. Taningher, P. Boero, and L. Santi (1982). *Mutat. Res.* 93:1.

Pastorino, U., F. Berrino, A. Gervasio, V. Presenti, E Riboli, and P. Crosignani (1984). "Proportion of lung cancers due to occupational exposure." *Int. J. Cancer* 33:231–237.

Pauling, L. (1970). Many public lectures.

Paustenbach, D.J. (1995). "The Practice of Health Risk Assessment in the U.S. (1975–1995)." *Human and Ecological Risk Assessment* 1:29–79.

Paustenbach, D.J. (2000). "The Practice of Exposure: A State-of-the-Art Review." *Journ. Toxic. and Envir. Health* 3:179–271.

Pearl, R. (1926). "Alcohol and Longevity." Alfred A. Knopf, New York.

Peers, F., and C, Linsell (1973). "Dietary Aflatoxins and Liver Cancer: A Population Based Study in Kenya." *British Journal of Cancer* 27:473.

Peto, R. (1985). In "Assessment of risk from low level exposure to radiation and chemicals." A.D. Woodhead, CJ Shellabarger, V Pond, A Hollaender, Eds., Plenum Press NY, 3–16.

Peto, R., and M. Schneiderman, Eds. (1981). "Quantification of Occupational Cancer." Cold Spring Harbor Laboratory Banbury Report 9, Cold Spring Harbor, NY.

Piattelli-Palmarini, M. (1991). "Probability Blindness: neither Rational nor Capricious." *Bostonia* March/April 28–35.

Pierce, D.A., Y. Shimuzu, D.L. Preston, M. Vaeth, and K. Mabuchi (1996). "Studies of the Mortality of Atomic Bomb Survivors-Report 12(1): Cancer 1950–1990." *Radiation Research* 146:1–27.

Pierce, D.A. and D.L. Preston (2000) "Radiation-related cancer risks at low doses among atomic bomb survivors." (RERF Report No. 21-99) *Radiation Research* 154:178-86.

Pirot, F., Y.N. Kalia, A.L. Stinchcomb, G. Keating, G., A. Bunge, and R.H. Guy (1997). "Characterization of the Permeability Barrier of Human Skin in vitro." *Proc. Natl. Acad. Sci. USA* 94:1562-1567.

Pochin, E.E., (1975). "The Acceptance of Risk." *British Medical Bulletin* 31:184.

Pochin, E.E. (1982). "Risk and Medical Ethics." *J. Medical Ethics* 8:180–4.

Poikolainen, K. (1995). "Alcohol and Mortality: A Review." *Clin. Epidemiology* 488:445–465.

Price, B., and R. Wilson (2001). "Trends in Mesothelioma Incidence and Asbestos Exposure Evaluation" in The Health Effects of Chrysotile Asbestos Contribution of Science to Risk Management Decisions. Eds. R.P. Nolan, A.M. Langer, M. Ross, F. Wicks & R.F. Martin. Canadian Mineralogist Special Publication 5 (2001).

Rabl, A. (1996). "Discounting of long term costs: what would future generations prefer us to do?" *Ecological Economics* 17:137–145 See also report of Sept. 1999, Centre d'Energétique, École des Mines, Paris. France.

Rabl, A. and J.V. Spadaro (2000). "Comparison of Health Risks from Routine Operation of Energy Systems." PSAM5 (to be published).

Raiffa, H., Schwartz W., and Weinstein M. (1977). "Evaluating Health Effects of Societal Decisions and Programs." In: Decision Making in the Environmental Protection Agency Vol. 2b. National Academy of Sciences.

Rappaport, E. (1974). "Economic Analysis of Life-and-Death Decision-Making." (Appendix 2 in UCLA-ENG-7478). Los Angeles: School of Engineering and Applied Science, University of California, CA.

Rasmussen, N.F. et al. (1975). "Reactor Safety Study." U.S. Atomic Energy Commission report, WASH 1400, NUREG 75/014. See also D. Okrent, *Science*, 236 296 (1987).

Red, J. (1973). Term paper in Harvard course on risks of energy systems.

Renn, O. 1983. "Technology, risk, and public perception." *Applied Systems Analysis* 4:50–65.

Renn, O., Burns W., Kasperson R.E., Kasperson J.X., Slovic P. (1992). "The social amplification of risk: theoretical foundations and empirical application." *Social Issues*, Special Issue: Public Responses to Environmental Hazards, 48(4): 137–160.

Resources (2000). News Item. 140:10-13.

Rhomberg, L.R. (1997). "A Survey of Methods for Chemical Health Risk Assessment Among Federal Regulatory Agencies." *Regulatory Toxicology and Pharmacology* 26:74–79.

Rhomberg, L.R., Cogliano V.J., Scott C.S., Barton H.A., Fisher J.W., Greenberg M., Kuntz K.M., Sorgen S.P., and Maul E.A. (1997). "Trichloroethylene Health Risk Assessment: A New and Improved Process." *Drug & Chemical Toxicology* 20(4):427–442.

Rhomberg, L.R., and Wolff S.K. (1998). "Empirical Scaling of Single Oral Lethal Doses Across Mammalian Species Based on a Large Database." *Risk Analysis* 18(6):741–753.

Ries, A.A., D.J. Vugia, L. Beingolea, A.M. Palacios , E. Vasquez, J.G. Wells, N. Garcia Baca, D.L. Swerdlow, M. Pollack, N.H. et al. (1992). "Cholera in Piura, Peru: a modern urban epidemic." *J. Infect. Dis.* 166(6):1429-33.

Rimmington, J. 1995. "A social regulator's use of science." *Transactions of the Institution of Chemical Engineers, Part B.* 73(B4):S5–S7.

Robins, J. and S. Greenland (1989). "The Probability of Causation Under a Stochastic Model for Individual Risk." *Biometrics* 45:1125–1138.

Rosenthal, A., Gray G.M., and Graham J.D. (1992). "Legislating Acceptable Cancer Risk from Exposure to Toxic Chemicals." *Ecology Law Quarterly* 19:269–362.

Rothman, K.J. (1977). Chapter 9 in "Persons at High Risk of Cancer." Ed J.F. Fraumeni Academic Press, NY.

Rothman, K.J. (1986). "Modern Epidemiology."

Rothman, K.J. (1990). "A Sobering Start for the Cluster Busters' Conference." *Amer. J Epidem.* 132(supp):S6–S13.

Ruckelshaus, W. (1983). "Science Risk and Public Policy." *Science* 231:1026–1028.

Ruckelshaus, W. (1984). "Risk in a Free Society." *Risk Analysis* 4:157–162.

Ruckelshaus, W. (1985). "Risk, Science and Democracy." *Issues in Science and Technology* 1:19–38.

Russell, K. and M. Meselson (1976). "Quantitative Measures of Carcinogenic and Mutagenic Potency." Proc. Cold Spring Harbor Conference on Origins of Human Cancer, New York.

Russell, M., and M Gruber (1987). *Science* 236:286.

Rutherford v. Owens-Illinois, Inc., (1997) 16 Cal.4th 953, 67 Cal.Rptr.2d 16, 941 P.2d 1203. Cal.

Sakaji, R.H. (1991). "Radon in California's drinking water: a water quality survey and exposure assessment." California Department of Health Services, Oakland, CA, October 1991, figure 4.

Samet, J.M. (1998). "Assessing Health Risks: The Relevance of Epidemiology." Newsletter of the Risk Sciences and Public Policy Institute, Johns Hopkins School of Public Health. 1–5.

Saracci,R. (1977)."Asbestos and lung cancer: an analysis of the epidemiological evidence on the asbestos-smoking interaction." *Int. J.Cancer* 20:323–331

Savage, I. (1993). "Demographic Influences on Risk Perceptions." *Risk Analysis* 13: 413–420.

Scheuplein, R.J. and I.H. Blank (1971). "Permeability of the skin." *Physiological Reviews* 51(4):702–747.

Scheuplein, R.J. and R.L. Bronaugh (1983). "Percutaneous Absorption." In *Biochemistry and Physiology of the Skin*, 2; VIII, (34);1237–1297 Ed. L. Goldsmith, O.U.P.

Scheuplein, R. (1990). "Perspectives on Toxicological Risk—An Example: Food-Borne Carcinogenic Risk." In: Progress in Predictive Toxicology, Part V, Chapter 17, Ed. Clayson, D.B., J.C. Monroe, P. Shubik and J.A. Swenberg, Elsevier.

Schneiderman, M.A. and N. Mantel (1973). "The Delaney Clause and a scheme for rewarding good experiments." *Preven. Med.* 2:165.

Schwing, R.C. (1979). "Longevity Benefits and costs of Reducing Various Risks." *Technological Forecasting and Social Change* 13:333–345.

Seidman, H, and I.J. Selikoff (1990). "Decline in death rates among asbestos insulation workers 1967–1986 associated with diminution of work exposure to asbestos." *Ann. N.Y. Acad. Sci. 609*: 300–317.

Selikoff, I.J., E.C. Hammond, and J. Churg (1968). "Asbestos exposure, smoking and neoplasia." *JAMA 204:106–112.*

Selikoff, I.J., E.C. Hammond, and H. Seidman (1979). "Mortality experience of insulation workers in the United States and Canada, 1943–1976." *Ann N Y Acad Sci.* 330: 91–116.

Selikoff, I.J., H. Seidman, and E.C. Hammond (1980). "Mortality effects of cigarette smoking among amosite asbestos factory workers." *JNCI* 65:507–513.

Shank, R., J. Gordon, E. Wogan, A. Nondasuta and B. Subhamani (1972). "Dietary Aflatoxins and Human Liver Cancer III: Field Survey of Rural Thai Families for Ingested Thai Families" *Food and Cosmetic Toxicology* 10:71.

Shihab-Eldin, A., A. Shlyakhter and R. Wilson (1992). "Is There a Large Risk of Radiation? A Critical Review of Pessimistic Claims." *Environment International* 18:117–151.

Shlyakhter, A.I, G. Goodman and R. Wilson (1992). "Monte Carlo Simulation of Rodent Carcinogenicity Bioassays" *Risk Analysis* 12:73-82.

Shlyakhter, A.I. (1994). "An improved framework for uncertainty analysis: accounting for unsuspected errors." *Risk Analysis* 14:441–447.

Shlyakhter, A., L.J. Valverde, Jr. and R. Wilson (1995). "Integrated Risk Analysis of Global Climate Change." *Chemosphere* 30:1585–1618.

Shlyakhter, A., K. Stadie and R. Wilson. (1995). "Constraints Limiting the Expansion of Nuclear Energy." Report to U.S. Global Strategy Council, pp. 1–41.

Slob, W. (1994). "Uncertainty Analysis in Multiplicative Models." Risk *Analysis* 14:571–576.

Slovic, P., B. Fischhoff, and S. Lichtenstein (1976). "Cognitive Processes and Societal Risk Taking." In J.S. Carrol and J.S. Payne, Cognition and Social Behavior, Potomac, MD: L. Erlbaum Associates.

Slovic, P., B. Fischoff, and S. Lichtenstein (1977). "Behavioral Decision Theory." *Annual Review of Psychology*, Vol. 28, Annual Reviews, Inc., Palo Alto, CA.

Slovic, P., H. Kunreuther, and G.F. White (1974). "Decision Processes, Rationality, and Adjustment to National Hazards." In G.F. White (Ed.) Natural Hazards, Local, National and Global, Oxford University Press, New York.

Slovic, P. (1987). "Perception of Risk." *Science* 236:280–285.

Slovic, P. (1993). "Perceived Risk, Trust and Democracy: a Systems Perspective." *Risk Analysis* 13(6):675–682.

Slovic, P. (1998). "The Risk Game." *Reliability and System Safety* 59(1):73-78.

Slovic, P. (1999). "Trust, Emotion, Sex, Politics, and Science: Surveying the Risk Assessment Battlefield." *Risk Analysis* 19:689–701.

Smith, A.E., Ryan P.B., and Evans J.S. (1992). "The Effect of Neglecting Correlations When Propagating Uncertainty and Estimating the Population Distribution of Risk." *Risk Analysis* 12:467–474.

Smith, A.H. et al. (1998). "Marked increase in bladder and lung cancer mortality in a region of Northern Chile due to arsenic in drinking water." *Am J Epidemiol.* Apr.

Solomon, K.A., R.C. Erdmann, and D. Okrent. (1975). "Estimate of Hazards to a Nuclear Reactor from Random Impact of Meteorites." *Nuclear Technology* 21(1):68.

Solomon, K.A., R.C. Erdmann, T.E. Hicks, and D. Okrent. (1974). "Airplane Crash Risk to Ground Population" (UCLA-ENG-7424). Los Angeles: School of Engineering and Applied Science, University of California.

Stamatelatos, M.G. (2001). "NASA's New Aggressive Approach in QRA." Talk at Special Symposium on Quantitative Risk Assessment, Irvine, CA; May 31st-June 2nd.

Starr, C. (1969). "Social Benefit versus Technological Risk: What is Our Society Willing to Pay for Safety." *Science* 165:1232.

Starr, C. (1972). "Benefit Cost Studies in Sociotechnical Systems." *Perspectives in Risk Benefit Decision Making,* National Academy of Engineering, pp. 17–42.

Stokinger, H.E. (1972). "Concepts of Thresholds in Standard Setting." *Archives of Environmental Health,* 25:153–157.

Sullivan, T. J., J.S. Ellis, C.S. Foster, K.T. Foster, R.L. Baskett, J.S. Nasstrom, and W.W. Schalk (1993). "Atmospheric Release Advisory Capability: Real-Time Modeling of Airborne Hazardous Materials." *Bulletin of the American Meteorological Society* 74:2343-2361.

Surgeon General. "Smoking and Health: a report of the surgeon general." PHS79-50066, Public Health service, Washington D.C. (many editions).

Tancrede, M., L. Zeise, R Wilson and E.A.C. Crouch (1987). "The Carcinogenic Risk of Some Organic Vapors Indoors: A Theoretical Survey." *Atmospheric Environment* 21:2187.

Taubes, G. (1995). "Epidemiology Faces Its Limits." *Science* 269:164–169.

Tengs, T.O., M.E Adams, J.S Pliskin, D G Safran, J.E Siegel, M.C. Weinstein and J.D. Graham. (1995). "Five hundred life saving interventions and their cost effectiveness." *Risk Analysis* 15:369–390.

Thaler, R. and S. Rosen. (1973). "The Value of Saving a Life: Evidence from the Labor Market." Department of Economics, University of Rochester, Rochester, New York.

Thun, M.J., C.A. Day-Lally, E.E. Calle, W.D. Flanders and C.W. Heath Jr. (1995). "Excess mortality among cigarette smokers: changes in a 20-year interval." *American J. Public Health* 85:1223–1230.

Thun, M.J., C. Day-Lally, D.G. Myers, E.E. Calle, W.D. Flanders, B-P. Zhu, M.M. Namboodiri, and C.W. Heath (1997a). "Trends in tobacco smoking and mortality from cigarette use in cancer prevention studies I (1959 through 1965) and II (1982 through 1988)." In *Changes in Cigarette-related disease risks and their implication for prevention and control.* Smoking and Tobacco Control Monograph No. 8, NIH Publication 97-4213, February 1997.

Thun, M.J., D.G. Myers, C. Day-Lally, M.M. Namboodiri, E.E. Calle, W.D. Flanders, S.L. Adams, and C.W. Heath (1997b). "Age and the exposure-response relationships between cigarette smoking and premature death in Cancer Prevention Study II." In *Changes in Cigarette-related disease risks and their implication for prevention and control.* Smoking and Tobacco Control Monograph No. 8, NIH Publication 97-4213, February 1997.

Thun, M.J., R. Peto, A.D. Lopez, J.H. Monaco, S.J. Henley, C. W. Heath and R. Doll (1997c). "Alcohol Consumption and Mortality in Middle-aged and Elderly U.S. adults." *New Engl J. Med* 337:1705–1714.

Toth, B. and J. Erickson (1986). "Cancer Induction in mice by feeding of the uncooked cultivated mushroom of commerce *Agaricus Bisporus.*" *Cancer Research* 46:4007–4011.

Toth, B., Gannett P., Visek W.J., and Patil K. (1998). "Carcinogenesis studies with the lyophilized mushroom Agaricus bisporus in mice." *In Vivo* 12(2):239–244.

Turoff, M. (1970). "The Design of a Policy Delphi." *Technological Forecasting and Social Change*, 2(2):84–98.

Tversky, A. (1975). "On the Elicitation of Preferences: Descriptive and Prescriptive Considerations." In: Proceedings of the Workshop on Decision Making with Multiple Conflicting Objectives. Laxenburg, Austria: International Institute for Applied Systems Analysis.

Tversky, A. and D. Kahneman. (1971). "Belief in the Law of Small Numbers." *Psychological Bulletin* 76:105–110.

Tversky, A.; and D. Kahneman. (1973). "Availability: A Heuristic for Judging Frequency and Probability." *Cognitive Psychology* 5:207–232.

Tversky, A., and D. Kahneman (1974). "Judgment Under Uncertainty: Heuristics and Biases," *Science*, 185, 1124–1131.

Tversky, A., and D. Kahneman (1981). "The Framing of Decisions and the Psychology of Choice *Science* 211:453–458.

Tversky, A. and Koehler D.J. (1994). "Support Theory: A Nonextensional Representation of Subjective Probability." *Psychological Review* 101:547–567.

Upton, A. (1988). Are there Thresholds for Carcinogens? The thorny Problem of Low Level Exposure." *Annals of the NY Academy of Sciences* 534:863–884.

Upton, A. (1989). "The Question of Thresholds for Radiation and Chemical Carcinogenesis." *Cancer Investigations* 7(3):267–276.

Upton, A. and R. Wilson (2000). "Compensating government workers exposed to radiation." *Risk in Perspective* 8 (7) September.

U.S.C. (1958). "The Food Additive Amendment of 1958." 21 U.S. Code 348(c)(3)(A) Section 408.

Van Rensberg, S., J. Van der Watt, I. Purchase, L. Pereira Coutinko and L Markham (1974). "Primary Liver Cancer and Aflatoxin Intake in a High Cancer Area." *South African Medical Journal* 38:2808A.

Vasallo, K.M., A.J. Ruttenberger, C.J. Garrett, and W.M Maine (1997). "Homicides in Colorado Workplaces, 1982–94." *Compensation and Working Conditions* 2(1)32-39. Also at: *http://stats.bls.gov/opub/cwc/1997/spring/art5abs.htm*

Vermont Yankee Nuclear Power Corp (1978). vs. U.S. National Resources Defense Council, Inc. 435 U.S. 519.

Wagoner, J.K., and V.E. Archer, F.E. Lundin Jr., D.A. Holaday and J.W. Lloyd (1965). "Radiation as the Cause of Lung Cancer Among Uranium Miners." *New England Journal of Medicine* 273:185.

Wakeford, R., B.A. Hutell, and W.J. Leigh (1998). "A review of probability of causation and its use in a compensation scheme for nuclear industry workers in the United Kingdom." *Health Physics* 74:1–9.

Walker, A.M. (1984). "Declining relative risks for lung cancer after cessation of asbestos exposure." *J. Occup. Med.* 26:422–426.

Walker, K.D., J.S. Evans, and D. MacIntosh (2001a). "Use of expert judgment in exposure assessment: Part I – Characterization of personal exposure to benzene." *Journal of the International Society for Exposure Assessment.* Accepted with Revision.

Walker, K.D., P. Catalano, J.K. Hammitt and J.S. Evans (2001b). "Use of expert judgment in exposure assessment: Part II – Calibration of expert judgments about personal exposure to benzene." *Journal of the International Society for Exposure Assessment.* Submitted

Webler, T., D. Levine, H. Rakel, and O. Renn (1991). "The Group Delphi: a novel attempt at reducing uncertainty." *Technological Forecasting and Social Change* 39(3):253–263.

Weisbrod, B.A. (1961). "The Valuation of Human Capital." *Journal of Political Economy* 69:425–436.

White, G.F. (1972). "Human Response to Natural Hazard." Perspectives on Benefit-Risk Decision Making, National Academy of Engineering, Council on Public Engineering Policy. Washington, D.C.

Whitman, C. vs. American Trucking Association Inc. (2001). 121 S.Ct. 903.

WHO (2000). "Evaluation and Use of Epidemiological Evidence for Environmental Health Risk Assessment: WHO Guideline Document." *Environmental Health Perspectives* 108(10):997–1002.

Wilkes, C.R., M.J. Small, C.I. Davidson, and J.B. Andelman (1996). "Modeling the effects of water usage and co-behavior on inhalation exposures to contaminants volatilized from household water." *J. Expos. Anal. Environ. Epidem.* 6:393–412.

Wilson, D.R. (1938). "Annual Report: of the H.M Chief Inspector of Factories for the year 1938" His Majesty's Stationary Office, London, UK.

Wilson, R. (1972). "Kilowatt Deaths." *Physics Today* 25:73.

Wilson, R. (1975). "Examples in Risk-Benefit Analysis." *Chemical Technology* 6:604–607.

Wilson, R. (1979). "The Daily Risks of Life," *Technology Review*, February pp. 41–46.

Wilson, R. (1985). "Risks Posed by Various Component of Hair Dyes." *Arch. Dermatol. Res.* 278: 165–170.

Wilson, R. (1988). Expert report for the Superfund Site at Midvale, UT.

Wilson, R. (1996). "Risk Assessment of EMF on Health." *Engineering in Medicine and Biology*, July/August 77–86.

Wilson, R. (1999a). "Effects of Ionizing Radiation at Low Doses on People." AAPT Resource Letter, *Am. J. Phys.* 67(5).

Wilson, R. (1999b). "The Nuclear Fuel Cycle and other Features of Nuclear Power—Reaching a Public Consensus." In: Technology for the Global Economic and Environmental Survival and Prosperity, B.N. Kursunoglu, Ed., Plenum Press, New York.

Wilson, R. (2000). "Comments to U.S. EPA on proposed arsenic regulations." Available on the web at *http://phys4.harvard.edu/~wilson/EPA3_2000.html*

Wilson, R. (2001a). "The Probability of Causation." *Nuclear News* June.

Wilson, R. (2001b). "The Proposed Arsenic regulations." *Regulation* (in press).

Wilson, R. and W. Clark (1991). "Risk Assessment and Risk Management: Their Separation Should Not Mean Divorce." In *Risk Analysis*, edited by C. Zervos, Plenum Press, New York pp. 187–196.

Wilson, R., E.A.C. Crouch and L. Zeise (1983). "The Risks of Drinking Water," *Water Resources Research*, 19, 1359.

Wilson, R., E.A.C. Crouch and L. Zeise (1985). "Uncertainty in Risk Assessment" in *Risk Quantitation and Regulatory Policy* Banbury Report 19, pp 33–147 Cold Spring Harbor Laboratory Press, Cold Spring Harbor, New York.

Wilson, R., A.M. Langer, R.P. Nolan, J.B.L. Gee, M. Ross (1994). "Asbestos in New York City Public School Buildings—Public Policy: Is there a Scientific Basis?" *Reg. Toxicol. Pharmacol.* 20 161–169.

Wilson, R., A.M. Langer and R.P. Nolan (1999). "A Risk Assessment for Exposure to Glass Wool." *Regulatory Toxicology and Pharmacology* 30:96-109.

Wilson, R., and Price B. (2001). "Risk Assessment for Asbestos and Management of Low Levels of Exposure." In The Health Effects of Chrysotile Asbestos Contribution of Science to Risk Management Decisions, Eds. R.P. Nolan, A.M. Langer, M. Ross, F. Wicks & R.F. Martin. Canadian Mineralogist Special Publication 5 (2001).

Wilson, R., and J.D. Spengler, Eds. (1996). "Particles in Our Air: Concentrations and Health Effects." Harvard University Press, Cambridge, MA.

Wogan, G., S. Papaliunga and P. Newbreme (1974). "Carcinogenic Effects of Low Dietary Levels of Aflatoxin B1 in Rats" *Food and Cosmetic Toxicology* 12:681.

Wu-Williams, A.H., L. Zeise and D. Thomas (1992). "Risk Assessment for Alflatoxin B1: a Modeling Approach." *Risk Analysis* 12(4)559–567.

Wynder, E.L., and G.B. Gori (1977). "Contribution of the environment to Cancer Incidence: An Epidemiological Exercise." *JNCI* 58:825–832.

Zeckhauser, R. (1975). "Procedures for Valuing Lives." *Public Policy* 23:419.

Zeckhauser, R. and D. Shepard (1976). 'Where now for saving lives?" *Law and Contemporary Problems* 40(5).

Zeise, L., E.A.C. Crouch and R Wilson (1986). "A Possible Relationship Between Toxicity and Carcinogenicity." *Journal of the Amer. Coll. of Toxic.* 5, 137.

Zeise, L., E.A.C. Crouch and R. Wilson (1984). "Use of Acute Toxicity to Estimate Carcinogenic Risk." *Risk Analysis* 4:187–189.

Zeise, L., E.A.C. Crouch and R. Wilson (1987). "The Dose Response Relationships for Carcinogens: A Review," *Environmental Health Perspectives* 73, 259.

Appendix *1*

Some Famous Quotations

"The Days of our Years are Three Score and Ten; if by reason of strength they be Four Score Years, yet is their strength Labor and Sorrow for It is Soon cut off and we Fly Away."
 —Psalm 90 Verse 10. The Holy Bible revised edition.

"As far as we know, God is not impatient for our lives to be lived soon"
 —H. Daly in 1982

"The desire for safety lies against any great and noble enterprise."
 —Tacitus; Annals XV c110.

"Once harm has been done, even a fool understands it."
 —Homer, The Iliad, Book XVII, 1.32.

"If a man cannot change direction, he can never avoid disaster."
 —Herbert Schofield, quoted by C. H. Rolph in "Living Twice," Gollancz, 1974, p. 212.

"Round Numbers are always false."
 —Samuel Johnson. 03/30/1778. Boswell "Life of Johnson" 3:226.

"You don't have to know where you are to be there but is helpful to know where you are if you wish to be someplace else."
 —W.H. Foege.

"It is unquestionably true that [rail travel] is safer than traveling by coach or horseback…if one wants anything safer he must walk."
—H.G. Prout, 1892. *The American Railway.* New York, Charles Scribner and Son, p 191.

"We are not prepared to go to limitless expense to save lives that could be saved on the basis of the technical knowledge we possess."
—Editorial, *The Observer* (London),14 January, 1968.

"If you protect your tooth brushes as well as you protect your diamonds, you will lose fewer tooth brushes, but you will lose more diamonds."
—Nobel Laureate John Hartsough Van Vleck, circa 1950.

"Any politician would prefer a dead body to a frightened voter."
—J.Dunster, UK Health and Safety Executive.

"Some ecologists harm their cause by overstating their case and by condemning any industrial development even if they do not hesitate to make use of the products of that industry! We need to recognize 'real' risks, and to concentrate on eliminating them while at the same time using our technology properly for the benefit of mankind."
—K. Mellanby, "Unwise Use of Chemicals," keynote address at 1st International Conference on the Environmental Future, Finland, 1971. K. Mellamby was Director of the Monks Wood Experimental Station of the (English) Nature Conservancy.

"Risk assessment is replacing total garbage by partial garbage."
—Richard Peto, Gatlinburg, TN, 1980.

"Setting a Standard Deviation on the Risk is Total Bullshit."
—Malcomb Pike, Cold Spring Harbor, NY, 1984.

"For a Successful Technology, reality must take precedence over public relations, for Nature cannot be fooled."
—Richard P. Feynman (Nobel Laureate), 1988.

"An important area for further research is the quantitative assessment of accident probability... The approach can be applied at various levels to a wide variety of problems as a contribution towards establishing priorities on an objective and systematic basis."
—Report of the Committee on Health and Safety at Work, 1972.

"Once the detailed risk and benefit analyzes are available, I must consider the extent of the risk, the benefits conferred by the substance, the availability of substitutes and the costs of control of the substance. On the basis of careful review, I may determine that the risks are so small or the benefits so great that no action or only limited action is warranted. Conversely, I may decide that the risks of some or all uses exceed the benefits and that stronger action is essential."
—Russell Train. *Federal Register*, 41FR41102, 25 May, 1976. This was written when Russell Train was Administrator of U.S. EPA.

"In accepting [risk] we should be guided by common sense and honesty. We should not subject others knowingly to risks that we would not accept for ourselves or for our families. The decisions on socially acceptable risks which imply the calculation of costs/benefits should not necessarily be confined to an elite group but rather be established through a consensus of society as a whole and/or its representatives assisted by experts."
—John Higginson. "A Hazardous Society? Individual Versus Community Responsibility in Cancer Protection." Third Annual B. Rosenhaus Lecture, *American Journal of Public Health*, 1976. John Higginson was Director of the International Agency for Research on Cancer (IARC)

"That's how I judge pain Lucille... Will it hurt more than a punch in the nose or less than a punch in the nose?"
—From a Charles Schulz "Peanuts" cartoon.

"Anyone who tries to deal with health in economic terms, which is a necessary part of a system-analytic point of view, is exposing himself to the risk of misunderstanding and even of bodily harm from outraged citizens"
—Nobel Laureate Joshua Lederberg.

"Some risks are clearly so unacceptable that they must be eliminated. Others, less severe or less likely should be reduced to the point where the benefits of the risky activity balance the costs of its ill effects. Striking the balance invariably involves compromise."
> —John Dunster. "The Risk Equations: Virtue in Compromise." *New Scientist*, May 1977. John Dunster was Director of the Health and Safety executive, UK.

"The consideration of [the] risk-benefit ratio is basic to any intelligent discussion of any problem involving technology and society, and is all to often ignored in the utterances of consumer advocates and industry spokesmen."
> —Jean Meyer 1976, in the forward to *Eaters Digest* by M.F.Jacobson, New York, Doubleday (Anchor Books).

"In skating over thin ice safety is our speed."
> —Ralph Waldo Emerson, Essays (iii).

"...it must be ethically insecure to propose or to use a procedure without some assessment, however approximate, of the hazards involved, and without some indication of whether those hazards will be clearly offset by the likelihood of benefit..."
> —Sir Edward Pochin, M.D., National Radiological Protection Board, UK, formerly Chairman, International Commission on Radiological Protection: Journal of Medical Ethics 1982.

"The responsibility of those who exercise power in a democratic society is not to reflect inflamed public feeling but to help form its understanding."
> —Felix Frankfurter, 1928. Carved in stone on the wall of the Federal Court House, Boston.

"Imperial Chemical Industries (ICI) has announced the discovery of a new fire-fighting agent to add to their existing capabilities. Known as WATER (Wonderful And Total Extinguishing Resource), it augments, rather than replaces, such existing agents as dry powder and BCF, which have been in use from time immemorial. The new agent is particularly suitable for dealing with fires in buildings, timber yards, and warehouses. Although large quantities are required, WATER is fairly cheap to produce, and it is intended that quantities of about a million gallons should be stored in urban areas and near other installations of high risk ready for immediate use. Powder and BCF are usually stored under pressure, but

WATER can be stored in open ponds or reservoirs and conveyed to the scene of the fire by hoses and portable pumps.

"ICI's new proposals are already encountering strong opposition from safety and environmental groups. Professor Connie Barrinner has pointed out that, if anyone immersed his head in a bucket of WATER, it would prove fatal in as little as 3 min. Each of ICI's proposed reservoirs will contain enough WATER to fill half a million 2-gal buckets. Each bucketful could be used a hundred times, so there is enough WATER in one reservoir to kill the entire population of the United Kingdom. Risks of this size, said Professor Barrinner, should not be allowed, whatever the gain. If the WATER were to get out of control, the results of Flixborough or Seveso would pale into insignificance by comparison. What use was a fire-fighting agent that could kill men as well as fires?

"A Local Authority spokesman said that he would strongly oppose planning permission for construction of a WATER reservoir in this area unless the most stringent precautions were followed. Open ponds were certainly not acceptable. What would prevent people from falling into them? What would prevent the contents from leaking out? At the very least the WATER would need to be contained in a steel pressure vessel surrounded by a leakproof concrete wall.

"A spokesman from the Fire Brigades said he did not see the need for the new agent because dry powder and BCF could cope with most fires. The new agent would bring with it risks, particularly to firemen, that would be greater than any possible gain. Did we know what would happen to this new medium when it was exposed to intense heat? It had been reported that WATER was a constituent of beer. Did that mean that firemen would be intoxicated by the fumes?

"The Friends of the World said that they had obtained a sample of WATER and found that it caused clothes to shrink. If it did this to cotton, what would it do to men?

"In the House of Commons recently, the Home Secretary was asked if he would prohibit the manufacture and storage of this lethal new material. The Home Secretary replied that, since the new agent was clearly a major hazard, Local Authorities would have to take advice from the Health and Safety Executive before giving planning permission. A full investigation of WATER is needed, and the Major Hazards Group was asked to make a report."

— T. A. Kletz, Division Safety Advisor, Imperial Chemical Industries, United Kingdom (1975). Note: as often happens when there is a really major risk, the public authorities are uncertain and hesitate to take action. Even 25 years later in the year 2000 the Major Hazards Group still has not reported.

Appendix 2

Application of EPA's Hazardous Waste Identification Rule

A very interesting example of many of the concepts in this book arise in an attempt by U.S. EPA to define a concentration for a particular hazardous substance that will distinguish "hazardous waste" from non-"hazardous waste" in such a way that under plausible disposal scenarios, non-"hazardous waste" will not pose an unacceptable risk. Given the variety of potential waste streams, and the number of possible ways of disposing of waste, attempting to identify a single concentration that is non-hazardous is obviously very difficult. However, it is almost as difficult to first define what is the problem to be solved. What are the uncertainties? What are the variabilities? (Chapter 3) What is the acceptable level of risk for each group or subgroup? (Chapters 4, 5 and 6)

Several problems of definition arise that should be resolved before any HWIR can be implemented because:

- there is uncertainty about the legislative mandate;

- there is variability in population characteristics, waste management unit characteristics, geographically related characteristics, local topographical characteristics, and other characteristics;

- there is uncertainty about various parameters that affect exposures, such as food intake rates, bioconcentration factors, rainfall rates, hydraulic conductivities, and so forth; and

- there are interactions between and among the above three factors.

Some characteristics may be both variable and uncertain, and the distinction between variability and uncertainty depends on the legislative mandate, as will be made clear below. Indeed, it is the presence of variability and uncertainty that introduces essentially all the problems, so we will start with them.

1. Variability

Various characteristics that affect exposures to wastes are variable—that is, they may be accurately measurable, and they may be known accurately, but they are not the same in all situations of interest. Examples of such variabilities are:

Geographic

Many characteristics of interest vary with location throughout the country on scales that vary from regional down to local. Examples of regional scale variations are rainfall, average temperatures, meteorology, agricultural practices (in types of animals and crops raised, and the husbandry of those animals and crops). At the more local scale, there are variations in such factors as soil characteristics, field slopes, distances to water bodies, types of water body, and so on.

Demographic

Population density, age distribution, sex distribution, racial distribution.

Personal

Different people have different characteristics and habits, leading to variability in ages, weights, surface areas, food and water consumption patterns, times spent performing various activities such as showering or gardening.

Source Characteristics

Different waste sources, even of the same general type, have different areas, waste quantities, management practices.

Waste Characteristics

Different waste streams, even containing similar chemicals, have differences in physical and chemical properties, including water content, density, particle size distribution, pH, organic carbon content, leachability, chemical form.

These variable characteristics can be represented mathematically by distributions that specify the extent to which they vary, how they co-vary (joint distributions), or how they depend on other factors.

2. Uncertainty

All characteristics that affect exposures to wastes are uncertain to some degree—that is, we do not know the correct value of the characteristic in the required situation—although the degree of uncertainty varies. For certain characteristics (e.g. molecular weight), the uncertainty is so small that it can be considered negligible for practical circumstances, while at the other extreme the uncertainties can be essentially infinite (e.g. how carcinogenic are low doses of 1,1-dichloroethene to humans), at least in one direction (we know some *upper* bounds on how carcinogenic 1,1-dichloroethene could be to humans, but it could also be non-carcinogenic or even anti-carcinogenic).

Our standard way of evaluating exposures (or the effects of such exposures) is to construct "physical" models (generally mathematical constructs in which mathematical entities represent physical quantities) based on theoretical ideas, and to evaluate the parameters of those models by fitting experimental data to those theoretical models.[1] All statements that are then made are strictly conditional on the validity of those models; all uncertainties are cited with respect to those models; and the degree of certainty in those models is extremely variable. Our model for molecular weight can be considered correct with a very high degree of certainty, but our model for the carcinogenicity of materials is almost infinitely uncertain (again, in a biased way). However, the uncertainty in carcinogenicity *conditional on the models we use* is finite, and can be handled in a straightforward way.

We thus usually split uncertainty into at least two components: model uncertainty and parameter uncertainty, the latter conditional upon the former. There may be very little that can be said about the former uncertainty. In some situations (notably, in some of the physical sciences) where there is a large amount of experimental data, and good theoretical knowledge, it may be possible to estimate the potential sizes of the model uncertainties. In particular, if the model is merely being used to interpolate between experimental measurements, it may be possible to make uncertainty statements that are practically independent of model uncertainties. More generally it may be possible to acknowledge the presence of biases and omissions that have been deliberately introduced in choice of models, e.g. the standard model for carcinogenicity is considered to be conservatively biased (to overestimate risks) and it omits the potential existence of inter-individual variations.

Once the models are chosen, the uncertainties in parameters lead to our estimated lack of knowledge of the situation. The parameter uncertainty should be evaluated statistically by fitting the models chosen to experimental data. Our uncertainty in the situation at hand (evaluation of hazardous waste exposures or effects, for example) then is estimated by using statistical procedures to extrapolate or interpolate with the model (including all its uncertain parameters).

3. Legislative Mandate and its Interpretation

Legislative mandates are generally, perhaps always and often deliberately, written in vague terms, leaving the details up to the implementors. The Hazardous and Solid Waste Amendments (HSWA) to the Resource Conservation and Recovery Act (RCRA), Section 3004(m)(1) has a mandate that says "...so that short-term and long-term threats to human health and the environment are minimized." Similarly vague is RCRA 1004(5) which defines "hazardous waste" as "a solid waste, or..., which...may (A) cause, or significantly contribute to an increase in mortality or an increase in serious irreversible, or incapacitating reversible, illness; or (B) pose a substantial present or potential hazard to human health or the environment when improperly treated, stored, transported, or disposed of, or otherwise managed."

EPA has interpreted these mandates in various, generally fairly ambiguous ways. The most coherent and apparently relevant statement of EPA's philosophy, interpretations, and intentions that we have located occurs in the *Hazardous Waste Management System: Land Disposal Restrictions—Proposed rule* at 51FR1602 (January 14, 1986), excerpts of which appear below. However, we am unsure as to how closely EPA intends to hew to this statement, or even whether they are still aware that they made it.

For the purposes of the HWIR, we need to evaluate what is the mandate with respect to the following, obviously inter-related, points of view:

■ Who (what population) is to be protected,

■ Against what is that population to be protected,

■ In what circumstances is the population to be protected,

■ What does "protect" mean in these circumstances, and

■ How certain should we be that the protection is achieved?

It seems obvious that any such mandate would direct protection for the whole population—until one starts to think of the equally obvious plausible exceptions. For example:

- Workers on site—they are covered by occupational exposure rules that are obviously much less stringent than general population rules.

- Certain hypersensitive (e.g. allergic) individuals—there is no way that one can have any degree of confidence that any individual allergic to a particular material will be protected. It should be noted that for non-carcinogenic materials, the current "standards" that are used (reference doses: RfDs) explicitly incorporate a factor designed to account for population variability in sensitivity to chemical exposures, and so are designed to protect sensitive individuals. The same is not true for the carcinogenic potency values used by EPA: there is no explicit incorporation of the possibility of particularly sensitive individuals.

- People with relatively unusual habits. There are reports that in some parts of the country, people still practice "earth eating," so that they are unusually exposed to soil. Are soil standards for hazardous waste disposal to be set based on this practice? Some people practice colonic irrigation regularly, while others require regular kidney dialysis, both leading to unusually large exposures to water. Are water standards for hazardous waste disposal to be based on these circumstances?

More generally, there is likely to be variability among the population with respect to various parameters that control exposure or response to a given exposure, and some decision has to be taken as to the fraction of the population that will generally be "protected" at any given level, or the fractions of the population that will be protected at various levels.

To take account of variability in exposures, EPA currently uses a "reasonably maximally exposed individual" (RMEI) as a standard approach to take account of variabilities in exposure, although they have never precisely defined this concept except insofar as is it supposed to be above some 90th percentile of exposure. Some relevant language in the *Hazardous Waste Management System: Land Disposal Restrictions—Proposed rule* at 51FR1624 (January 14, 1986) that indicates that the EPA would also like to incorporate an alternative is:

"The Agency is also considering an alternative method…"

"…the Agency would choose a cutoff percentile such that the target protection level (e.g. 10^{-6}) is achieved in most cases and the risk to individuals falling beyond the cutoff also falls in the acceptable risk range."

"…the maximum risk posed in cases beyond the percentile cutoff (which can be no greater than the risk of directly ingesting full strength leachate) is required to fall within the Agency's acceptable risk range of 10^{-4} to 10^{-7}."

"Thus the maximum risk can be assured to remain within the Agency's acceptable risk range of 10^{-4} to 10^{-7} by selecting a leachate limit (screening level) that itself is associated with a risk no greater than 10^{-4}…"

and also (at a time when the Agency's standard approach was to evaluate a "maximally exposed individual"):

"…the Agency would prefer to consider expanding the basis for these protective thresholds to include total population risk as a factor in conjunction with risk to the maximum exposed individual in setting screening levels." (51FR1635)

RCRA mandates protection against "short-term or long-term threats to human health and the environment," and is elsewhere similarly vague. In practice, this has always meant that exposures have to be kept sufficiently low that they are below reference doses or doses that correspond to carcinogenic risk estimates that fall within or below the Agency's acceptable risk range of 10^{-4} to 10^{-7}. This combination of requirements helps to take account of the variability in sensitivity in the population, since reference doses themselves are designed so that it is highly unlikely that such doses would lead to any harm to any individuals (they explicitly incorporate population variability in their derivation), while the models upon which the carcinogenic risk estimates are based were designed to estimate an upper bound on risk.

In what circumstances should this protection be achieved? It cannot be in every circumstance, since everything (even water, oxygen, *etc.*) may be toxic in extreme circumstances. For HWIR, EPA/RTI have examined a subset of the ways in which wastes may be managed, namely ash monofills, land application units, waste piles, surface impoundments, and aerated tanks. Even for this subset of possible ways of dealing with waste, one still has the problem of deciding how extreme the circumstances to be examined have to be. Some potentially relevant language from the *Hazardous Waste Management System: Land Disposal Restrictions—Proposed rule* (51FR1602) is:

"Because these levels are intended to identify levels that are protective, to the best of EPA's knowledge, at *all existing and future land disposal sites,* and thereby define when wastes can be land disposed without prior treatment, the assumptions used in modeling must be conservative, i.e., representing a reasonable worst case." (51FR1623, emphasis added)

However, other language (in the context of modeling the effect of ground-water) may mitigate this:

"As a matter of policy, the Agency proposes to select the 90 percent level of the Monte Carlo probability distribution as the appropriate regulatory level. In this case, the level of treatment selected will ensure that down gradient concentrations will not exceed the specified target concentration in more than 10 percent of all possible settings for RCRA Subtitle C land disposal units."

"The Agency believes that selection of the 90 percent level is reasonable because of the extreme unlikelihood that hazardous waste land disposal facilities would be sited in the very worst locations. EPA believes that selection of a level higher than 90 percent would result in setting screening levels on highly improbable scenarios."

"Rather the exposure point must represent a point of potential exposure both during the active life of the facility, as well as after the closure and the post-closure care periods." (51FR1624).

This recognizes (to some extent) the problem of combining the variability of siting (which is covered by the Monte Carlo analysis mentioned in the above excerpts) with the uncertainty inherent in estimating any particular site (which is dealt with by using conservative parameter estimates), but the approach taken is still not rigorous. The variability across sites is inextricably mixed up with the uncertainty at a particular site, so that there is no predetermined confidence level for achieving a particular degree of protection at any given site.

4. Precise Definitions

A precise definition of the problems to be analyzed in any HWIR can be specified by selection of the:

■ Scenario(s) to be evaluated,

■ Measure(s) of risk to be evaluated,

■ Confidence levels to be achieved, and

■ Comparison value(s) for that(those) measure(s) of risk.

In general, all measures (and possibly also the comparison values) must be considered as distributions, in order to be able to incorporate uncertainties. The exact specification of the measure(s) of risk to be evaluated should be sufficient to eliminate any variability, although it may be desired to evaluate a complete variability distribution in addition—examples are described below.

a. Scenarios

The scenarios to be evaluated correspond to the placing of any or all of the five source types (ash monofill, land application unit, waste pile, surface impoundment, aerated tanks) in possible locations, with each source type handling waste streams appropriate for that type. Various options for the scenarios include:

(a) Current sources with current waste streams in their current locations.

(b) Current sources with current waste streams in any location currently occupied by another of the sources of the same type, or of different types, subject to physical constraints.

(c) (a), but with potential waste streams.

(d) (b), but with potential waste streams.

(e) Current sources with current waste streams in any (random) location throughout the (contiguous or whole) U.S., subject to physical constraints.

(f) (e), but with potential waste streams.

(g) Potential sources with potential waste streams in any (random) location throughout the whole U.S.

"Physical constraints" here are supposed to include consideration of the sizes of the sources and the sizes of the sites available for them, and any other engineering constraints deemed relevant.

"Sources" here refers to the combination of characteristics that define a source, including:

■ Physical dimensions

■ Containment parameters, if any (e.g. for surface impoundments)
■ Waste disposal rates

while "waste stream" refers to the combination of characteristics that define the waste stream, including density, water content, and organic carbon content.

The varying characteristics of each type of source define a variability distribution for the sources; the varying characteristics of each waste stream define a variability distribution for the waste streams; and the variation of characteristics associated with location define variability distributions for each location. Of course, for any individual source, waste stream, or location, one could only measure each characteristic with some degree of uncertainty; but that uncertainty is, for most characteristics, very small compared with the variation expected between different sources, so that there is no particular need to deal with any but the variability distributions—the uncertainties can be thought of as simply shifting analysis to a slightly different source, waste, or location than the one first considered.

Scenarios (a) and (b) have the advantage that all locations and characteristics of current sources and their locations are (or could be) known, and that the computational procedures are in principal finite (since there are only finite numbers of sources and locations). In practice, the locations of the current sources have not been assembled, and the characterization of current sources is not really complete.

Scenario (f) is the procedure we recommend. It is both comprehensive and feasible. Sources will be characterized by the distributions of current source characteristics, insofar as they have been measured, including the correlations between those characteristics. Waste streams will be characterized by distributions of current waste stream characteristics, but these will be allowed to be disposed in any source of the same type (so that any current correlations between source characteristics and waste stream characteristics will be ignored, except those induced by engineering considerations). We would limit the analysis to the contiguous U.S. because we suspect that Alaska and Hawaii present special problems of characterization.

Scenario (g) corresponds approximately to the current implementation of HWIR, since potentially important correlations between characteristics of current sources have been omitted (leading to an extension of the possible characteristics of current sources—i.e. potential sources). We suspect that the resulting extended characteristics are in some cases mutually exclusive (i.e.

either are not physically possible, or do not satisfy engineering constraint), or at least highly unlikely.

b. Measures of Risk

The choice of measure of risk determines how one has to deal with variability and uncertainty, and the best way that I can explain is to give examples.

Example 1

Consider the problem of evaluating the risks from a single site to individuals living near that site. Such risks will obviously depend (among other things) on where the individual lives with respect to the site, and on characteristics of the individual. We may wish to know how the individual risks vary with respect to distance from the site, or with respect to some other indicator of location with respect to the site. To account for this, we introduce a parameter that indicates location (e.g. distance from the site, a set of annular distance ranges around the site, a two-dimensional coordinate locator, a set of mutually exclusive areas defined on a map) and evaluate risk estimates (including all the uncertainty evaluations) separately for each parameter value. The variation in risk estimates with these parameter values then provides the variability distribution.[2] Any identifiable variability remaining at fixed values of the distance parameter selected (e.g. variability of soil type within an annular distance range from the site) must be treated as an uncertainty at that fixed parameter value.

As an example of the (correct) treatment of variability as an uncertainty, we do not know exactly who the individual is for whom we are estimating risks,[3] nor what his/her characteristics are. We therefore might demand to know what would be the risks to a random individual (implicitly, chosen from some population). In that case, the characteristics for the individual would be uncertain to the degree to which those characteristics vary among that population—the variability distribution among the population has to be considered an uncertainty distribution for this case.

The measure of risk being evaluated in this case is: the complete uncertainty distribution of risk to a randomly chosen individual (from some defined population) at some defined location with respect to the site, as a function of that location. A special case of this measure is the uncertainty distribution to a randomly chosen individual within some defined distance from the site. This last is the simplest case to evaluate, since there is only one location, and all variability distributions become uncertainty distributions for a random individual.

Example 2

Suppose we wish to evaluate a similar situation to that in Example 1, but wish to evaluate the variability between individual farmers around a site, no matter whether that variability is due to location with respect to the site or to personal characteristics. In that case, we may select a location (presumably within some pre-defined set of locations close to the site in some way) and an individual farmer (represented by whatever personal characteristics define an individual farmer), and evaluate the uncertainty distribution for that individual. In principal, the same procedure may be repeated for every location and every possible individual farmer, giving an infinite set of uncertainty distributions for risk, each labelled by location and personal characteristics.

It would then be possible to make certain probability statements about the risks for individual farmers: for example, one could find some value x such that, for 95% of the set of uncertainty distributions obtained, the 85th percentile of the uncertainty distribution for risk was less than x. Indeed, one could (for example) construct a variability distribution for the 85th percentile of the set of uncertainty distributions—this corresponds to imposing an ordering on the infinite set of uncertainty distributions. It should be clear, however, that there is no "natural" ordering of this set—it allows answering of certain questions, but those questions have to be carefully formulated, and the interpretation of the answers has to be strictly limited.

To illustrate this limitation on interpretation, consider the same problem as just defined, except that now we include the variability in the milk yield of the cows that are providing milk for the farmers as a variability, rather than as an uncertainty (as we implicitly assumed previously, since we did not specify it explicitly as a variability). Differing milk yields of cows certainly contribute to the variability of farmers' exposures,[4] and such differing milk yields are in principal measurable. Incorporating this variability, we will now (probably) get a different result for the value x defined above—for each individual member of the set of risk estimates, the uncertainty will smaller; but the variability will be larger. However, we are now measuring the variability of farmers' intakes due to location, personal characteristics, and the characteristics of their cows; and this is a slightly different problem than was originally specified for this example.

The measures of risks evaluated in this example are first: the set of uncertainty distributions for individual risk for a farmer at a specified location and with specified personal characteristics; and second, the set of uncertainty distributions for individual risk for a farmer at a specified distance, with specified characteristics, and with cows of specified characteristics. In other respects than those explicitly specified, the farmers are chosen at random (so that other characteristics are chosen at random, although incorporating any correlations with specified characteristics).

Example 3

The logical extension of Example 2 is to treat every variability distribution in any parameter in the whole risk assessment as a variability. However, this may not be the correct approach if what is required is some other measure of risk. The simplest example is evaluation of many measures of total population risk—there can be no variability in total population risk due to variability in the characteristics of members of that population. That does not mean that population risk estimates may not vary. They may differ because of site location, population distribution, or population characteristics,[5] for example.

Requirements for the HWIR program

The HWIR program is complex in that, for each source type, it requires consideration of geographic location, local topography, local demography, source characteristics, and waste characteristics. One can obviously devise many measures of risk that are plausible candidates for evaluation; but since the legislative mandate is unclear, no unambiguous choice can be made. It seems clear, based on the SAB comments and on the high correlations of other parameters with geographic location, that variability with respect to site location should be considered explicitly. In view of the recent NRC report (Science and Judgement in Risk Assessment, National Research Council, 1994), variability for any reason between individuals in exposed populations should be explicitly taken into account. Finally, the excerpts in Section 4 suggest that both individual risks and total population risks should be evaluated.

Variability between sites may be considered by evaluating sites one by one, leading to our formulation of the single-site problem as an initial requirement:

(a) For a given site and type of source, and for a list of chemicals in a waste with certain characteristics, obtain uncertainty distributions for the standard[6] (i.e., using EPA RfD and potency slope estimates) calculated, upper bound, excess lifetime carcinogenic risk estimates and hazard index estimates as a function of the concentration of each chemical in the waste.

These uncertainty distributions should be evaluated for individuals; and the choice of individuals to evaluate is a policy decision. Plausible examples are:

(i)   an individual living at the worst possible location with respect to that source;

(ii) an individual living as close as may be expected to the facility;

(iii) a random individual anywhere within Z km of the facility (with Z probably about 2 to 5 km); or

(iv) all individuals anywhere within Z km of the facility (with Z probably about 2 to 5 km)—i.e., obtain the variability distribution for individuals within this range.

Case (i) or (ii) corresponds most closely to what is attempted in the current HWIR program. Case (iii) is probably easiest to implement. Case (iv) is the most informative, but also the most difficult to do.

(b) Since population risk estimates are also required, perform the same analysis as in (a), but evaluate total population risk (i.e. total number of cancers in the population, and total number of non-cancer health effects expected). There can be no variability in these estimates (for a single site), only uncertainty.

Once the single-site problem has been evaluated, the multi-site problem is straightforward (in principal):

(c) For all feasible sites in the contiguous U.S., and for each (alternatively, any) type of source, do the same analysis as in (a) and (b).

c. Confidence Limits to be Achieved

Having obtained sets of uncertainty distributions, as outlined in Section 5.2, what is to be done with them? The usual approach is to select a single value from the uncertainty distributions and compare them with some single standard value (see Section 5.4). The spirit of the excerpts in Section 4 would be something like:

Find the value x (of concentration in waste) such that for 90% of sites, the risk estimate for the maximum exposed individual is less than the standard value Y.

The more precise statement and well-defined requirement using uncertainty and variability distributions would be something like:

Find the value x (of concentration in waste) such that for 90% of the sites, the upper 85th percentile of the uncertainty distributions is less than the standard value Y for at least 95% of the population.

(Note: We have chosen the 85th and 95th percentiles arbitrarily, simply as fairly conservative ones. The 90th percentile comes from Section 4).

In view of the language in recently proposed legislation (in particular, bills S 343 and HR 1022), this last may be considered too stringent, in view of the calls for a "best estimate." However, what "best estimate" means is ambiguous; it may be argued that it is a call for a mean estimate of uncertainty distributions, in which case the statement would become:

Find the value x (of concentration in waste) such that for 90% of the sites, the mean estimate of the uncertainty distributions is less than the standard value Y for at least 95% of the population.

This statement would probably be very little different from the previous one—it may even be more stringent[7]. Obviously other interpretations of the proposed legislative language are possible.

d. Comparison Values for the Selected Measures of Risk

What are the standard values against which the selected measures of risk will be compared (the values Y in Section 5.3)? The HWIR program appears to be taking the approach of selecting a hazard index estimate of 1.0 and a carcinogenic risk estimate value of 10^{-6}, with similar single point values for the ecologic criteria. This corresponds to the usual EPA approach of selecting a hazard index of 1.0 as a standard for non-carcinogenic materials, and a risk estimate of 10^{-4} to 10^{-7} for carcinogenic risk, although they have sometimes considered adequate risk estimates as high as 10^{-3} or more for small populations. The choice of comparison value is independent of how the risk assessment is performed, and the stringency of requirements is an interaction between the measures of risk selected (see Section 5.3) and the comparison value(s).

It is not necessary to limit comparisons to fixed point values. One obvious extension is to define a point comparison value for individual risks as a function of total population risk, with (usually) larger individual risks allowed with smaller population total risk. It is also possible to specify a comparison distribution in such a way that the shape of the uncertainty distribution for risks is taken into account in performing the comparison. With variability distributions available, it would be possible to specify comparison distributions rather than point estimates.

Notes

1 This fitting procedure uses a statistical model, based wherever possible on the physical model, but possibly introduced in an *ad hoc* way and so introducing further model assumptions.

2 If the location parameter is continuous, or has continuous pieces, this is strictly not a distribution until we define an order relation on the continuous pieces of the location parameter, or on each component of the location parameter if that parameter is multi-dimensional. See Example 2.

3 Even if we did know this, our models are not really good enough to be used on an individual basis.

4 Cows that differ in milk yields likely produce milk that differs in concentrations of certain contaminants.

5 In some cases, the uncertainty in population characteristics will be related to the variability of similar characteristics among individuals of that population, so that the same distributions may be used in a different way in the evaluation of different risk measures.

6 This corresponds to the relegation to "model uncertainty" of all the uncertainty in evaluation of toxicity.

Appendix 3

Procedure Used for Age Adjustment by NCHS

Age adjustment, using the direct method, is the application of age-specific rates in a population of interest to a standardized age distribution in order to eliminate differences in observed rates that result from age differences in population composition. This adjustment is usually done when comparing two or more populations at one point in time or one population at two or more points in time.

Age-adjusted death rates are calculated by the direct method as follows:

$$\sum_{i=1}^{n} r_i \times (p_i/P)$$

where

$r_i =$ age-specific death rates for the population of interest,

$p_i =$ standard population in age group i

$P = \sum_{i=1}^{p_i}$ for the age groups that comprise the age range of the rate being age adjusted,

$n =$ total number of age groups over the age range of the age-adjusted rate.

Mortality Data

Death rates are age adjusted to the U.S. standard million population (relative age distribution of 1940 enumerated population of the United States totaling 1,000,000) (Table A3-1). Age-adjusted death rates are calculated using age-specific death rates per 100,000 population rounded to 1 decimal place. Adjustment is based on 11 age groups with 2 exceptions. First, age-adjusted death rates for black males and black females in 1950 are based on nine age groups, with under 1 year and 1–4 years of age combined as one group and 75–84 years and 85 years of age and over combined as one group. Second,

TABLE A3-1

Standard million age distribution used to adjust death rates to the U.S. population in 1940

Age	Standard Million
All ages	1,000,000
Under 1 year	15,343
1–4 years	64,718
5–14 years	170,355
15–24 years	181,677
25–34 years	162,066
35–44 years	139,237
44–54 years	117,811
55–64 years	80,294
65–74 years	48,426
75–84 years	17,303
85 years and over	2,770

age-adjusted death rates by educational attainments for the age group 25–64 years are based on four 10-year age groups (25–34 years, 35–44 years, 45–54 years, 55–65 years).

The rate for years of potential life lost (YPLL) before age 75 is age adjusted to the U.S. standard million population (Table A3-1) and is based on eight age groups (under 1 year, 1–14 years, 15–24 years, and 10 year age groups through 65–74 years).

Appendix 4

Are Mushrooms Safe to Eat, or Should They Be Considered Toxic Waste?

The problem of interpretation of the results of bioassays of synthetic organic chemicals is not straightforward. It was originally considered that such bioassays would turn up a few chemicals that were overtly toxic, and that banning the use of such chemicals might substantially reduce the incidence of cancers, at least in some populations. However, these bioassays actually show that a large fraction of the chemicals tested are carcinogens under the conditions of the bioassays in the rodents (mice and rats) typically studied. The following analysis of a perfectly ordinary food that happens to have been studied in a bioassay perhaps indicates the problems of interpretation that can arise.

The Problem

Raw commercial mushrooms have recently been shown to be carcinogenic in a mouse bioassay that is equivalent in most respects to similar bioassays of synthetic organic chemicals. Here is a naive analysis that parallels the analysis that the FDA or EPA might perform on a synthetic organic chemical food additive (FDA) or a potentially toxic waste (EPA). The problem then arises as to whether raw mushrooms should be banned from stores as being an imminent hazard (FDA), and whether their disposal (if not eaten) should be governed by hazardous waste regulations (EPA). Subsequently, a few of the problems of interpretation that have been skipped over in this analysis are discussed.

Materials and Methods

Raw commercial mushrooms, obtained from the supplier of local food stores, have been tested in a bioassay (Toth and Erickson, 1986) similar to those used for synthetic organic chemicals. We can therefore perform a risk assessment on raw mushrooms similar in all respects to the risk assessments performed on synthetic organic chemicals. In the mushroom experiment, there was one control group of 50 mice for each sex and one experimental group of 50 mice for each sex, the former kept on a normal diet and the latter fed the material under test at an average rate of about 157,000 mg/kg-day for their lifetime (assuming mice weigh 30 g, typical for the mice used). Feeding of the dosed group was *ad lib* mushrooms (without other feed) 3 days/week, normal diet 4 days/week; while the control group received the normal diet. Average mushroom consumption was 11 g/day/mouse during days on which mushrooms were the only food available (mushrooms are about 90% water, accounting for the apparently huge weight of mushrooms eaten).

The experiment was continued for the natural lifetime of the animals, and no differences were seen in the lifetime of the dosed animals versus the control groups. However, the average weight of the dosed animals was substantially lower than the average weight of the control groups. There were increased incidences of tumors in several organs, as indicated in Table A4-1. The last column of the table indicates the probability of seeing the differences between control group and dosed group purely by chance, assuming that the two groups are otherwise equal.

Results

As can be seen from the table, there is a very large and very significant increase in the rate of tumors of the forestomach, a more modest but still

TABLE A4-1

Tumor Site: Type	Sex	Control Group	Dosed Group	Significance
Bone: various	F	0/50	8/50	0.003
Bone: various	M	0/50	8/50	0.003
Forestomach: various	F	0/50	19/50	2.3×10^{-7}
Forestomach: various	M	2/50	14/50	0.00094
Liver: hepatoma	F	0/50	4/50	0.059
Liver: hepatoma	M	1/50	6/50	0.055
Lung: all tumors	F	13/50	20/50	0.1
Lung: adenoma	F	6/50	12/50	0.096
Lung: adenocarcinoma	F	7/50	11/50	0.22
Lung: all tumors	M	17/50	31/50	0.0045
Lung: adenoma	M	12/50	24/50	0.006
Lung: adenocarcinoma	M	9/50	13/50	0.23

significant increase in the rate of various bone tumors, and statistically significant increases in the rate of some lung tumors.

From these results we can construct the following maximum likelihood and 95th upper percentile estimates for potency (q_1 and $q_1{}^*$) in mice (Table A4-2), following the standard method adopted by the EPA (Anderson et al., 1983).

Using the EPA methodology, the value usually chosen as a protective indicator of the carcinogenic potential for mushrooms would be the highest value of $q_1{}^*$ that corresponds to a statistically significant result—5.8×10^{-6} kg-d/mg— and this value would then have to be extrapolated to humans using an extrapolation factor of $(70 \text{ kg}/30 \text{ g})^{1/4} = 6.95$ (that is, the ¼ power of the ratio of bodyweights). This extrapolation is in accordance with the recommendations of an EPA/FDA/CPSC interagency task force (EPA, 1992) that these agencies modify their procedures to use a common factor corresponding to the ¼ power of the body weight ratio (in contrast to the previous situation, where EPA would use a ⅓ power, and FDA would use a zero power). The result is an upper bound estimate for the carcinogenic potency of mushrooms in humans of 4×10^{-5} kg-d/mg.

Implications

What does this imply for eating raw mushrooms in your salad or on your pizza?

■ A upper bound estimate of potency of 4×10^{-5} kg-d/mg implies that the dose rate required to give an upper bound estimate of risk of 10^{-6} (one in a million in a lifetime) is 0.025 mg/kg-d, or about 45 g (1.6 oz) per lifetime using the standard 70 year lifetime, 70 kg body weight assumption usually adopted by EPA. You would probably accumulate substantially more than this from the small quantities of mushrooms used as flavoring agents in various foods (like gravies and sauces), even if you consciously avoided eating mushrooms.

T A B L E A 4 - 2			
Tumor site:type	Sex	q_1 (kg-d/mg)	$q_1{}^*$ (kg-d/mg)
Bone: various	F	1.1×10^{-6}	1.9×10^{-6}
Bone: various	M	1.1×10^{-6}	1.9×10^{-6}
Forestomach: various	F	3.0×10^{-6}	4.4×10^{-6}
Forestomach: various	M	1.8×10^{-6}	2.9×10^{-6}
Lung: total	F	1.3×10^{-6}	2.9×10^{-6}
Lung: total	M	3.5×10^{-6}	5.8×10^{-6}

■ A consumption of 1 oz/month (13.3 mg/kg-d) of raw mushrooms corresponds to an upper bound estimate of lifetime risk of 5×10^{-4}. This is above the range that EPA (for example) generally considers as acceptable (that range being 1×10^{-6} to 1×10^{-4}).

■ According to Toth and Erickson (1986), estimated annual U.S. consumption of these mushrooms was 340×10^{6} kg in 1984–1985. This was an annual average per capita consumption of about 55 mg/kg-d, corresponding to an upper bound estimate of lifetime risk of 2×10^{-3} for the whole U.S. population. Presumably not all the mushrooms would be eaten raw, but we have no idea what would be the effect on the carcinogenicity of the mushrooms of cooking them. However, not everyone partakes of mushrooms, so the eaters would be at proportionately greater risk.

■ With the figures given in (3), the upper bound estimate of the annual number of cancers expected in the U.S. to be due to mushrooms is about 4000!

■ It is estimated that in Russia, Belarus and the Ukraine, near Chornobyl, adults gather forest products (Bruk et al. 1999) for their own use and consume 10 kg of mushrooms per year or 27 gms (390 mg/kg) per day— 7 times the U.S. figure. The lifetime risk from the chemicals therefore exceeds 10^{-2} which is large but still unmeasurable by any epidemiological study. A radiation dose of 50 mrems per year gives a smaller risk of 10^{-3}. Yet 50 mrems/yr (calculated using the same 27 gms per day) is the "intervention level" for ^{137}Cs in mushrooms, at which level people are not allowed to eat the mushrooms.

Mushrooms are known to contain various compounds, including hydrazine analogs, that are mutagenic *in vitro* and/or carcinogenic in laboratory animals under certain conditions. An extract of mushrooms of the type tested has also been shown to be mutagenic. However, the spectrum of tumors found in this experiment on raw mushrooms was not what might be expected from the known carcinogenic compounds present in the mushrooms. It is plausible that there are different carcinogenic compounds are also present, or that there was an interaction with other chemicals present.

The questions that now arise are manifold. These risk estimates correspond to risks much higher than would usually be regulated by EPA and FDA. Should FDA ban raw mushrooms as being immediately hazardous? Should EPA start regulating the disposal of mushrooms under RCRA statutes? If a Superfund site contains a building with a damp basement in which mushrooms are growing, should the risk assessment have to consider those mushrooms?

Modifying Comments

The reader is probably aware that mushrooms have not been removed from the market (at least at the time of writing). The question as to whether our food supply would be safer and more wholesome if they were to be removed from the market is not so simple as the above analysis would seem to suggest. Here are some of the complications

This bioassay is just one experiment of many on mushrooms. There have been others since then, on this type of mushroom and others, and on extracts of and known compounds in mushrooms. An experiment in which dried mushroom of the same type were fed to rats (making up 30% of the diet) failed to observe any carcinogenic activity (Matsumoto et al., 1991). However, more recently the original authors have also shown possible carcinogenic activity in mice of lyophilized mushrooms of the same type (Toth et al., 1998) fed at 2.5%, 5% and 10% of the diet, although no dose-response relation was established. Whether even this type of mushroom is a carcinogen in other animal species, or at dose levels corresponding to human consumption, must be considered an open question.

The experimental conditions of the first experiment, with the dramatic increases in some tumors, also introduce many problems in extrapolating the results to other circumstances. The animals were fed mushrooms only for 3 days/week, then the control diet for 4 days. Despite the large quantity of mushrooms eaten, they did not supply an adequate diet—the body weight of the mice cycled down and up as the mice went on and off the mushroom-only diet (personal communication between E. Crouch and B. Toth), and the average bodyweight was depressed. The incidence of many tumor types is likely to be affected by the substantial alterations in body chemistry implied by this cycling of body weight.

These are just two of the many reasons that confirmatory bioassays in other species and under different conditions are generally required before anything is declared to be carcinogenic—and even then, it must be borne in mind that the conditions of the experiment or exposure situation may be as important, or more so, than the agent being tested. While follow-up testing may show that *Agaricus Bisporus* is indeed carcinogenic, possibly even in humans, it is still questionable as to whether the human food supply would be made more wholesome by removal of mushrooms from it. A large number of human foods contain carcinogenic components, and are probably carcino-genic under certain conditions. Similarly, a large number of foods contain anti-carcinogenic components. The two sets of food are not mutually dis-tinct—it is likely that many foods contain both carcinogenic and anti-carci-nogenic components.

For what it is worth, the authors of this book still enjoy eating mushrooms in every form, including in their salad and on pizza (and one of us has enjoyed eating mushrooms near Chornobyl).

For references see Chapter 8.

Appendix 5

Evaluating the Lung-Cancer Risks Due to Smoking, Exposure to Asbestos, and Their Combination

This appendix is designed to give the reader some idea of the complexities involved in fairly detailed dose-response analyses using data from epidemiological studies. The results of this appendix are supposed to be useful—to allow as accurate as possible an assignment of the risk of lung cancer in humans who choose to smoke and who may also be exposed to asbestos. The object is to obtain dose-response curves for smoking and asbestos exposure effects on lung cancer death rates, so that given an individual's history of both, that individual's age-specific risk of lung cancer may be computed. The human epidemiology of smoking and lung cancer is now so extensive that a relatively complex dose-response curve may be estimated that takes account of average smoking rate (cigarettes/day), age, and age at starting smoking. For asbestos, much less information is available—for example, there are essentially no adequate data in women. In addition, smoking and asbestos exposure interact in the causation of lung cancer, making for a much more complex analysis.

While this appendix evaluates smoking and asbestos, it does not do a complete job. Only lung cancer is evaluated. Other causes of mortality and morbidity are not examined, so that the full effects of smoking and asbestos exposure are not captured here. In particular, the other very extensive and very large effects of smoking on health, including other lung diseases and other cancers, are not examined; and the effect of asbestos on mesothelioma is not included.

Smoking

Previous literature

In a paper applying a similar approach to that used here, Chase et al., (1985) used the results of Doll and Peto (1978). The latter authors summarized lung cancer incidence at age t among smokers (male British doctors) in the age range 40 through 79 as:

$$0.273 \times 10^{-12} \, (d + 6)^2 \, (t - 22.5)^{4.5} \qquad \text{(A5-1)}$$

for persons who continuously smoked a self-reported average of d (≤ 40) cigarettes/day since age 16 to 25. The average age of beginning smoking was 19.2 years. This formula represents a dose-response model that has been estimated from human data, but it has some obvious drawbacks. It is based on data in another country, for cigarettes different from those on the U.S. market, at a time when smoking habits may have been different. Moreover, this formula cannot adequately incorporate non-smokers.

Application of relatively old data on British doctors to U.S. populations is not ideal. More recent, and larger, studies have generated extensive data on U.S. populations. In particular, the most up-to-date, extensive, and well-documented studies are those of the American Cancer Society in their Cancer Prevention Studies I and II (CPS-I and CPS-II). These are studies of smoking and mortality, begun in 1959 and 1982, respectively, each involving more than 1 million American adults.

CPS (Cancer Prevention Study)-I and CPS-II data

This relies on data about lung-cancer in current smokers and non-smokers from the CPS-I and CPS-II studies, most recently reported extensively in *Changes in cigarette-related disease risks and their implication for prevention and control, Smoking and Tobacco Control Monograph 8* (NIH, 1997), in particular from chapter 3 (Burns et al., 1997), chapter 4 (Thun et al., 1995, 1997a), and chapter 5 (Thun et al., 1997b) of that volume.

The data on lung cancer (observed deaths, and person-years observed) come specifically from the following locations within CDC (1997):

CPS-I data

White Male Non-smokers:	Chapter 3, Appendix C, Table 1
White Female Non-smokers:	Chapter 3, Appendix C, Table 4
White Male Smokers:	Chapter 3, Appendix A
White Female Smokers:	Chapter 3, Appendix A

The published data are grouped into 5 year intervals of age (from 25 to 110 years for non-smokers, 40 to 85 years for smokers), 5 year intervals of duration of smoking (from 0 to 80 years), and self-reported cigarette smoking of 1–9, 10–19, 20, 21–39, 40+ cigarettes per day. There are a total of 955 (sex) × (age) × (duration) × (cigarette exposure) cells in which there are reported death and person-year-exposed data. All 955 cells were used in this analysis.

CPS-II data

The data for CPS-II are not so well arrayed as for CPS-I. Some has to be stitched together from different locations within CDC (1997). Chapters 4 and 5 deal with CPS-II (chapter 4 also examined CPS-I). Chapter 4 explicitly examines white males and females in most tables (page 310, para 1). Chapter 5 appears to look at the whole cohort (93% white, page 306, para 1).

Male Non-smokers	Chapter 4, Appendix 3 & 19 and Chapter 5, Appendix 4. Chapter 5, appendix 2 gives slightly different (higher) numbers of death, but that is for "lung cancer as any mention on death certificate" (see page 386, last para) rather than as an underlying cause of death.
Female Non-smokers	Chapter 4, appendix 4 & 20 and Chapter 5, appendix 4 (see comment above).
Male smokers	Deaths: Chapter 5, appendix 6 supplemented by Chapter 4, appendix 3. Person-years were obtained by combining deaths, death rates and marginal totals for person-years.
Female smokers	Deaths: Chapter 5, appendix 7 supplemented by Chapter 4, appendix 4. Person-years were obtained by combining deaths, death rates and marginal totals for person-years.

For non-smokers, usable data were available for ages 30 through 85 in 5-year intervals. For smokers, the data were grouped in 10 year intervals of age (50 through 80 years), 10 year intervals of duration of smoking (20 through 50 years), and self-reported cigarette smoking categories of 1–19, 20, 21–39, 40, and 41+ cigarettes/day. Additional data provided for 50+ years of duration and 85+ years of age categories could not be used because of the open-endedness of the categories. The number of deaths were available for all cells, but person-year-exposed data had to be computed by using the reported rates combined with marginal totals. For cells with zero deaths, the person-year-exposed data was obtained where possible by using marginal totals, although some could not be so re-constructed. Such cells are not used in the analysis. A total of 185 (sex) × (age) × (duration) × (cigarette exposure) cells could be constructed in which there are reported and usable death and person-year-exposed data, and all these are used in the analysis.

Dose-Response Analysis

Various simple dose-age-duration models were fitted to the available data. By extensive empirical evaluation of the data, coupled with theoretical ideas, it was discovered that the following model form fits all the data exceedingly well:

$$r = a\,(t/t_0)^{\alpha}\,(1 + bf(d)\,g(\tau/t)) \tag{A5-2}$$

where
$r =$ Mortality rate from lung cancer (deaths per 100,000 per year)
$t =$ Age (yrs)
$t_0 =$ A nominal age, taken to be 50 yrs, to normalize results
$a =$ A measure of background rate (deaths/100,000 per year)
$\alpha =$ Power law dependence
$b =$ A measure of potency (day/cigarette)
$d =$ Dose rate of cigarettes (self-reported cigarettes/day)
$f =$ Reported exposure-response shape for exposure to d cigarettes/day, normalized so that $f(20\ \text{cigs/day}) = 20\ \text{cigs/day}$
$\tau =$ Period of exposure (yrs)
$g =$ Duration-response shape for fractional-lifetime exposure, with $g(0) = 0$, $g(1) = 1$

The disaggregate data in CPS-I allows a good specification of the shape function g, while the aggregate data in CPS-II allows for obtaining parameters for that more recent cohort.

A subsidiary analysis showed that the background mortality rate (in the absence of smoking) has the same power law (α) age-dependence for men and women in CPS-I and CPS-II, and that the data are consistent with a pure power law up to the largest ages (approximately 110) in the data on non-smokers. The multiplying coefficients (a) are different for men and women, but the same for CPS-I and CPS-II. These observations were confirmed using the full model on all the non-smoker and smoker data combined.

To get some idea about the shape of $g(x)$, empirical estimates were made for each dose, sex and study, together with combinations over sexes and studies, by accumulating observed deaths in smokers and expected deaths (for non-smokers of the same age range) over ranges of x = (duration of smoking)/age, and plotting the ratio observed/expected versus x. The expected deaths were estimated from the excellent power-law fits to the non-smoker-data, together with the person-years-exposed data. These empirical plots suggested that the function g should be similar for males and females, and for CPS-I and CPS-II, in agreement with the prior belief that the mechanisms ought to be similar in males and females and over time. The common function g was then empirically parameterized by 10 values at $x = 0$, 0.1, 0.2, ... , 0.9, 1 (the values at 0 and 1 being held fixed at 0 and 1), with linear interpolation used between these values. Maximum likelihood estimates were obtained for the values at $x = 0.1, 0.2, ... , 0.9$ by requiring $f(d = 20) = 20$, where d and f are in cigarettes/day, but allowing all other values of f required at the nominal doses in CPS-I and CPS-II to be estimated by the maximum likelihood procedure, and demanding that g be monotonic increasing.

The likelihood was maximized by maximizing its logarithm. The loglikelihood was the usual poisson loglikelihood:

$$L = \sum_i (o_i \ln(e_i/o_i) - e_i + o_i) \tag{A5-3}$$

where the index i runs over all the available (sex) × (age) × (duration) × (cigarette exposure) cells, the observed number of deaths in cell i is o_i, and the expected number e_i is obtained as $100,000 r_i P_i$, where P_i is the person-years-exposed for that cell and r_i the expected rate per 100,000 given by the model in Equation A5-2. The arbitrary additive constant in Equation A5-3 is chosen so that the loglikelihood vanishes for an exact fit for every cell entry; and the loglikelihood behaves approximately as half a chi-squared variate indicating lack of fit of the model. All estimates for significance in what follows were obtained by likelihood ratio tests using this loglikelihood.

The nominal exposures used for CPS-I and CPS-II are:

CPS-I		CPS-II	
Reported Exposure (cigarettes/day)	Nominal Exposure (cigarettes/day)	Reported Exposure (cigarettes/day)	Nominal Exposure (cigarettes/day)
1–9	5	1–19	10
10–19	10	20	20
20	20	21–39	30
21–39	30	40	40
40+	50	41+	50

The resulting empirical estimates for g were examined and various functional forms used, while still allowing the values of f at the nominal doses to be set by the maximum likelihood procedure. The best-fitting functional form (one that resulted in non-significant change in likelihood from the 8-free-parameter empirical fit) was:

$$g(x) = \frac{\exp(\beta x) - 1}{\exp(\beta) - 1} \qquad \text{(A5-4)}$$

where the parameter was not significantly different for males, females, CPS-I, or CPS-II.

With g given by Equation A5-4, maximum likelihood estimates for f at the nominal doses for males, females, CPS-I, and CPS-II were obtained. These values guided the selection of a dose-response shape of the form:

$$\begin{aligned}
f(d) &= d\sqrt{20/\min(20,d_b)} \quad &\text{for } d \le d_b \\
&= \sqrt{d \max(20,d_b)} \quad &\text{for } d \le d_b
\end{aligned} \qquad \text{(A5-5)}$$

where d is the nominal reported exposure in cigarettes/day; d_b is a "breakpoint" below which the dose-response curve is linear, and above which it has square-root behavior. This form is chosen so that $f(20) = 20$.

With the above choices, using the empirical dose function f (16 parameters; 4 for each sex for each of CPS-I and CPS-II) and the empirical duration/age function g (8 parameters), a common power law for age-dependence, but with different coefficients for males and female (3 parameters) gave a loglikelihood of -475.9 for 1140 total cells (approximately 1113 degrees of freedom, indicating an excellent fit). With the parameterizations described, the loglikelihood decreased to -507.8 (12 parameters—a common power law [1], overall rate coefficients for males and females [2], a common duration parameter [1], and potency estimates [4] and break points [4] for distinct for males and females, CPS-I and CPS-II, again an excellent fit). The maximum likelihood estimates (MLE) are:

a (male)	5.2967 per 100,000 per year
a (female)	3.6193 per 100,000 per year
α	5.1877
β	2.8154
b (male, CPS-I)	1.5920 per cigarette/day
b (female, CPS-I)	0.8847 per cigarette/day

b (male, CPS-II)	2.6123 per cigarette/day
b (female, CPS-II)	2.6226 per cigarette/day
d_b (male, CPS-I)	27.934 cigarettes/day
d_b (female, CPS-I)	46.814 cigarettes/day
d_b (male, CPS-II)	8.6409 cigarettes/day
d_b (female, CPS-II)	26.537 cigarettes/day

The five digit precision provided here is for comparison purposes only; the accuracy of these values in representing the data is limited by the available data. The uncertainty in the dose response curve was estimated by evaluating the uncertainty in b (which is essentially interpretable as a cancer potency factor for relative risk). The multiplicative uncertainty factors obtained for b for CPS-II are:

b (male, CPS-II), uncertainty factor	1.0682
b (female, CPS-II), uncertainty factor	1.0665

These were obtained by finding upper and lower 95% confidence limits (90% confidence interval) on b (while keeping and d_b fixed) using standard asymptotic likelihood estimates, taking the logarithm of the ratio (upper limit)/(lower limit), dividing by 2×1.644854 (inverse normal of 0.95), and exponentiating. The upper and lower 95% confidence limits are almost exactly symmetrical around the MLE on a logarithmic scale.

Decline of relative risk after cessation of smoking

The relative risk for lung cancer declines after cessation of smoking. Empirical evidence indicates that the decline is adequately modeled by an exponential decrease in the excess relative risk with time since cessation, although the rate of decrease appears to differ for different average cigarette consumption rates. For men, data from the CPS-II indicate a decay constant for relative risk of 0.11018 yr^{-1} for cigarette consumption no greater than 20 cigarettes/day, and 0.08839 yr^{-1} for cigarette consumption over 20 cigarettes/day. These estimates were obtained as maximum likelihood fits (assuming poisson distributions for the number of deaths observed) to an exponentially declining excess RR, based on data provided in CDC (1990, Table 3).

The same analysis applied to CPS-II data on females gives: 0.22573 yr^{-1} for cigarette consumption no greater than 20 cigarettes/day, and 0.09873 yr^{-1} for cigarette consumption over 20 cigarettes/day.

There are data on the decline of relative risk in several other groups also, as given in Table 3 of CDC (1990) (prospective studies), together with Chapter 7, Table 4 (page 509) of NIH (1997). All give decay rates for excess relative risk of 0.06 through 0.23 yr^{-1}. CPS-II is the only prospective study in Table 3 of CDC (1990) reporting on RR for females.

Selection of Values to Use in a Current Population

The CPS-II study has greatest relevance for the computations required in evaluating current and recent populations. Of available studies with sufficient data to allow analysis, CPS-II most closely corresponds to the probably time periods of interest, reports results in Americans, and has high data quality and the most extensive reporting. Thus the best available dose-response model for the relative risk of death from lung cancer due to smoking is:

$$s = 1 + bf(d)g(\tau/t)e^{-\lambda\xi} \qquad (A5\text{-}6)$$

where b, f, d, g, τ, and t have the meanings assigned in Equations (2), (4), and (5), the value of b is:

Males:	2.6123 per cigarette/day
Females:	2.6226 per cigarette/day

g involves a parameter β that takes the value 2.8154127, f contains a parameter d_b that takes the values:

Males	8.6409 cigarettes/day,
Females:	26.537 cigarettes/day,

and the others parameters are:

t_q quitting age (in years),
ξ the larger of 0 and $t-t_q$, and
λ coefficient with values:

Males:	$\lambda_1 = 0.11018$ yr^{-1} for $d \le 20$ cigs/day	
	$\lambda_2 = 0.08839$ yr^{-1} for $d > 20$ cigs/day	
Females:	$\lambda_1 = 0.22573$ yr^{-1} for $d \le 20$ cigs/day	
	$\lambda_2 = 0.09873$ yr^{-1} for $d > 20$ cigs/day	

The values given above for males are the defaults. The uncertainty in the relative risk value is estimated by using an uncertainty factor on the coefficient b. This uncertainty factor was also estimated using the combined CPS-I and CPS-II data (with β and d_b held fixed), using likelihood methods. The value obtained was a factor of 1.068 for males, 1.067 for females.

Some Limitations and Caveats

The dose-response curve described above, while the most comprehensive available, suffers from several drawbacks. For one thing, it strictly was derived for a constant self-reported cigarette smoking rate between the starting and quitting times, but probably is adequate to estimate the effect of an average self-reported cigarette smoking rate. Smoking histories may be used to estimate an average self-reported consumption rate for cigarettes between starting and quitting the use of cigarettes (or lung cancer occurrence, whichever is earlier).

The smoking data do not extend beyond about age 80, so that use of the dose-response curve above that age is a substantial extrapolation. There is some evidence (from the British Doctors' Study) that at greater ages, the shapes of the absolute and relative risk curves alter, and it would probably be inaccurate to extrapolate the dose-age-exposure duration curves much.

The dose-response curve has limitations at high self-reported cigarette consumption rates. The CPS-II study had a cigarette exposure group defined as 41+ cigs/day, and this group is well-represented in our analysis by 50 cigs/day. There is no adequate reported information on relative risks for average consumption of more than 50 cigs/day. For strict matching of any particular smoker to the exposure groups of the CPS-II study, self-reported cigarette smoking of 1–19 cigs/day should be considered to be 10 cigs/day, 20 cigs/day as 20 cigs/day, 21–39 cigs/day as 30 cigs/day, 40 cigs/day as 40 cigs/day, and 41+ cigs/day as 50 cigs/day. Any other assignment (such as the actual self-reported values) must be recognized as interpolations.

The shape of the dose-response curve as a function of self-reported cigarette consumption is linear at low doses and square root at high doses. The linear low-dose regime is incorporated on general principles—there really are inadequate reported data disaggregated to doses below 10 cigarettes per day to decide on the shape of the curve at low doses. The shape at high doses was a surprise, particularly since it is completely different from the British Doctor's study (Doll and Peto, 1978). Because the dose-response shape cannot be adequately represented by an exponential function, and because the range of lung cancer relative risks induced by smoking is so large, the common practice of attempting to correct for smoking in epidemiological studies by using a standard linear term in an exponential relative risk model is likely to be substantially in error.

Asbestos

Potency of asbestos

To estimate relative risk from exposure to asbestos, 15 epidemiologic cohorts reported in 22 publications have been analyzed. The methods and results of analysis (using maximum likelihood) have been detailed in a published paper (Lash et al., 1997). The model used was:

$$R = A(1 + kM)$$ (A5-7)

where R = relative risk of lung cancer
          A = a background relative risk (relative to the population standard), different for each cohort
          M = cumulative exposure to asbestos, measured in fiber-yrs/ml
          k = the estimated coefficient for cumulative exposure, per fiber-yr/ml

Different epidemiologic studies are likely to give different estimates of k for several reasons, including differences in absolute calibration of measurement instruments, problems in inter-conversion of measurements made with different measurement methods, and different distributions of fiber size, type, and other characteristics. Similarly, different studies give different estimates for A, probably due to differences between the cohorts and standard populations in cigarette smoking and perhaps other exposures. The results reported (Lash et al., 1997) indicate that estimates of k and A obtained from different studies are distributed approximately lognormally. The different estimates of k obtained from the different epidemiologic studies were combined using a random effects model on both k and A with the assumption of lognormal distributions of values. The resulting best estimate were $k = 0.0026$ per fiber-yr/ml, with an uncertainty of a factor of 1.776 (95% confidence interval 0.00065 to 0.0074 per fiber-yr/ml).

The Effect of Selikoff's Cohort on the Potency Estimate

The analyses in the paper (Lash et al., 1997) did not include the Selikoff et al. (1979) insulation cohort, because the original publications made no attempt to estimate exposures. This cohort was the basis for many current estimates of the risk of asbestos, including that performed by OSHA. In his OSHA risk assessment, Nicholson (OSHA & Nicholson, 1983) used this cohort to estimate a value for k_L of 0.02 ml/f-yr. The data he used are listed in a table of SMRs versus years from onset of employment (Table 3 in OSHA & Nicholson,

1983) for those aged 25–45 at time of employment over the time period 1967–1980. He picks the highest SMR, 7.83, occurring at 30–35 years from onset of employment. He associates with this an exposure of 15 f/ml for a period of 22.5 (= 32.5 – 10) years, where the 15 f/ml is his estimate of the average exposure, and he assumes a lag period of 10 years for exposures to become effective. He then assumes that the SMR for zero exposure is unity. Thus he obtains (7.83–1)/(15*22.5) = 0.02 ml/f-yr.

To test the effect of such an assumption about exposures on the estimates given (Lash et al., 1997), this cohort was added into the fixed and random effects models. All the data were used up to the peak of the curve in Selikoff et al.'s (1979) data, at 30–34 years from onset of employment. To estimate exposures, the center of each age range was taken, minus a delay period of 10 years, and multiplied by the 15 f/ml average exposure. Nicholson provides observed numbers of lung cancers and an SMR, so the expected numbers were calculated, and the observed and expected numbers used as in the other cohort analyses. There are 5 exposure groups in the cohort, corresponding to 10–14, 15–19, 20–24, 25–29, and 30–34 years from onset of employment.

Inserting this extra cohort has very little effect on either fixed or random effects models. The fixed model without the cohort gives 0.000423 ml/f-yr; with the cohort, 0.000468 ml/f-yr. The random effects model without the cohort gives 0.002606 ml/f-yr; with the cohort 0.002801 ml/f-yr.

The reason for the small effect, despite Nicholson's high estimate for the coefficient, is not difficult to find. The lowest dose group has an SMR of 5.27, and no group (up to 30–34 years from onset of employment) has an SMR of less than 4.71. Thus Nicholson makes a huge leap in assuming that the SMR would have been 1 had this cohort not been exposed to asbestos. The correct approach is to use Poisson regression (to correctly take account of the small numbers of deaths in each group) on a relative risk model, with the possibility for an SMR different from 1 at zero asbestos exposure.

Using Poisson regression on the relative risk model $RR = A(1+kM)$ (where A is the background relative risk, k the coefficient, and M the effective exposure, equal to the period of exposure above a delay of 10 years multiplied by the average exposure of 15 fibers/ml), the best estimate of the coefficient is 0.0041 (again, only the data on exposures up to 35 years were used). Nicholson's approach (solid line) is contrasted with the Poisson regression approach (dashed line) in Figure A5-1. The intercept of the Poisson regression is at a relative risk of 3.05.

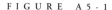

FIGURE   A 5 - 1

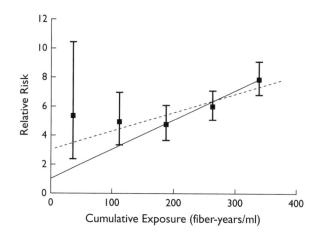

Cumulative Exposure (fiber-years/ml)

In fact, the situation is more complicated. The approaches described so far do not account for the probable differences in cigarette smoking in the various cohorts of asbestos insulators who started work at different times and ages. Some idea of the effect of such differences can be examined by using Table 1 of OSHA & Nicholson (1983). There Selikoff and Seidman have provided observed rate, expected rate, and numbers of deaths by 5 year interval of period of exposure, and by age groups 15–25, 25–35, and 35+ at age of first employment. Evaluating these separately and together using Poisson regression (again, only up to a total of 35 years of exposure—the peak of relative risk in all age groups), one finds that the k coefficient is indistinguishable for the three age groups, with value 0.0033 ml/fiber-yr, but that the intercept terms are significantly different (with values of 4.28, 3.08, and 2.32 respectively for 15–25, 25–35, and 35+ at age of first employment), as illustrated in Figure A5-2 (lines are Poisson regression fits, error bars are 90% poisson confidence intervals on the RR, assuming no uncertainty in the expected rates). The different intercept terms are presumably explained by differences in average smoking habits for these groups of men, but once the differences in intercept are taken into account, asbestos has the same multiplicative effect on relative risk in each group.

This finding of different intercepts for the different age groups shows that it is unhelpful to simply sum the results for differing age groups, as done by Nicholson. The effect of such summing is to mix up the effect of differing

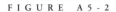

F I G U R E   A 5 - 2

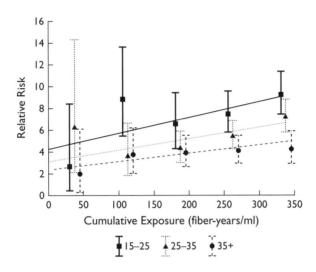

baseline risks (presumably due to smoking) with the effect of asbestos on multiplying those risks.

Decline in Relative Risk After Cessation of Exposure

It has also been observed that the relative risk for lung cancer does not increase until some time after exposure begins, and probably continues to increase for some time after exposure terminates. Nicholson et al. (1982) used this approach with a delay period of 10 years, and Chase et al. (1985) chose a delay period of 7.5 years. The majority of the studies included in the analysis of Lash et al. (1997) included a similar delay period.

Some time after termination of exposure, there appears to be a decline in relative risk (Walker, 1984). This decline has been inferred from the declines in relative risk found in epidemiologic studies at large times since first employment, rather than from a direct measurement of such an effect—principally in the cohort studied by Selikoff et al. (1979). It has been noted (Walker, 1984) that the decline after presumed elimination of asbestos exposure is slower than that observed after termination of cigarette smoking.

To estimate the rate of decay of relative risk after exposure, the data of Seidman and Selikoff (1990) were analyzed. Those authors provide person-years-exposed by 5-year intervals of age and 10 year intervals of period of exposure for the three calendar time periods 1967–1972, 1973–1979 and 1980–1986, and deaths by the 10-year intervals of period of exposure. The lung cancer rates in the latter two periods are affected by two effects—the increase in lung cancer rates with age, and the reduction in relative risks due to an increase in time since cessation of exposure. Implicitly, this analysis assumes that asbestos exposure was so much lower after about 1970 compared with before that it can be considered to have effectively ceased in this cohort between the latter two time periods; and the analysis also assumes that smoking habits did not change between these two time periods. The rate of lung cancer was assumed to increases with age according to the power law fitted to the CPS-II data (Equation A5-2). Then the Seidman and Selikoff (1990) data were approximated with a model for the distribution of exposure periods of the form

$$G(t) \propto (\tau/t_0)^\theta \exp(-\omega(\tau/t_0)^\varsigma) \tag{A5-8}$$

where τ = exposure period
          t_0 = an arbitrary age selected as a normalization constant
          $\theta, \omega, \varsigma$ = parameters describing the shape of the exposure period distribution

   This functional form was simply chosen to fit the data adequately. With this parameterization, the age-dependent rates during 1973–1979 were estimated as

$$r = a (\tau/t_0)^\alpha (A + BG(\tau)) \tag{A5-9}$$

and the 1980–1986 rates were estimated by

$$r = a (\tau/t_0)^\alpha (A + BG(\tau - \Delta t)e^{-\eta \Delta t}) \tag{A5-10}$$

where the terms a, t, t_0, and α have their previously defined meanings (Equation A5-2) of a rate coefficient, age, an arbitrary normalizing age, and the age-power law for lung cancer. The parameter is the rate of decline of relative risk after cessation of exposure to asbestos, Δt is the time shift (7 years) between observation periods, and A, B are fixed parameters. All the parameters were fitted to the observed numbers of deaths in both periods using maximum likelihood, assuming the numbers of deaths were poisson-distributed, and the resultant estimated decline rate estimated to be 0.02118 yr^{-1}.

   This estimate is probably an overestimate, because it neglects two effects that work in the same direction. First, if there were a decline of cigarette smoking between the two periods, as seems likely, then the estimated rate of decline of relative risk due to asbestos would include some of the reduction in relative risk due to the change in cigarette smoking. Second, there appears to have been differential mortality with length of exposure to asbestos in the examined cohort, as would be expected, so that the shape of the person-years versus length of exposure curve appears to be shifted only about 3.5 years rather than 7 years. In such circumstances, the assumption that the shape of the curve did not change between the two periods corresponds to overestimating the decline rate .

Assigning Causation of Lung Cancer to Smoking and Asbestos— the Logic of the Approach

In epidemiologic studies of exposure to an agent that may cause a particular disease, it is typical to estimate the relative risk (RR) for those exposed compared to those unexposed. This RR is the ratio of incidence of the disease in those exposed to the agent to the incidence in those not exposed. Ideally, the RR is a direct measure of the probability of causation in those with the disease. With sufficient data, the variation of relative risk with exposure variables, such as dose and period of exposure, may be obtained.

For smoking and asbestos exposure taken one-at-a-time, this last is the case. As described above, it is possible to evaluate the relative risk of lung cancer as a function of:

1. age,
2. age at termination of exposure,
3. age at first exposure, and
4. average intensity of exposure

for smoking, with a slightly simpler set of variables (age, cumulative exposure) for asbestos. In each case, for any individual with lung cancer incident at a given age and with a history of exposure corresponding to a relative risk r at that age, one may unambiguously attribute causation to exposure or natural background (strictly, anything other than the particular exposure) as the ratio r–1:1, since r is directly proportional to the probability for lung cancer.

For smoking and asbestos exposure taken both together, there is a fundamental ambiguity. One may compute the relative risk (s) for smoking acting alone, and the relative risk (a) for asbestos acting alone, according to the respective exposure circumstances. If there were no interaction between smoking and lung cancer, the relative risk (c) of both acting together would be given by:

$$c = 1 + (a - 1) + (s - 1) \qquad \text{(A5-11)}$$

and, for any individual so exposed and found to have lung cancer, there would be an unambiguous attribution of causation in the proportions $(a-1){:}(s-1){:}1$ to asbestos, smoking, and natural background. However, the relative risk (c) of both acting together is not given by this equation—there is an interaction between smoking habit and asbestos exposure—and the ambiguity arises in dealing with the relative risk due to this interaction.

Empirical studies initially indicated that, approximately, the total relative risk c is given by the product of the relative risks for smoking and asbestos separately, so that $c \approx as$. This relation is not important to the logic of the discussion, however, and is discussed further below.

Chase et al. (1985) wrote down one way of apportioning the relative risk to asbestos and smoking. They demanded that the apportionment satisfy several "self-evident" properties, and then wrote down the simplest formula that would satisfy these properties[1]. Grimson (1987) pointed out that one could write:[2]

$$c = (1) + (a - 1) + (s - 1) + (c - a - s + 1) \qquad \text{(A5-12)}$$

and treat the four terms on the right as proportional to the attributable fractions for natural background, asbestos, smoking, and the interaction. The interaction term could then be attributed explicitly to smoking or asbestos in any proportion one chooses. The attribution of Chase et al. corresponds to the choice that the interaction term is attributed to asbestos and smoking in proportion to the attribution that would occur if there were no interaction— that is, in the ratio $(a-1){:}(s-1)$.

To formalize the above discussion, extend the nomenclature of Chase et al. as follows:

a	is the relative risk due to the asbestos exposure alone,
s	is the relative risk due to smoking alone,
c	is the relative risk due to the combined effects of smoking and asbestos,
$P_A(a,s)$	is the fraction apportioned to asbestos,
$P_S(a,s)$	is the fraction apportioned to smoking, and
$P_0(a,s)$	is the fraction apportioned to background.

Chase et al. (1985) required the following properties (among others that are not important here—they have to do with the exposures before and after a cut-off date[3]).

1. Each fraction apportioned is a number between 0 and 1.
2. P_A increases with a, and is non-increasing with s; P_S increases with s, and is non- increasing with a.
3. $P_A + P_S + P_0 = 1$.
4. $P_A \rightarrow 1$ as $\alpha \rightarrow \infty$, $P_S \rightarrow 1$ as $s \rightarrow \infty$.
5. $P_A(1,s) = 0$, $P_S(a,1) = 0$.

Chase et al. (1985) wrote down "simple" expressions that satisfy these requirements, and then assumed that $c = as$. Grimson (1987) modified the expressions by explicitly apportioning the interaction term using arbitrary weights, again assuming that $c = as$. The formulae of Chase et al. (1985), without the assumption $c = as$, can be expressed as:

$$P_A = \frac{a - 1}{a + s - 2} \frac{c - 1}{c}$$

$$P_S = \frac{s - 1}{a + s - 2} \frac{c - 1}{c} \qquad \text{(A5-13)}$$

$$P_0 = \frac{1}{c}$$

In the absence of interaction, these formulae are strictly unique (although the requirements 1 through 5 are not enough to specify this uniqueness). This uniqueness arises because what are being dealt with are relative risks, proportional to probabilities, and the calculus of probabilities is additive. For example, if in Equation A5-13 one replaces a by $1 + F(a-1)$, s by $1 + F(s-1)$, and c by $1 + F(c-1)$, where F is a monotonically increasing function that satisfies $F(0) = 0$, properties 1 through 5 remain valid. However, in the absence of interaction, the result of such a substitution does not in general result in attributable fractions in proportion to probabilities. Thus we add the extra requirement:

6. The apportionment shall be by probabilities in the absence of interaction.

To make the assignments clear, we follow the approach of Grimson. The total relative risk may be written as:

$$c = 1 + (a - 1) + (s - 1) + (c - a - s + 1) \qquad \text{(A5-14)}$$

where the four terms on the right correspond respectively to background (RR of 1), the effect of asbestos alone, the effect of smoking alone, and the interaction term. This equation is a probability equation—each term is proportional to the probability of an effect, and so if the interaction term is zero, the three remaining terms on the right provide the unique probability apportionments for the three causes.

If the interaction term is not zero, then we may assign it to asbestos and smoking using a weight w ($0 \le w \le 1$) that has to be chosen:

$$c = [1] + [(a - 1) + w(c - a - s + 1)] + [(s - 1) + (1 - w)(c - a - s + 1)] \quad \text{(A5-15)}$$

With each such assignment (i.e. for each choice of weight w), the three terms on the right in brackets correspond to the relative apportionments for background, asbestos, and smoking. Grimson reaches this point, but then does not comment on the weight function w.

An assignment that is compatible with some approaches to equity occurs when the weight w is chosen so that the interaction term is assigned to smoking and asbestos in proportion to the probabilities in the absence of any interaction. We have excluded the attribution of any part of the interaction term to the background for the same reason. That is, we may choose:

$$w = \frac{a - 1}{a + s - 2} \qquad \text{(A5-16)}$$

This assignment corresponds exactly to the apportionment given by Equation A5-13. Other assignments might be considered equitable in other circumstances. For example, one might assign a value of w of 0.5 (that is, 50%), assigning the indirect risks 50:50 to asbestos and to smoking.

Interaction between Smoking and Cigarettes

The analysis of the asbestos cohorts discussed here makes use of an exactly multiplicative relative risk model for the risk of lung cancer due to asbestos. Of course, the major factor affecting lung cancer rates in most cohorts is smoking, as also previously discussed. Thus it is worth examining whether a pure multiplicative model for the relative risks of lung cancer due to smoking and asbestos is valid.

A 1990 report of the Industrial Disease Standards Panel (IDSP, 1990) reported that there are essentially three major sources for evaluation of the interaction between asbestos RR and lung cancer RR: Berry et al. (1972), Hammond et al. (1979), and McDonald et al. (1980). The IDSP cites Enterline (1983) as providing an analysis of the Selikoff et al. (1979) study, and also mentions Hilt et al. (1985) as showing multiplicativity, while Berry et al. (1985) suggest a larger effect on non-smokers than on smokers.

Saracci (1977) attempted to evaluate the interaction by examination of various published studies. He examined:

- Braun and Truan (1958). This is at Thetford Mines and Asbestos.

- Selikoff's small and large insulator cohorts.

- Elmes and Simpson (1971) (Saracci gives an incorrect citation). This has an update (not cited by Saracci) in Elmes and Simpson (1977).

- Berry et al. (1972). This has an update in Berry et al. (1985).

Saracci (1977) makes an error in computing expected rates for the Braun & Truan (1958) study. Moreover, it is impossible to calculate expected rates by length of exposure using the data provided by Braun & Truan (1958), as would be required for a reasonable evaluation of multiplicativity. Setting up the age × length of exposure matrix requires estimating about 18 cell entries using 10 marginal values for each of smokers, non-smokers, and unknowns (all deaths can be exactly located, because age and length of exposure and smoking status is known for each). Thus the Braun & Truan (1958) study cannot be used.

The study by Elmes and Simpson (1971, 1977) is small (170 men total), has very few non-smokers (5 total), and has no analysis by duration of exposure. The last rules out its effective use, and the first two indicate that inclusion of this study would have little effect on any result.

Berry et al. (1985) combined multiple studies to estimate that the relative risk of lung cancer due to asbestos was 1.8 times greater in non-smokers than in smokers (95% CI 1.1 to 2.8). This corresponds to any interaction effect being less than multiplicative. However, Berry et al. (1985) gave a reasoned caution against accepting this estimate at face value, and do not consider that the data they examined establish that non-smokers have a higher relative risk due to asbestos than smokers.

Erren et al. (1999) examined 12 epidemiologic studies for the synergistic effect of asbestos and lung cancer, using three indices of such synergistic effects, and calculations based on summary statistics. They estimated that approximately ⅓ of cancer cases among smokers could be attributed to the synergistic behavior of the two carcinogens. However, Erren et al. (1999) incorporated no dose-response modeling.

We have performed a meta-analysis for the interaction between smoking and asbestos effects on lung cancer that includes data from the thirteen cohorts:

- Berry et al. (1972, 1985)—female factory workers, 1960–70

- Berry et al. (1985)—male factory workers, 1971–1980

- Berry et al. (1985)—female factory workers, 1971–1980

- Selikoff et al. (1968)—the 370 NY insulators (1963–67)

- Hammond et al. (1979)—the U.S. and Canadian insulators (1967–76)

- Selikoff et al. (1980)—workers in an amosite factory

- Liddell et al. (1984)—chrysotile miners and millers in Quebec (pre-1976)

- Martischnig et al. (1977)—admissions to a thoracic surgical center

- Blot et al. (1978)—coastal Georgia, shipyard exposures

- Blot et al. (1980)—coastal Virginia, shipyard exposures

- Pastorino et al. (1984)—occupational exposures in Lombardy region of Italy

- Kjuus et al. (1986)—two Norwegian regional hospitals, occupational exposure

- de Klerk et al. (1991)—workers at Wittenoom asbestos factory, Western Australia

Berry et al. (1985), used the first seven of these, except that they combined male and female factory workers for the period 1971–1980. Erren et al. (1999) rejected the use of Selikoff et al. (1968) since that cohort is included in the cohort studied by Hammond et al. (1979), although Erren et al. (1999) failed to note that these papers report data for non-overlapping time periods. They combined the data from men and women in Berry et al. (1985), and used in addition data from the six other studies listed above. In addition, Erren et al. (1999) used data from Cheng and Kong (1992), but estimated the standard errors associated with the reported relative risks, a procedure that we consider incorrect. Further papers by Acheson et al. (1984), and Hilt et al. (1985), mentioned by Erren et al. (1999) provide too few data to allow a likelihood function to be written, and Berry et al. (1972, 1985) similarly provide too few data to include the 1960–1970 cohort of male factory workers.

McDonald et al. (1993) provide further follow-up (1976–1988) of the chrysotile miners and millers in Quebec analyzed by Liddell et al. (1984). They provide observed numbers and SMRs relative to the population, but not relative to non-smokers, so providing too few data to allow a likelihood to be constructed. Similarly, Liddell et al. (1998) provide yet further follow-up of this cohort to 1992, including results of an analysis of the smoking-asbestos interaction, but again too few data are provided to allow construction of a likelihood.

We fitted a relative risk model of the form

$$c = 1 + (a - 1) + (s - 1) + \mu(a - 1)(s - 1) \qquad \text{(A5-17)}$$

where as before c is the total relative risk, and a and s are the relative risks that would be realized due to exposure to asbestos or smoking alone. We found that a single value of μ was adequate (p = 0.077). The MLE for was 0.72, with 90% CI of 0.44 to 1.23 (an uncertainty factor of 1.37).

This result agrees with those found by Berry et al. (1985) and Erren et al. (1999), although it is stated in a different way and using somewhat different assumptions and analysis methods. Berry et al. (1985) also gave cogent arguments as to why the confidence limits are likely to be larger than indicated. Thus, although the best estimate for the interaction term corresponds to a non-multiplicative model, the pure multiplicative model is not ruled out by available data.

For references, see Chapter 8.

Epilog

A cartoon some years ago suggested that calculating the risk-benefit ratio might be inappropriate when considering a young man's proposal of marriage.

While indeed each of us is glad that our spouses did not keep us waiting on tenterhooks while the full panoply of options were subjected to Monte Carlo analysis, we suggest that the astute parents in earlier times did make some sort of risk-benefit calcualation when they arranged marriages for their children.

We suggest that the more one calculates risks, the more automatic becomes the procedure for guarding against them.

That enables hazardous behavior to be easily avoided. On the other hand it also enables a person to safely engage in activities others might consider too risky. For example, those scientists (such as RW) who have spent a limited time inside the sarcophagus of the Chornobyl reactor measure their dose and calculate their risk. The only bravery in their actions is that they believe their own measurements and calculations.

Index

Absolute risk, 17
Acceptability of risks, 109
Accidents, 2-3, 9, 16, 20, 26, 28-29, 36, 39-41, 46, 56, 68, 73, 76-77, 85-86, 105, 107, 110, 123, 126, 130, 136, 172, 174, 179, 194, 196-197, 199, 201, 208, 210, 218, 224-225, 228, 238, 266-267, 271, 277, 281-282, 290, 292
Accident initiators, 28
Acute toxicity, 59, 63, 117, 121, 161, 309
Aflatoxin, 84, 120-122, 156, 163, 182, 214, 236, 307, 309
Age, 3-4, 8, 11, 16, 36, 50, 56, 66, 76, 129-130, 146, 156, 192-195, 198-199, 203, 208, 210, 252-258, 260-262, 284, 305, 318, 333-334, 341-346, 348-349, 351-355, 359
Age adjustment, 8, 333
Aircraft, accidents, 281
Air pollution, 18, 30-31, 34-35, 51, 69-70, 72-74, 96, 107, 123, 136, 157, 170, 186, 189, 202, 209-210, 233-234, 272-273, 285, 298
Air travel, 107, 225
Alcohol, 38, 46, 52, 54-56, 87, 129, 199, 202, 204-205, 209, 213-214, 231, 237-238, 247, 255, 289, 297-298, 300-301, 306
    consumption, 38, 52, 55, 70, 87, 204-205, 209, 231, 238, 242, 289, 306, 318, 336, 338-339, 347, 349
    risk, 1-7, 9, 11, 13-15, 25-36, 38, 41, 44-45, 47-53, 56, 58-60, 62-68, 70-71, 75-97, 100-105, 107-116, 118-128, 131-133, 135-153, 155-169, 171, 173-182, 184-189, 192-210, 212, 218-220, 223-241, 251, 258-260, 262, 265-278, 280-289, 291-309, 312-315, 317, 321-324, 326-331, 335-339, 341-363
Ammonia, 45
Ammonium Nitrate, 45
Arsenic, 51-53, 61, 199, 202, 209, 237, 248, 270, 286, 289, 298, 304, 308
As low as reasonably achievable criterion (ALARA) 152, 157, 159, 178, 220
Asbestos, 7-8, 46, 53, 63, 67, 163, 170-171, 174-176, 198, 205, 231-232, 249, 283-285, 287, 290, 292-297, 299, 301, 303, 307-309, 341, 350-356, 358-361
Asteroids, 270, 287, 291
Automobile accidents, 46, 85-86, 105, 225, 238
Availability of alternatives, 104
Averages, 11, 35, 66, 72, 74, 192, 213
Background risk, 17, 50, 198
Bears, 226-227
Benefits and risks, 100, 108-110, 136-139, 267, 291
Beneficial, 5, 48, 53-56, 67, 77, 130, 238
Benzene, 15, 46, 53, 63, 71, 180, 185-186, 215, 249-250, 268, 289, 294, 296, 307
Best available control technology, 6, 23, 154, 157-158, 178, 186
Bibliography, 7, 23, 265, 267
Black Lung, 12, 15, 29, 32, 198, 202, 208, 218, 230
Boundary, 5, 18-19, 73, 75, 139, 202

Cancer, 2, 6, 8, 10, 12-13, 16, 43, 46-51, 53-56, 59-62, 64, 66, 68, 70, 74, 77, 82-85, 90, 92, 95, 104, 107, 116, 118-121, 124-130, 134, 136, 142,

146, 150, 155-156, 162, 164-165,
167-171, 174, 177, 182-183, 188,
198-199, 202, 205, 209-210, 217,
219, 223, 227-242, 253-256, 258,
263, 265-267, 270-271, 276, 279-
280, 282-297, 300, 302-307, 309,
313, 341-363
and air pollution, 30, 107, 285
and radiation, 107, 131, 155, 287
Carcinogenesis and carcinogens
Evaluation of, 5, 15, 27, 33, 62, 70,
74, 145-146, 155, 228, 266, 280,
287, 320, 328, 331, 344, 359
Management of, 176, 185, 252, 256,
267, 278, 309
New risk, 27
Carbon dioxide, 102, 180, 296
Carson, Rachel, 177
Catastrophes, 7, 21, 218-219, 221, 259,
272
Causal chains, 38
Causal connections, 33
Causes of death, 36, 203, 274
Charcoal broiling, 234
Chloroform, 13, 117-120, 158, 160,
202, 209, 216, 233, 251, 291
Chornobyl, 40, 76, 115, 124, 130, 171-
173, 221, 241-242, 338, 340, 363
Chronic, 30, 59, 62, 164, 199, 228,
233, 261-262, 284, 293, 296
Risks, 1-3, 5-12, 14-23, 25-29, 31-
32, 34-36, 38-39, 41, 45-49, 56-58,
64, 68, 70, 74-75, 77-79, 81-84, 87,
92-93, 95, 99-100, 102-105, 107-
110, 112-117, 120, 122, 124, 126,
131-133, 136-139, 141-148, 150-
152, 154-155, 158, 162-166, 173-
177, 182-186, 189, 191-203, 205-
212, 218-219, 222-225, 227-229,
231, 235-236, 238-239, 242, 265-
268, 271, 274-275, 277, 279-280,
282, 286-287, 290-291, 293-294,

296, 298-303, 305, 307-308, 312-
315, 319, 326-328, 331, 338, 341-
342, 349, 353-354, 356-358, 360-
361, 363
Exposure, 5, 8, 15, 8, 10-11, 26, 30,
46-48, 54, 57-59, 62, 64-68, 70-71,
77, 88-89, 92, 110, 115-116, 118,
127-128, 132, 146, 156-157, 159,
163-164, 167-171, 174-180, 185,
198, 210, 212-217, 228, 230-232,
235, 239-241, 249-251, 269, 283-
290, 292-303, 306-307, 309, 321,
323, 339, 341, 343-346, 349-356,
359-361
Cigarette smoking, 35, 46-47, 85, 103,
124-125, 128-129, 168, 199, 230,
289, 292-293, 303, 305, 343, 349-
350, 352-353, 355
Cirrhosis of the liver, 55-56, 87, 199,
204-205, 231
Classes of risk, 26
Coal mining, 13, 15-16, 30-32, 108,
136, 142, 183, 196, 218
Cohen, B. L., 287
Confounding variables, 30
Congress, 3, 4, 7, 14, 154, 156, 158,
166, 168-169, 178, 182-184, 287-
288, 299
Cost, 1, 5, 6, 52, 104, 122, 136, 138-
139, 141-143, 145-146, 149, 152,
154-155, 158-159, 166-167, 175,
177, 182, 184, 186, 198, 219-220,
244-263, 267, 305
Effectiveness, 6-7, 22, 122, 146, 154,
184, 305
Benefit, 1, 6, 15, 23, 47, 107-110,
120, 122, 124, 135-138, 146, 165,
173, 175, 177-178, 238, 267, 289,
305, 312-314
Crump, K., 288

Daubert, 187-189, 289
Decision analysis, 21, 158, 272, 274, 284
Decision making, 14, 109, 137, 189, 271, 273-274, 301, 305-307
  criteria for, 6, 152, 183, 269
Delaney amendment, 1-7, 9, 11, 13-15, 25-36, 38, 41, 44-45, 47-53, 56, 58-60, 62-68, 70-71, 75-97, 100-105, 107-116, 118-128, 131-133, 135-153, 155-169, 171, 173-182, 184-189, 192-210, 212, 218-220, 223-241, 251, 258-260, 262, 265-278, 280-289, 291-309, 312-315, 317, 321-324, 326-331, 335-339, 341-363
Differential risk, 18-19
Dioxin, 7, 46, 58, 63, 107, 120-122, 163, 174, 176, 202, 251, 287
Disaggregation of averages
  reactor safety study, 89, 301
Discount factor, 145
Dose response, 48-49, 51, 53, 56, 59-61, 63, 66-67, 70, 115-117, 122, 124-125, 130, 164-166, 174, 176, 178-179, 182-183, 185-186, 198, 205, 209, 228, 232-233, 242, 309, 347

Elements of risk assessment, 150
Elicitation, 5-6, 67, 95, 306
Emergency Core Cooling System, 39, 44, 90
Engineering system, 5
Epidemiology, 5, 46-47, 126, 228, 238, 270, 279, 290, 293, 301-302, 305, 341
Error estimates, 94
  See also Uncertainties
European Commission, 20, 75-76, 122-123, 142, 290
Event tree analysis, 44, 172-174

Expected value of risk, 38
Expressed preference method, 107-110
Expert opinion, 5, 67
Exposure, 5, 8, 10-11, 15, 26, 30, 46-48, 54, 57-59, 62, 64-68, 70-71, 77, 88-89, 92, 110, 115-116, 118, 127-128, 132, 146, 156-157, 159, 163-164, 167-171, 174-180, 185, 198, 210, 212-217, 228, 230-232, 235, 239-241, 249-251, 269, 283-290, 292-303, 306-307, 309, 321, 323, 339, 341, 343-346, 349-356, 359-361
  pathways, 65, 68

Fault tree, 43-44, 172
Fischoff, B., 291
Food additives, 129, 155
Food and Drug Administration, 14, 156, 165, 182, 271, 276-277, 291
FDA, 62, 87-88, 121, 156, 162-163, 177, 182, 236, 291, 335, 337-338

Hazard identification, 150
HERP, 62, 212-217, 235-236, 238
Hill, Sir Austen Bradford, 47
Historical risks, 5, 26-27
Hormesis, 5, 48, 53-54, 56

Immeasurable, 5, 78
Impact pathway, 5, 69, 75, 151
Implied preference method, 107
Impossible, 5, 19, 64, 77, 120, 126, 151, 295, 359
Incentives, 7, 23, 150, 156, 159, 176, 179, 183
Incremental risk, 5, 17
Influenza, 3, 199, 258
Injuries, 11-12, 15, 38, 152, 196-198, 248, 266, 295
Iron production, 19-20

Lave, B. L., 272, 277
Life expectancies
  USA, 14, 125, 221, 298, 300
  UK, 45, 53, 61, 99, 164, 173, 200-201, 266, 271-276, 278, 282-283, 293-295, 308, 312, 314
  Sweden, 3, 7, 278
  Japan, 3, 7, 13-14, 66, 74, 221, 225, 274
  France, 3, 7, 197, 220-221, 266, 272, 274, 294, 301
  Russia, 74, 130, 195, 285, 338
Lijinsky, W., 297
Lists, 7, 23, 63, 108, 161, 191, 195, 218, 228
LOLE, 7, 12, 210
Lowrance, W., 273

Magnitude of perceived risks, 109
Management of risks, 267
Managers, risk, 148, 151, 218
Mantel, 157, 159, 303
Market, 142-143, 154, 175, 180, 187, 296, 305, 339, 342
Measures of risk, 5, 11-18, 109, 136, 186, 192, 326, 328, 330
Meselson, M., 63, 302
Methodology, 68, 108, 137, 283, 337
Mining industry, 31
Models, 6, 19, 27, 33-35, 38, 47, 50, 66, 68, 71-74, 91-92, 94-95, 140, 175, 223, 237, 285, 297, 304, 319, 322, 331, 344, 351
Monte Carlo models, 6, 92
Morbidity, 12, 30, 290, 341
Morgan, M.G., 273, 298
Motor vehicle accidents, 28, 110
Mountain climbing, 28, 111, 227, 284, 290
Mushrooms, 8, 235, 335-340

Natural, 26, 28, 45, 50-51, 61-62, 64-65, 95, 104, 108, 116, 121, 123, 179, 182, 221, 233, 235, 242, 246, 268, 304, 307, 327, 336, 355-356
Carcinogens, 46, 49, 61-63, 70, 85, 90, 93, 117, 120-121, 155-158, 161-162, 165, 213-217, 223, 233-237, 283-284, 288, 292, 306, 309, 335, 360
New risks, 5, 26-27, 38, 46, 57-58, 155
Nuclear Regulatory Commission (NRC), 67, 112, 174, 178-179, 181, 186, 198, 220, 299, 328
Nuclear reactor accidents, 172, 224

Objectives, 1, 77, 149, 268, 272, 306
Occupational risk, 13, 136, 163, 224-225
Oil, 15, 20-21, 29, 45, 74, 90, 123, 188, 242, 252
Overconfidence, 6, 96-97

Particulates, 34, 72
Perception, 2-3, 5-6, 6-10, 22, 96, 99-100, 102-105, 107-110, 112-114, 116, 118, 120, 125-126, 131, 140, 146, 151-152, 169, 187, 274, 277, 291, 301, 304
Permeability of skin, 300, 303
Precautionary principle, 77, 159
Prediction, 32, 55, 59, 73, 102, 174, 271, 281, 286, 289, 292
Probability of causation, 5, 7, 10-11, 64, 66-67, 167, 183, 189, 239, 302, 307-308, 355
POC, 10, 64-67, 167-171
Probabilistic risk analysis, 89, 173
PRA, 77, 89, 123, 173

Radiation, 7, 10, 41, 43, 46-47, 49, 53, 56, 64, 66, 69-70, 78, 104-105, 107, 115-116, 123-124, 129-131, 142-

143, 146, 151, 155, 159, 168-171, 177-179, 181, 209, 221, 224, 228-229, 239, 242, 251-252, 266, 273, 278, 285, 287-288, 299-300, 303, 306-308, 338

Exposure, 5, 8, 15, 8, 10-11, 26, 30, 46-48, 54, 57-59, 62, 64-68, 70-71, 77, 88-89, 92, 110, 115-116, 118, 127-128, 132, 146, 156-157, 159, 163-164, 167-171, 174-180, 185, 198, 210, 212-217, 228, 230-232, 235, 239-241, 249-251, 269, 283-290, 292-303, 306-307, 309, 321, 323, 339, 341, 343-346, 349-356, 359-361

Protection, 7, 14, 69, 88, 142-143, 150, 152, 157, 178-179, 183, 201, 245, 266, 269, 272, 277-278, 280, 283-285, 287-288, 294, 299, 301, 313-314, 320-323

Reduction, 11, 29, 32, 35, 38, 101, 109, 118, 124, 163, 166, 173, 176-179, 184, 201-202, 212, 218, 228, 238, 244, 248, 251, 254, 284, 354-355

Reactor safety study, 89, 301

Recreational risks, 206-207, 225

Red Book, 150-151, 278

Reducing risk, 7, 101, 173, 176, 178

Risk-averse behavior, 141

Risk cost benefit analysis, 267

Risk-prone behavior, 141

Risks, 1-3, 5-12, 14-23, 25-29, 31-32, 34-36, 38-39, 41, 45-49, 56-58, 64, 68, 70, 74-75, 77-79, 81-84, 87, 92-93, 95, 99-100, 102-105, 107-110, 112-117, 120, 122, 124, 126, 131-133, 136-139, 141-148, 150-152, 154-155, 158, 162-166, 173-177, 182-186, 189, 191-203, 205-212, 218-219, 222-225, 227-229, 231, 235-236, 238-239, 242, 265-268, 271, 274-275, 277, 279-280, 282, 286-287, 290-291, 293-294, 296, 298-303, 305, 307-308, 312-315, 319, 326-328, 331, 338, 341-342, 349, 353-354, 356-358, 360-361, 363

Ruckelshaus W., 302

Russell, K., 302

Saccharin, 136, 156, 163, 177, 182, 209, 215, 232, 291

Saccharin and its salts; Proposed rule and hearing, 62, 87-88, 121, 156, 162-163, 177, 182, 236, 291, 335, 337-338

Safety, 1, 7, 13-15, 28, 32, 34, 39, 41, 44-46, 67, 76-77, 88-90, 93, 97, 99, 104, 108, 117, 120, 155, 157, 166, 172-174, 179, 183, 185-186, 191, 197, 201, 207, 218-220, 226, 232, 244-245, 247-248, 252, 265, 270-271, 273-275, 278, 280-282, 288, 293, 297, 299, 301, 304-305, 311-315

Culture, 2, 7, 76, 183, 277

Schwing, R.C., 274, 303

Silent Spring, 177, 275

Size of establishment as variable, 29

Slovic P., 274, 278, 295, 301, 304

Soda machines, 207, 225

Spacecraft, 225-226, 239

Space probes, 239-240

Starr, C., 305

Subpopulations, 138

See also Disaggregation of averages

Superfund, 13, 169, 183, 202, 268, 308, 338

System boundaries, 18-21, 25, 122

Taboo, 6, 23, 155

(see ban)

Technologies, 20, 38, 107-109, 111, 124, 172, 183, 226
    Improvement of, 179
Threshold dose, 48, 116, 209
Time, 1-3, 6-8, 10, 13, 22, 28-29, 32, 35-36, 38, 40-41, 43-44, 48, 59-60, 64, 71, 73-75, 79, 82, 85-86, 88, 97, 100, 103, 107, 109, 116, 118, 123-124, 132, 134, 136-137, 141-146, 150-151, 155, 157-158, 167, 170, 178, 180, 184, 191, 193-196, 203, 208-210, 228-229, 232, 237, 240, 253-254, 256, 286, 289, 297, 312, 314, 322, 333, 339, 342, 345, 347-348, 351, 353-354, 360, 363
Time horizon, 137
Time trends, 28
Tornadoes, 26, 36-38, 108, 200, 208
Tversky, A., 274, 306

Uncertainties, 2, 6-7, 13, 21-23, 49, 52, 82-86, 88-97, 100, 102, 105, 133, 145, 159, 209, 223, 298, 317, 319, 324-325
    Statistical, 12, 32-33, 47, 49, 83, 89, 93-94, 103, 107, 123-124, 128, 140, 160, 162, 184, 187, 195, 197, 200-201, 207, 220, 225, 230, 265-266, 279, 282, 288, 320, 331
    Model uncertainty, 2, 6, 92-93, 95, 319, 331

U.S. Supreme Court, 15, 167, 185-188
Upton, Arthur, 11, 49
Utility function, 139

Variability, 2, 6, 8, 38, 61, 81-82, 86-89, 93, 151, 196, 285, 293-294, 298, 317-318, 321-331

Waste, 8, 68, 123, 142-144, 167, 220, 237, 239, 248, 250, 269, 271, 283, 298, 317-318, 320-325, 328-330, 335
Water pollution, 158, 228
Websites, 7, 241, 279-281, 283
Weight, 10, 59-60, 86, 88, 117, 232, 235, 246, 259, 286, 319, 336-337, 339, 358
Weighting factors, 15

X-rays, 111, 116, 145-146, 170, 177-178, 288